Eosinophil-Associated Disorders

Editors

AMY D. KLION
PRINCESS U. OGBOGU

IMMUNOLOGY AND ALLERGY CLINICS OF NORTH AMERICA

www.immunology.theclinics.com

August 2015 • Volume 35 • Number 3

ELSEVIER

1600 John F. Kennedy Boulevard • Suite 1800 • Philadelphia, Pennsylvania, 19103-2899
http://www.theclinics.com

IMMUNOLOGY AND ALLERGY CLINICS OF NORTH AMERICA Volume 35, Number 3
August 2015 ISSN 0889-8561, ISBN-13: 978-0-323-39338-6

Editor: Jessica McCool
Developmental Editor: Barbara Cohen-Kligerman

Immunology and Allergy Clinics of North America (ISSN 0889–8561) is published quarterly by Elsevier Inc., 360 Park Avenue South, New York, NY 10010-1710. Months of issue are February, May, August, and November. Periodicals postage paid at New York, NY and additional mailing offices. Subscription prices are $320.00 per year for US individuals, $454.00 per year for US institutions, $150.00 per year for US students and residents, $395.00 per year for Canadian individuals, $220.00 per year for Canadian students, $577.00 per year for Canadian institutions, $445.00 per year for international individuals, $577.00 per year for international institutions, $220.00 per year for international students. To receive student/resident rate, orders must be accompanied by name of affiliated institution, date of term, and the *signature* of program/residency coordinator on institution letterhead. Orders will be billed at individual rate until proof of status is received. Foreign air speed delivery is included in all *Clinics* subscription prices. All prices are subject to change without notice. **POSTMASTER**: Send address changes to *Immunology and Allergy Clinics of North America,* Elsevier Health Sciences Division, Subscription Customer Service, 3251 Riverport Lane, Maryland Heights, MO 63043. **Customer Service: 1-800-654-2452 (U.S. and Canada); 314-447-8871 (outside U.S. and Canada). Fax: 314-447-8029. E-mail: journalscustomerservice-usa@elsevier.com (for print support); journalsonlinesupport-usa@elsevier.com (for online support).**

Reprints. For copies of 100 or more, of articles in this publication, please contact the Commercial Reprints Department, Elsevier Inc., 360 Park Avenue South, New York, New York 10010-1710. Tel. 212-633-3874, Fax: 212-633-3820, E-mail: reprints@elsevier.com.

Immunology and Allergy Clinics of North America is covered in MEDLINE/PubMed (Index Medicus), Current Contents/Life Sciences, Science Citation Index, ISI/BIOMED, Chemical Abstracts, and EMBASE/Excerpta Medica.

Contributors

EDITORS

AMY D. KLION, MD
Clinical Investigator, Laboratory of Parasitic Diseases, National Institute of Allergy and Infectious Diseases, National Institutes of Health, Bethesda, Maryland

PRINCESS U. OGBOGU, MD
Assistant Professor of Medicine, Section of Allergy and Immunology, Division of Pulmonary, Allergy, Critical Care and Sleep Medicine, Wexner Medical Center at the Ohio State University, Columbus, Ohio

AUTHORS

PRAVEEN AKUTHOTA, MD
Assistant Professor of Medicine, Division of Pulmonary, Critical Care, and Sleep Medicine; Division of Allergy and Inflammation, Beth Israel Deaconess Medical Center, Harvard Medical School, Boston, Massachusetts

HELMUT BELTRAMINELLI, MD
Department of Dermatology, Inselspital, Bern, Switzerland

BRUCE S. BOCHNER, MD
Samuel M. Feinberg Professor of Medicine, Division of Allergy-Immunology, Department of Medicine, Northwestern University Feinberg School of Medicine, Chicago, Illinois

SOUMYA CHATTERJEE, MD, MS, FRCP
Department of Rheumatic and Immunologic Diseases, Cleveland Clinic, Cleveland, Ohio

CASEY CURTIS, MD
Assistant Professor of Medicine, Section of Allergy and Immunology, Division of Pulmonary, Allergy, Critical Care and Sleep Medicine, Wexner Medical Center at the Ohio State University, Columbus, Ohio

ELISABETH DE GRAAUW, MD
Department of Dermatology; Institute of Pharmacology, University of Bern, Inselspital, Bern, Switzerland

LORENZO FALCHI, MD
Department of Leukemia, The University of Texas MD Anderson Cancer Center, Houston, Texas

ALEXANDRA F. FREEMAN, MD
Staff Clinician, Immunopathogenesis Section, Laboratory of Clinical Infectious Diseases, National Institute of Allergy and Infectious Diseases, National Institutes of Health, Bethesda, Maryland

GLENN T. FURUTA, MD
Professor of Pediatrics, Gastrointestinal Eosinophilic Diseases Program, Section of Pediatric Gastroenterology, Hepatology, and Nutrition, Department of Pediatrics, Digestive Health Institute, Children's Hospital Colorado, University of Colorado School of Medicine, Aurora, Colorado; University of Colorado School of Medicine, Denver, Colorado

CAROL A. LANGFORD, MD, MHS
Department of Rheumatic and Immunologic Diseases, Center for Vasculitis Care and Research, Cleveland Clinic, Cleveland, Ohio

POOJA MEHTA, MD
Gastrointestinal Eosinophilic Diseases Program, Section of Pediatric Gastroenterology, Hepatology, and Nutrition, Department of Pediatrics, Digestive Health Institute, Children's Hospital Colorado, University of Colorado School of Medicine, Aurora, Colorado

JOSHUA D. MILNER, MD
Chief, Genetics and Pathogenesis of Allergy Section, Laboratory of Allergic Diseases, National Institute of Allergy and Infectious Diseases, National Institutes of Health, Bethesda, Maryland

THOMAS B. NUTMAN, MD
Head, Helminth Immunology Section; Head, Clinical Parasitology Section, Laboratory of Parasitic Diseases, National Institute of Allergy and Infectious Diseases, National Institutes of Health, Bethesda, Maryland

ELISE M. O'CONNELL, MD
Clinical Fellow, Helminth Immunology Section, Laboratory of Parasitic Diseases, National Institute of Allergy and Infectious Diseases, National Institutes of Health, Bethesda, Maryland

PRINCESS U. OGBOGU, MD
Assistant Professor of Medicine, Section of Allergy and Immunology, Division of Pulmonary, Allergy, Critical Care and Sleep Medicine, Wexner Medical Center at the Ohio State University, Columbus, Ohio

FLORENCE ROUFOSSE, MD, PhD
Department of Internal Medicine, Hôpital Erasme, Institute for Medical Immunology, Université Libre de Bruxelles, Brussels, Belgium

DAGMAR SIMON, MD
Department of Dermatology, Inselspital, Bern, Switzerland

HANS-UWE SIMON, MD
Institute of Pharmacology, University of Bern, Inselspital, Bern, Switzerland

HIROMICHI TAMAKI, MD
Department of Rheumatic and Immunologic Diseases, Cleveland Clinic, Cleveland, Ohio

SRDAN VERSTOVSEK, MD, PhD
Professor of Medicine, Department of Leukemia, The University of Texas MD Anderson Cancer Center, Houston, Texas

ANDREW J. WARDLAW, MD, PhD
Professor of Allergy and Respiratory Medicine; Director of the Leicester Institute for Lung Health; Director of the NIHR Leicester Respiratory Biomedical Research Unit, Department of Infection Immunity and Inflammation, Institute for Lung Health, University of Leicester; Department of Respiratory Medicine and Allergy, University Hospitals of Leicester NHS Trust, Leicester, United Kingdom

PETER F. WELLER, MD
Professor of Medicine, Division of Allergy and Inflammation; Division of Infectious Diseases, Beth Israel Deaconess Medical Center, Harvard Medical School, Boston, Massachusetts

KELLI W. WILLIAMS, MD, MPH
Allergy and Immunology Clinical Fellow, Laboratory of Clinical Infectious Diseases, National Institute of Allergy and Infectious Diseases, National Institutes of Health, Bethesda, Maryland

KERRY WOOLNOUGH, MBChB, MRCP(resp)
Clinical Research Fellow, Department of Infection Immunity and Inflammation, Institute for Lung Health, University of Leicester; Department of Respiratory Medicine and Allergy, University Hospitals of Leicester NHS Trust, Leicester, United Kingdom

Contents

> Peripheral blood eosinophilia is commonly encountered in clinical prac-
> tice. The causes of peripheral blood eosinophilia are varied, ranging
> from benign eosinophilia to malignancy. A careful history and physical
> examination along with directed clinical evaluation may help determine
> the cause. When uncontrolled, peripheral blood eosinophilia may result
> in end-organ damage and life-threatening complications. This article sum-
> marizes the differential diagnosis and evaluation of persistent marked
> eosinophilia.

> Eosinophil-associated disorders can affect practically all tissues and or-
> gans in the body, either individually or in combination. This article provides
> an overview of end-organ manifestations of eosinophilia and discusses
> selected organ systems, including the upper and lower respiratory, cardio-
> vascular, gastrointestinal, nervous, dermatologic, and renal systems.
> Mechanisms by which eosinophilia leads to end-organ damage are also
> considered.

> The gastrointestinal (GI) tract provides an intriguing organ for considering
> the eosinophil's role in health and disease. The normal GI tract, except for
> the esophagus, is populated by eosinophils that are present throughout
> the mucosa, raising the possibility that eosinophils participate in innate
> mechanisms of defense. However, data from clinical studies associates
> increased numbers of eosinophils with inflammatory GI diseases, promp-
> ting concerns that eosinophils may have a deleterious effect on the gut. We
> present clinical features of 4 disease processes that have been associated
> with eosinophilia and suggest areas requiring investigation as to their clin-
> ical significance and scientific relevance.

> Eosinophilia in the peripheral blood can be the manifestation of various
> medical conditions, including benign or malignant disorders. There are 3
> main types of eosinophilia-associated myeloid neoplasms (MN-eos):

myeloid and lymphoid neoplasms, chronic eosinophilic leukemia not otherwise specified, and idiopathic hypereosinophilic syndrome (HES). Imatinib mesylate has revolutionized the treatment of molecularly defined MN-eos, and novel agents have been successfully used to treat HES. The discovery of new, recurrent molecular alterations in patients with MN-eos may Improve their diagnosis and therapy. This review focuses on the hematologist's approach to a patient with eosinophilia and treatment options for those with eosinophilic myeloid neoplasms.

Peripheral and tissue eosinophilia can be a prominent feature of several unique rheumatologic and vascular diseases. These diseases span a wide range of clinical features, histologic findings, therapeutic approaches, and outcomes. Despite the rare nature of these entities—which makes large-scale studies challenging—knowledge has continued to grow regarding their epidemiology, pathophysiology, and management. This review compares and contrasts 5 rheumatologic and vascular conditions in which eosinophilia can be seen: eosinophilic granulomatosis with polyangiitis (Churg-Strauss), immunoglobulin G4–related disease, diffuse fasciitis with eosinophilia, eosinophilia-myalgia syndrome, and eosinophilic myositis.

Lung disease associated with marked peripheral blood eosinophilia is unusual and nearly always clinically significant. Once recognized, it is generally easy to manage, albeit with long-term systemic corticosteroids. A failure to respond to oral steroids in the context of good compliance suggests a malignant cause for the eosinophilia. An important development is the introduction of antieosinophil therapies, particularly those directed against the interleukin 5 pathway, which is hoped to provide benefit in the full spectrum of eosinophilic lung disease as well as asthma, reducing the burden of side effects and resultant comorbidities.

In determining the etiology of eosinophilia, it is necessary to consider the type of patient, including previous travel and exposure history, comorbidities, and symptoms. In this review, we discuss the approach to the patient with eosinophilia from an infectious diseases perspective based on symptom complexes.

Increased serum eosinophil levels have been associated with multiple disorders of immune deficiency or immune dysregulation. Although primary immunodeficiency diseases are rare, it is important to consider these in the differential diagnosis of patients with eosinophilia. In this review, the clinical features, laboratory findings, diagnosis, and genetic basis of disease of several disorders of immune deficiency or dysregulation are discussed. The article includes autosomal dominant hyper IgE syndrome, DOCK8 deficiency, phosphoglucomutase 3 deficiency, ADA-SCID, Omenn syndrome, Wiskott-Aldrich syndrome, Loeys-Dietz syndrome, autoimmune lymphoproliferative syndrome, immunodysregulation, polyendocrinopathy, enteropathy, X-linked syndrome, Comel-Netherton syndrome, and severe dermatitis, multiple allergies, and metabolic wasting syndrome.

Elisabeth de Graauw, Helmut Beltraminelli, Hans-Uwe Simon, and Dagmar Simon

Eosinophil infiltration can be observed in skin disorders, such as allergic/immunologic, autoimmune, infectious, and neoplastic diseases. Clinical presentations are variable and include eczematous, papular, urticarial, bullous, nodular, and fibrotic lesions; pruritus is a common symptom in all. In this review, we present representative eosinophilic skin diseases according to their clinical pattern, together with histologic findings and diagnostic procedures. We also discuss the potential roles of eosinophils in the pathogenesis of dermatologic disorder. Current pathogenesis-based diagnostic and therapeutic approaches are outlined.

Florence Roufosse

The symptomatic hypereosinophilic patient must be approached in a stepwise manner, with thorough assessment to determine whether the hypereosinophilia itself is contributing to damage and disease manifestations (thereby defining a hypereosinophilic syndrome), and to identify an eventual cause of hypereosinophilia, followed by initiation of treatment directed against the underlying condition or deleterious hypereosinophilic state. Situations encountered in the clinic are extremely heterogeneous because of the numerous potential causes of hypereosinophilia and the variable spectrum of eosinophil-mediated organ damage. A practical approach to many of these situations is presented in this review.

Bruce S. Bochner

Current therapies for eosinophilic disorders are limited. Most treatment approaches remain empirical, are not supported by data from controlled clinical trials, involve the off-label use of agents developed for treatment of other diseases, and tend to rely heavily on the use of glucocorticoids and other agents with significant toxicity. Great progress has been made in the discovery, preclinical development, and clinical testing of a variety of biologics and small molecules that have the potential to directly or indirectly influence eosinophils, eosinophilic inflammation, and the consequences of eosinophil activation.

Eosinophil-Associated Disorders

IMMUNOLOGY AND ALLERGY CLINICS OF NORTH AMERICA

THE CLINICS ARE AVAILABLE ONLINE!
Access your subscription at:
www.theclinics.com

Preface

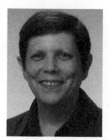 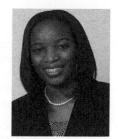

Amy D. Klion, MD   Princess U. Ogbogu, MD
Editors

Eosinophilia may be present in a wide variety of disorders, including but not limited to, allergic, immunologic, and neoplastic disorders, infectious diseases, and rare hypereosinophilic syndromes. Identification of the cause of eosinophilia is not only crucial with respect to choice of therapy and prevention of eosinophil-mediated end-organ damage, but also has important implications with respect to prognosis. Due to the wide array of organs affected, clinical presentations, and complications, patients with peripheral eosinophilia may present to a variety of specialists. The goal of this issue *of Immunology and Allergy Clinics of North America* is to provide approaches to the diagnosis and treatment of eosinophilic disorders from the perspective of the varied specialists to whom these patients present. The information in this issue is intended to aid clinicians in the differential diagnosis of patients who present with peripheral eosinophilia (absolute eosinophil count $>1500/mm^3$) and/or marked tissue eosinophilia. This issue also reviews the evaluation of persistent eosinophilia, end-organ manifestations, and highlights advancements in disease classification and novel therapies for eosinophilic disorders. It is our hope that this unique focus on the clinical presentations of these patients to various subspecialists will promote better understanding of the heterogeneity of these disorders and help clinicians more readily identify and care for patients presenting with eosinophilia.

Immunol Allergy Clin N Am 35 (2015) xi–xii
http://dx.doi.org/10.1016/j.iac.2015.06.001
0889-8561/15/$ – see front matter © 2015 Published by Elsevier Inc.

immunology.theclinics.com

We would like to thank all of the authors who graciously contributed their time and expertise; and Stephanie Wissler, Susan Showalter, and Jessica McCool at Elsevier, for their patience and editorial support.

Amy D. Klion, MD
Laboratory of Parasitic Diseases
National Institute of Allergy
and Infectious Diseases
National Institutes of Health
Bethesda, MD 20892, USA

Princess U. Ogbogu, MD
Section of Allergy & Immunology
Division of Pulmonary, Allergy
Critical Care and Sleep Medicine
Wexner Medical Center
at the Ohio State University
Columbus, OH 43210, USA

E-mail addresses:
AKLION@niaid.nih.gov (A.D. Klion)
Princess.Ogbogu@osumc.edu (P.U. Ogbogu)

Evaluation and Differential Diagnosis of Persistent Marked Eosinophilia

Casey Curtis, MD*, Princess U. Ogbogu, MD

KEYWORDS

- Eosinophilia • Hypereosinophilic syndrome • *FIP1L1-PDGFRA*
- Lymphocytic hypereosinophilic syndrome (L-HES)
- Myeloproliferative hypereosinophilic syndrome (M-HES)

KEY POINTS

- The causes of peripheral blood eosinophilia are varied, ranging from benign eosinophilia to malignancy; a careful history and physical examination along with directed clinical evaluation may help determine the cause.
- Although drug allergy is the most common cause of hypereosinophilia in the United States, parasitic diseases are the most common cause worldwide.
- Hypereosinophilic syndrome is a diagnosis of exclusion; however, it should be considered in patients with peripheral eosinophilia of unknown cause, because delay in diagnosis may result in end-organ damage.
- In recent years, advances in molecular diagnostics have improved the ability of physicians to identify and treat hypereosinophilic syndrome.

EOSINOPHIL BIOLOGY

In order to better appreciate the implications of eosinophilia and eosinophilic tissue infiltration, it is helpful to have an understanding of eosinophil development, structure, and function. Eosinophils are terminally differentiated granulocytes derived in the bone marrow from CD34+ hematopoietic stem cells.[1] Cytokines integral to the transition from progenitor cells to eosinophils include interleukin (IL)-3, IL-5, and granulocyte-macrophage colony–stimulating factor (GM-CSF); IL-5 also participates in regulation of other aspects of eosinophil function, including release of mature cells from the

Conflicts of Interest: The authors have no significant financial, personal, or organizational interests that could inappropriately influence the content of this review.
Section of Allergy & Immunology, Division of Pulmonary, Allergy, Critical Care and Sleep Medicine, Wexner Medical Center at the Ohio State University, 410 West 10th Avenue, Columbus, OH 43210, USA
* Corresponding author. 201 Davis Heart & Lung Research Institute, 473 West 12th Avenue, Columbus, OH 43210.
E-mail address: curtis.159@osu.edu

Immunol Allergy Clin N Am 35 (2015) 387–402
http://dx.doi.org/10.1016/j.iac.2015.04.001
0889-8561/15/$ – see front matter © 2015 Elsevier Inc. All rights reserved.

immunology.theclinics.com

bone marrow and migration into tissue.[2] Progression toward the eosinophil lineage is directed by several key transcription factors, including GATA-binding protein 1 (GATA-1), PU.1, interferon consensus–binding protein, and CCAAT-enhancer binding proteins.[3] The half-life of eosinophils in the peripheral blood is approximately 18 hours, and under normal circumstances they represent only 1% to 5% peripheral blood leukocytes. However, their survival is significantly prolonged after recruitment into tissue, where they represent a more substantial proportion of the cellular population.[3,4]

Eosinophils have a characteristic morphology, with bilobed nuclei and numerous cytoplasmic granules that bind to the dye eosin, leading to a distinct pink coloration of the cytoplasm on microscopy.[5,6] Their specific granules contain hydrolytic enzymes and cationic granule proteins including major basic protein (MBP), eosinophil peroxidase, eosinophil-derived neurotoxin (EDN), and eosinophil cationic protein.[6] These proteins are responsible for many fundamental activities of eosinophils. Specific granules also contain cytokines, chemokines, and growth factors, such as CC chemokine ligand 5 (CCL5)/regulated on activation, normal T cell expressed and secreted (RANTES), CCL11/eotaxin, GM-CSF, IL-2, IL-4, IL-5, IL-6, IL-13, transforming growth factor alpha, and tumor necrosis factor alpha.[6] As these mediators are preformed and do not require de novo synthesis, activated eosinophils can respond rapidly to changes in the environment, promoting efficient cellular recruitment and coordinated immune responses.

Understanding the normal mechanisms of eosinophil development and proliferation is essential for identifying the derangements in these pathways that lead to eosinophilia. Similarly, knowledge of eosinophil function provides a framework for comprehension of the abnormalities that can occur in the setting of increased eosinophil number or activity.

EOSINOPHILIA

Eosinophilia is defined as an increase in the peripheral absolute eosinophil count (AEC). There are defined categories including mild (AEC from 500–1500/mm^3), moderate (AEC 1500–5000/mm^3), and severe (AEC >5000/mm^3).[7] The clinical impact of eosinophilia is variable. The severity of symptoms does not always correlate with the degree of eosinophilia; some patients with substantial peripheral eosinophil increases remain asymptomatic, whereas others with mild eosinophilia have severe complications.[8] The fact that blood eosinophil counts may not be representative of eosinophilic tissue infiltration may be partially responsible for this. Eosinophil counts in tissue are generally higher than those present in peripheral blood, and the release of preformed mediators in associated tissue often leads to the clinical manifestations and complications of eosinophilia.[9] The discrepancy between degree of eosinophilia and manifestation of clinical symptoms may also be explained by differences in the degree of eosinophil activation. Studies of members of an asymptomatic family with hypereosinophilia (2000–5000 eosinophils/mm^3) showed that they had relative lack of eosinophil activation (decreased serum levels of EDN and MBP, and decreased surface expression of CD25) compared with those with nonfamilial hypereosinophilic syndrome (HES).[10]

The causes of eosinophilia are varied, and are further explored later in this article. It is essential to systematically approach patients who present with unexplained eosinophilia, because the treatments may vary by cause and the urgency of management may be guided by the presence or absence of end-organ manifestations. A detailed discussion of end-organ manifestations associated with eosinophilia is provided by Akuthota and Weller elsewhere in this issue.

CAUSES OF HYPEREOSINOPHILIA
Drug Hypersensitivity

Medications are a frequent cause of eosinophilia, and are likely the most common cause in areas with a low prevalence of parasitic infection.[11] Although prescription medications can cause increased eosinophil counts, any medication, including over-the-counter drugs, herbal therapies, and dietary supplements, can be implicated and should be considered as part of the diagnostic evaluation. As such, a detailed medication history should be obtained in any patient presenting with eosinophilia.

Drug-induced eosinophilia may be asymptomatic and found incidentally, as is commonly the case with cephalosporins, quinine, and quinolones.[12] Eosinophilia does not necessarily require cessation of a causative medication; the prescribing physician must take into account the necessity of the medication, available alternatives, and presence of end-organ complications related to eosinophilia. In some situations, the medication may be continued under close monitoring.[9]

In other cases, eosinophilia related to medication use may lead to organ-specific complications. For instance, eosinophilic pulmonary infiltrates have been well described during treatment with multiple medications, including sulfasalazine, nitrofurantoin, and nonsteroidal anti-inflammatory drugs (NSAIDs).[13] Acute interstitial nephritis (AIN) is another condition associated with organ-specific eosinophilic complications. This condition has been noted secondary to semisynthetic penicillins, cephalosporins, NSAIDs, sulfonamides, phenytoin, cimetidine, and allopurinol, among others.[14] Although renal interstitial eosinophilic infiltration is a characteristic of AIN, eosinophiluria is considered to lack diagnostic sensitivity, with one study of 51 patients with suspected AIN showing a positive predictive value of less than 40%.[14,15] Treatment of these conditions involves cessation of the causative medication, but patients may also require additional supportive care specific to the organ system involved.

Eosinophilia with multiorgan system involvement secondary to medication use has also been described. Eosinophilia-myalgia syndrome (EMS) is a disorder in which increased eosinophil counts are associated with severe myalgias, neuropathy, dermatologic induration, and varied multisystem complaints. EMS has been most commonly reported secondary to impurities of ingested L-tryptophan linked specifically in the United States to a company producing contaminated L-tryptophan supplements.[16] A similar deadly epidemic, known as toxic oil syndrome, occurred with the ingestion of contaminated rapeseed oil in Spain.[17] L-tryptophan–induced EMS is now rarely seen, and toxic oil syndrome has not recurred.[18]

Drug rash with eosinophilia and systemic symptoms syndrome, also known as drug-induced hypersensitivity syndrome (DIHS), warrants specific mention because mortality may be as high as 10% to 20% in affected patients.[19] DIHS generally develops around 4 to 12 weeks after initiation of a causative medication, and may persist for weeks beyond cessation of the drug. Patients frequently present with fevers, lymphadenopathy, and hematologic abnormalities, including AEC greater than 1500/mm³. End-organ involvement may include hepatitis, interstitial nephritis, pneumonitis, and carditis.[19] Medications are not the only known cause, and DIHS can result from reactivation of latent viruses such as human herpesvirus (HHV)-6, HHV-7, Epstein-Barr virus, and cytomegalovirus.[20,21]

Some medications commonly associated with eosinophilia and DIHS are shown in **Box 1**; this list is not comprehensive. Any prescription medication, supplement, or over-the-counter medication can lead to eosinophilia.

Box 1
Medications commonly associated with eosinophilia and DIHS

Antibiotics

- Penicillins
- Cephalosporins
- Fluoroquinolones
- Tetracyclines
- Doxycycline
- Linezolid
- Nitrofurantoin
- Metronidazole

Antiepileptics

- Phenytoin
- Carbamazepine
- Phenobarbital
- Lamotrigine
- Valproate

Antidepressants

- Desipramine
- Amitriptyline
- Fluoxetine

Antiinflammatories

- Piroxicam
- Naproxen
- Diclofenac
- Ibuprofen

Sulfonamides/sulfones

- Dapsone
- Sulfasalazine
- Trimethoprim-sulfamethoxazole

Antihypertensives

- Hydrochlorothiazide
- β-Blockers
- Angiotensin-converting enzyme inhibitors

Other

- Abacavir
- Nevirapine
- Allopurinol
- Ranitidine
- Cyclosporine

Allergic Disorders

Eosinophilia can be observed in the setting of conditions such as atopic dermatitis, allergic rhinitis, and asthma, although generally the AEC is less than 1500/mm^3 in the setting of these conditions. Severe atopic dermatitis and marked eosinophilia may prompt evaluation for rare causes of immune deficiency and immune dysregulation such as hyper–immunoglobulin (Ig) E syndrome and Omenn syndrome (reviewed by Williams and colleagues elsewhere in this issue).

Allergic bronchopulmonary aspergillosis (ABPA) and allergic bronchopulmonary mycoses (ABPM) are hypersensitivity reactions to fungi resulting in increased total IgE levels, presence of IgE and IgG to *Aspergillus fumigatus* (or other fungi), bronchiectasis, and pulmonary infiltrates in the setting of asthma.[22] Pronounced eosinophilia in the setting of asthma also raises concern for eosinophilic granulomatosis with polyangiitis (EGPA), formerly known as Churg-Strauss syndrome, which is further explored later in this article.

Infection

Tissue invasive parasitic helminth infection is the most common cause of eosinophilia worldwide.[23] *Strongyloides stercoralis*, a helminthic parasite found in tropical and subtropical climates, including the southeastern United States, can cause variable degrees of eosinophilia. Strongyloides infection may be prolonged, having been documented to persist for decades, and may be asymptomatic.[24] Importantly, some individuals with strongyloidiasis do not have associated eosinophilia.[25] Treatment with corticosteroids in the setting of strongyloidiasis can lead to a disseminated and fatal infection, so screening for this condition is indicated before treatment if possible.[26] Less commonly, eosinophilia can be found in the setting of infection with other parasites, such as *Isospora belli* and *Sarcocystis hominis*.[27,28] Ectoparasites, such as scabies, are also known to cause eosinophilia.[29]

Bacterial infection generally leads to low peripheral eosinophil counts.[30] Eosinophilia in the setting of a significant bacterial infection warrants evaluation for another cause, such as an antibiotic being used to treat the infection. Alternatively, viral infections such as human T-cell leukemia virus (HTLV) and human immunodeficiency virus (HIV) can be associated with eosinophilia. HTLV has been associated with eosinophilia in the setting of dermatologic disorders including induration and ulceration of the skin with a CD8 predominant cellular infiltration; it has been theorized that eosinophilia in this setting may be related directly to skin damage versus induction of a cytokine profile promoting eosinophilia.[31] Patients coinfected with HTLV-1 and *Strongyloides* have a modified immune response to the parasite, consisting of increased levels of interferon gamma and decreased production of IL-4, IL-5, IL-13, and IgE; the efficacy of strongyloidiasis treatment is decreased in these individuals.[32] Eosinophilia can be associated with HIV infection; factors that may contribute to eosinophilia in this population include immune dysregulation, increased medication use, and HIV-associated eosinophilic folliculitis.[33,34] Fungal infections can also be a cause of eosinophilia. Primary coccidioidomycosis can be associated with eosinophilia, with more significant increases associated with disseminated disease.[35] Eosinophilia associated with *Aspergillus* is primarily seen in ABPA, as outlined earlier. A more extensive review of infectious causes of eosinophilia is provided by O'Connell and Nutman elsewhere in this issue.

Overall, there are several factors that may suppress eosinophilia in the setting of infection, such as hyperthermia, acute illness, and treatment with corticosteroids. When these situations are remedied, eosinophilia may become apparent. Adrenal insufficiency may also result in eosinophilia, particularly in acutely ill patients, because of the loss of endogenous glucocorticoids.[36]

Neoplasm

Eosinophilia may be found in association with various types of malignancy. Solid tumors may be associated with peripheral eosinophilia and may lead to infiltration of eosinophils into the area immediately involved with the mass.[37] Local eosinophilic infiltration may be more common in carcinoma of the lung, squamous cell carcinoma of the vagina, penis, skin, and nasopharynx, and transitional cell carcinoma of the bladder. Peripheral eosinophilia has been reported in the setting of carcinoma of the kidney, adrenal glands, thyroid, liver, gallbladder, pancreas, and breast; peritoneal mesothelioma; and liposarcoma.[37] Mechanisms contributing to the eosinophilia in this setting may include eosinophilotactic responses to tumor necrosis, increased eosinophil production in the bone marrow caused by tumor cell dissemination, and increased tumor production of eosinophilopoietins such as IL-3, IL-5, and GM-CSF.[38]

Eosinophilia may also result from hematologic malignancies of both myeloid and lymphoid origins. Examples include chronic myelogenous leukemia (CML), Hodgkin and non-Hodgkin lymphoma, and peripheral T-cell lymphomas, such as Sézary syndrome, adult T-cell leukemia/lymphoma, and angioimmunoblastic T-cell lymphoma.[39]

Other

EGPA, formerly known as Churg-Strauss syndrome, is a condition of necrotizing vasculitis and extravascular granulomatous disease that can be associated with asthma and prominent eosinophilia. Patients may show sinusitis or other paranasal abnormalities, migratory lung infiltrates, peripheral neuropathy, and eosinophilic end-organ complications involving the heart, gastrointestinal (GI) tract, and lungs.[40] Antineutrophil cytoplasmic antibodies (ANCAs), typically antimyeloperoxidase, can be associated with EGPA, although these are found in only approximately 40% of patients.[41] The presence of ANCA may have implications regarding disease phenotype. Although there is overlap between clinical presentations, ANCA-positive EGPA tends to be associated with features such as necrotizing glomerulonephritis, pulmonary hemorrhage, and mononeuritis multiplex. ANCA-negative EGPA often shows more significant eosinophilic tissue infiltration, including eosinophilic gastritis/enteritis and complications associated with toxic products of eosinophils.[41]

Eosinophilia can be found in association with rheumatologic diseases, including IgG4-related disease, eosinophilic myositis, diffuse fasciitis with eosinophilia, and various systemic autoimmune disorders such as systemic lupus erythematosus, Sjögren syndrome, rheumatoid arthritis, and Bechet's disease. Rheumatologic conditions associated with eosinophilia are further explored elsewhere in this issue by Tamaki and colleagues. Systemic mastocytosis (SM) may also be associated with eosinophilia, with up to 28% of patients showing eosinophilia greater than 650 eosinophils/mm^3.[42] Eosinophilia in SM has been reported in patients with the D816V mutation in the *KIT* gene, and shows overlapping features with myeloproliferative variant HES such as splenomegaly and increased serum tryptase and vitamin B$_{12}$ levels.[42] However, despite these similarities, the dysfunction caused in SM is thought to be secondary to the mastocytosis rather than clonal eosinophilia.[43]

As previously mentioned, eosinophilia accompanied by unusual or recurrent infections should prompt evaluation for certain immune deficiencies (see O'Connell and Nutman elsewhere in this issue). Examples of primary immune deficiencies associated with eosinophilia include autoimmune lymphoproliferative syndrome (ALPS), Omenn syndrome, and hyper-IgE syndromes (related to mutations in signal transducer and activator of transcription 3 [*STAT3*] or dedicator of cytokinesis 8 [*DOCK8*]). Characteristic features, such as an expanded CD4$^-$CD8$^-$, T cell receptor (TCR)αβ$^+$, CD3$^+$ T-cell population (also known as double-negative T cells), lymphadenopathy, and hepatosplenomegaly, should prompt further evaluation for ALPS. In contrast, high levels of serum IgE and severe eczema are suggestive of hyper-IgE syndrome.

There are several distinct syndromes associated with eosinophilia, including Kimura disease, Gleich's syndrome, and nodules, eosinophilia, rheumatism, dermatitis, and swelling (NERDS) syndrome. Kimura disease is a rare inflammatory condition that presents primarily, but not exclusively, in Asian men. It is associated with subcutaneous nodularity and lymphoid infiltrates involving the salivary glands. There is often lymphadenopathy of the head and neck, although the axillae and groin may be involved as well. Eosinophilic microabscesses may be seen histologically, and serum abnormalities include increased IgE levels and eosinophilia. This condition has been associated with nephrotic syndrome, bronchial asthma, ulcerative colitis, and aortitis. The cause remains unknown; treatment consists of surgical resection of nodules or involved lymph nodes, with some reports indicating a benefit of corticosteroids.[44]

Gleich's syndrome, also known as episodic angioedema with eosinophilia (EAE), consists of cyclic episodes of eosinophilia with associated symptoms including fevers, weight gain, and angioedema. Khoury and colleagues[45] recently studied 4 patients with this rare condition. In addition to variable eosinophilia, these patients showed multilineage cell cycling, with episodic changes in neutrophil and lymphocyte counts with a periodicity of 25 to 35 days. All patients studied had aberrant populations of $CD3^-CD4^+$ T cells, with 3 of 4 showing clonal populations of T cells. Intracellular cytokine profiles in these patients suggest that eosinophilia and eosinophil activation may be lymphocyte driven. Other characteristic features of EAE include increased IgM levels and variable hypocomplementemia; EAE is generally steroid responsive and has a good prognosis.[46]

The initial patients described presenting with NERDS showed pronounced eosinophilia, articular nodules on extensor tendons, dermatitis, and intermittent swelling of the hands and feet. Rheumatologic complaints included myalgias and stiffness in the hands, knees, and elbows. One patient showed a positive rheumatoid factor with a high titer as well as borderline hypocomplementemia. She responded well to long-term prednisone therapy, whereas the second patient did not require steroid therapy; the condition is considered largely benign.[47]

Marked peripheral eosinophilia may also be seen in association with organ-restricted eosinophilic disorders, such as eosinophilic gastrointestinal disorder (EGID), chronic eosinophilic pneumonia, and Wells syndrome. EGIDs, including eosinophilic esophagitis, eosinophilic gastritis, eosinophilic gastroenteritis, eosinophilic enteritis, and eosinophilic colitis, are characterized by tissue eosinophilia that primarily affects the gastrointestinal tract. Presenting symptoms vary depending on the affected organ and may include dysphagia, reflux, nausea/vomiting, abdominal pain, diarrhea, and failure to thrive.[48] The diagnosis is made through endoscopy and biopsies showing abnormal eosinophilic infiltration; for example, although eosinophils are not typically found in Peyer's patches or the intraepithelial region, they can be present in these locations in the setting of EGID.[49] Many patients with EGID are atopic; the associated gastrointestinal diseases show features of both IgE-mediated and non-IgE–mediated hypersensitivity.[50] Peripheral eosinophilia may be present at levels of greater than 1500/mm^3 in patients with EGID. However, limited studies have shown that these patients may be at lower risk of cardiac or bone marrow involvement; despite this, surveillance for end-organ complications is recommended in this setting.[51]

Although not a comprehensive list, selected causes of eosinophilia are outlined in Fig. 1.

Hypereosinophilic Syndrome

The criteria for HES were established by Chusid and colleagues[52] in the mid-1970s to better characterize a cohort of patients with increased AECs without a clear secondary cause. At the time, the diagnostic criteria included AEC greater than 1500/mm^3 for more than 6 months, evidence of end-organ complications of eosinophilia, and lack of a known secondary cause. It was apparent even then that there were phenotypic differences within this patient population, with significant variability in clinical course and response to therapy.

The definition of HES has undergone revisions as understanding of disease processes and efficacy of treatment have advanced. In 2006 the term HES was expanded to include other systemic conditions known to cause eosinophilia, including EGID, EGPA, and chronic eosinophilic pneumonia.[2] A working group further refined the definition in 2010, with new considerations for disease variability and defined molecular subtypes. With recognition that significant complications could occur with low levels of peripheral eosinophilia, the absolute cutoff of 1500 eosinophils/mm^3 was eliminated

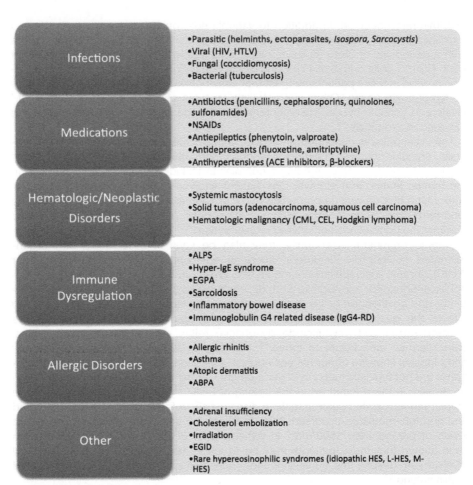

Infections	•Parasitic (helminths, ectoparasites, *Isospora, Sarcocystis*) •Viral (HIV, HTLV) •Fungal (coccidiomycosis) •Bacterial (tuberculosis)
Medications	•Antibiotics (penicillins, cephalosporins, quinolones, sulfonamides) •NSAIDs •Antiepileptics (phenytoin, valproate) •Antidepressants (fluoxetine, amitriptyline) •Antihypertensives (ACE inhibitors, β-blockers)
Hematologic/Neoplastic Disorders	•Systemic mastocytosis •Solid tumors (adenocarcinoma, squamous cell carcinoma) •Hematologic malignancy (CML, CEL, Hodgkin lymphoma)
Immune Dysregulation	•ALPS •Hyper-IgE syndrome •EGPA •Sarcoidosis •Inflammatory bowel disease •Immunoglobulin G4 related disease (IgG4-RD)
Allergic Disorders	•Allergic rhinitis •Asthma •Atopic dermatitis •ABPA
Other	•Adrenal insufficiency •Cholesterol embolization •Irradiation •EGID •Rare hypereosinophilic syndromes (idiopathic HES, L-HES, M-HES)

Fig. 1. Selected causes of eosinophilia. ACE, angiotensin-converting enzyme; CEL, chronic eosinophilic leukemia; L-HES, lymphocytic HES; M-HES, myeloproliferative HES.

if eosinophilic complications were present. Further, because some forms of HES can be rapidly progressive, the requirement of persistently elevated AEC over a 6-month time frame was removed in favor of increases of greater than 1500 eosinophils/mm^3 on 2 occasions. End-organ damage was also discarded as a diagnostic parameter, because patients with significant eosinophilia may never show complications secondary to tissue damage. In addition, exclusion of secondary causes remains a diagnostic necessity, although it was recommended that secondary causes be amended to include molecularly defined disease subtypes that had been established since the initial description of HES.[53]

By following the evolution of the definition of HES, it becomes clear that understanding of the condition has advanced significantly since it was initially recognized. This improved knowledge base has been established through monitoring the natural history of cohorts of patients, technological advancements allowing molecular characterization of disease subtypes, and observing responses to therapy. Established clinical variants of HES include myeloproliferative HES (M-HES) and lymphocytic HES (L-HES), as well as other defined categories. The HES subtypes are outlined in **Fig. 2**.

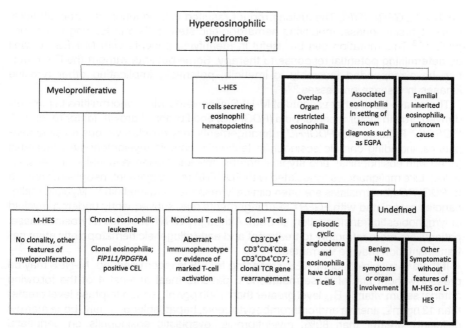

Fig. 2. Variants of HES. The heavy outline connotes conditions that may be associated with T cell–driven eosinophilia. (*Adapted from* Simon H-U, Rothenburg ME, Bochner BS, et al. Refining the definition of hypereosinophilic syndrome. J Allergy Clin Immunol 2010;126:45–9; and Cogan E, Roufosse F. Clinical management of the hypereosinophilic syndromes. Expert Rev Hematol 2012;5(3):275–90.)

Lymphocytic Hypereosinophilic Syndrome

In L-HES, aberrant populations of activated T cells generate eosinophilopoietins, resulting in marked peripheral eosinophilia. These T cells show abnormal patterns of cell surface markers, with the most common being CD3$^-$CD4$^+$; other atypical patterns that have been characterized include CD3$^+$CD4$^-$CD8$^-$ and CD3$^+$CD4$^+$CD7$^-$. The presence of these irregular cells allows these lymphocyte populations to be identified via T-cell receptor rearrangement studies and flow cytometric analysis.[54] Other abnormal laboratory parameters include increased levels of thymus and activation-regulated chemokine (TARC)/CCL17 and increases in serum IgE.[55,56] Although IL-5 has been implicated in the generation of eosinophilia in L-HES, increased IL-5 levels neither correlate with the presence of L-HES nor predict therapeutic response.[57]

Myeloproliferative Hypereosinophilic Syndrome

Patients with M-HES show eosinophilia in the setting of features consistent with myeloproliferative disorders, including anemia, thrombocytopenia, hepatosplenomegaly, and eosinophilic tissue damage and/or fibrosis.[53] Initial descriptions of M-HES included young male patients with aggressive disease that proved refractory to standard treatments. It was later discovered that these patients showed marked clinical improvement with imatinib, a tyrosine kinase inhibitor.[58] Many of these patients were found to have a deletion of an 800-kb region on chromosome 4q12 containing the *CHIC2* gene; this led to an abnormal fusion of Fip1-like 1 (*FIP1L1*) and platelet-derived growth factor receptor alpha (*PDGFRA*), or

FIP1L1-PDGFRA (F/P). The fusion product resulted in production of a constitutively active tyrosine kinase, modifying hematopoietic stem cells and leading to eosinophilia.[7,58] This mutation can be useful in identifying patients with M-HES, as well as determining potential response to therapy. Some patients without the F/P mutation have responded favorably to imatinib, potentially implicating other tyrosine kinases in disease processes.[59]

There have been other variants of M-HES associated with abnormalities in platelet-derived growth factor receptor beta *(PDGFRB)* and fibroblast growth factor receptor 1 *(FGFR1)*.[9] Patients with *PDGFRB* rearrangements may develop various myeloid neoplasms, including chronic eosinophilic leukemia, chronic myelomonocytic leukemia (often with eosinophilia), and atypical chronic myeloid leukemia (usually with eosinophilia). Like malignancies associated with *PDGFRA* rearrangement, neoplasms related to *PDGFRB* abnormalities are often clinically responsive to imatinib.[60] Myeloid malignancies associated with *FGFR1* rearrangements may subsequently undergo myeloid or lymphoblastic transformation, or both. Although *FGFR1* encodes a tyrosine kinase, patients are more refractory to treatment and early allogeneic hematopoietic stem cell transplantation may be warranted.[60]

If there is suspicion for M-HES, screening for F/P is recommended. M-HES may be present without any of these mutations if patients meet at least 4 of the following criteria: serum vitamin B_{12} level greater than 1000 pg/mL, serum tryptase level greater than 12 ng/mL, anemia and/or thrombocytopenia, hepatosplenomegaly, bone marrow cellularity greater than 80%, myelofibrosis, dysplastic eosinophils on peripheral smear, or spindle-shaped mast cells in the bone marrow.[9]

Myeloproliferative features may also coexist with eosinophilia in the setting of chronic eosinophilic leukemia (CEL), which is discussed in detail elsewhere in this issue.

Other Categories of Hypereosinophilic Syndrome

There are other clinically defined subgroups of HES, including associated, overlap, familial, and undefined; many conditions comprising these subgroups are discussed earlier. Associated HES is characterized by an AEC greater than $1500/mm^3$ and is associated with another known condition.[53] These conditions include EGPA, SM, and sarcoidosis. Overlap HES consists of organ-specific eosinophilic disorders associated with peripheral eosinophilia, with examples including EGID and eosinophilic pneumonia. Familial HES is a rare autosomal dominant condition in which marked eosinophilia presents in successive generations. The eosinophilia may be asymptomatic, but some affected individuals develop complications, including cardiac fibrosis and neurologic abnormalities.[61] Although the exact cause is unknown, the responsible gene has been localized to 5q31-q33, in the region of the cytokine gene cluster. This area also contains genes encoding IL-3, IL-5, and GM-CSF, all of which are important to eosinophil development and function.[62]

Undefined HES consists of benign eosinophilia, episodic eosinophilia, and other eosinophilia that does not fit distinctly into another category. Episodic HES presents with intermittent eosinophilia and angioedema, and was discussed earlier in the article as Gleich's syndrome. Benign eosinophilia, also known as hypereosinophilia of unknown significance (HE_{US}), is prolonged eosinophilia that does not result in significant clinical manifestations. A recent retrospective study by Chen and colleagues[63] found that of 210 patients referred for unexplained eosinophilia, 8 of the 36 subjects who were *FIP1L1-PDGFRA* negative with unexplained eosinophilia greater than 1500/mm^3 on no therapy at the time of referral remained asymptomatic without clinical or laboratory evidence of end-organ dysfunction for at least 5 years. The eosinophilia had been identified on routine blood work in all 8 subjects. Levels of IL-5, GM-CSF, IL-9, and IL-17A were similar in subjects with HE_{US} and symptomatic HES.

Approach to the Evaluation of Patients with Persistent, Marked Eosinophilia

In any patient with eosinophilia, the first step is to determine the urgency of evaluation. Patients with exceptionally high peripheral eosinophil counts or end-organ damage that may be attributable to eosinophilic infiltration may require inpatient admission with supportive care and expedited work-up. If these factors are not present, evaluation may occur in the outpatient setting in a stepwise fashion.

Given the myriad of secondary causes, obtaining a thorough history is vital. Because eosinophilic tissue infiltration can affect nearly any organ, a review of systems with particular attention to hematologic, neurologic, dermatologic, cardiovascular, and pulmonary systems should be obtained.[64] Organ-specific symptoms may be present, such as abdominal pain and nausea in the setting of EGID. Inquiries regarding constitutional or B symptoms should also be made to assess for any signs of malignancy or lymphoproliferation. Any family or personal history of chronic medical conditions known to be associated with eosinophilia including autoimmune disease, atopy, and malignancy, should be addressed. It is important to take a detailed travel history, with a focus on any tropical or developing areas that may be endemic for causative parasites or infectious agents. It is necessary to review medication lists with specific attention to supplements, over-the-counter medications, and any recent medications that may have had a transient course, such as antibiotic or nonsteroidal anti-inflammatory drug (NSAID) use. Note that the causative medication need not be initiated recently, because even those that have been used consistently for years have been implicated in causing eosinophilia. An occupational history may reveal potential environmental exposures leading to eosinophilia as well.

The physical examination is also important in narrowing the differential diagnosis in the setting of eosinophilia. Examination of the skin can help to assess for evidence of external causes of eosinophilia, such as scabies. There may also be evidence of cutaneous malignancies, such as Sézary syndrome. Some eosinophilic phenotypes have more characteristic skin findings; for instance, patients with L-HES often have generalized pruritus, urticaria, and erythroderma.[65] Lymphadenopathy may be an indicator of a specific disease entity, such as Kimura syndrome or lymphoma. The presence of hepatosplenomegaly may indicate the presence of a malignancy. Eosinophilic infiltration of the heart can lead to valvular dysfunction with resultant murmurs, arrhythmias, and evidence of heart failure.[66] Pulmonary involvement in eosinophilic disease can result in variable findings, including weight loss, lung infiltrates, and fibrosis.[67] Eosinophilic end-organ damage may be evident in other ways as well, such as jaundice in the setting of liver damage, or edema with renal disease.

If no clear cause of eosinophilia is ascertained by history or physical examination, laboratory assessment can be a helpful tool to assess for the cause. Laboratory evaluation should be considered in any patient with AEC greater than $1500/mm^3$ on 2 or more occasions, patients with AEC 500 to $1500/mm^3$ with potential exposure to infectious agents, or AEC greater than $500/mm^3$ in the setting of end-organ dysfunction.[68] A recommended diagnostic approach is provided in **Fig. 3**. Depending on the urgency of evaluation, clinical suspicion, and the results of the initial laboratory work-up, a more focused set of tests may be indicated. If HES is confirmed, monitoring for evidence of end-organ complications is of the utmost importance. The type and frequency of these evaluations depends on previous end-organ complications, degree of eosinophilia, and existing comorbidities.

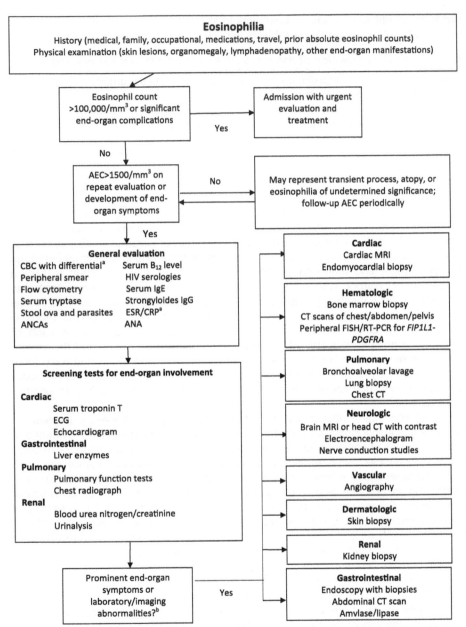

Fig. 3. Algorithm for evaluation of hypereosinophilia. [a] Studies that may be affected by concurrent steroid use. [b] Other studies for end-organ involvement may be warranted based on clinical presentation. ANA, antinuclear antibody; CBC, complete blood count; CRP, C-reactive protein; CT, computed tomography; ECG, electrocardiogram; ESR, erythrocyte sedimentation rate; FISH, fluorescent in situ hybridization; RT-PCR, reverse transcription polymerase chain reaction.

SUMMARY

Identifying the cause of persistent eosinophilia is vital; implications of an increased AEC may range from a benign finding to an aggressive malignancy. Clinical history, physical examination, and laboratory studies can all aid in distinguishing reactive causes of eosinophilia, such as medications and parasites, from primary causes, such as HES. Treatment is highly variable depending on the underlying basis of disease. Although advances in molecular diagnostics and therapies have ushered in changes in the diagnosis and treatment of eosinophilia, the importance of determining the underlying cause remains the same.

REFERENCES

1. Uhm TG, Kim BS, Chung IY. Eosinophil development, regulation of eosinophils-specific genes, and role of eosinophils in the pathogenesis of asthma. Allergy Asthma Immunol Res 2012;4(2):68–79.
2. Khoury P, Grayson PC, Klion A. Eosinophils in vasculitis: characteristics and roles in pathogenesis. Nat Rev Rheumatol 2014;10:474–83.
3. Jung Y, Rothenberg ME. Roles and regulation of gastrointestinal eosinophils in immunity and disease. J Immunol 2014;193:999–1005.
4. Davoine F, Lacy P. Eosinophil cytokines, chemokines, and growth factors: emerging roles in immunity. Front Immunol 2014;5(570):1–17.
5. Parmley RT, Crist WM, Roper M, et al. Intranuclear crystalloids associated with abnormal granules in eosinophilic leukocytes. Blood 1981;58(6):1134–40.
6. Spencer LA, Bonjour K, Melo RC, et al. Eosinophil secretion of granule-derived cytokines. Front Immunol 2014;5(496):1–9.
7. Gotlib J. World Health Organization-defined eosinophilic disorders: 2011 update on diagnosis, risk stratification, and management. Am J Hematol 2011;86:678–88.
8. Klion AD, Bochner BS, Gleich GJ, et al. Approaches to the treatment of hypereosinophilic syndromes: a workshop summary report. J Allergy Clin Immunol 2006;117:1292–302.
9. Roufosse F, Weller PF. Practical approach to the patient with hypereosinophilia. J Allergy Clin Immunol 2010;126(1):39–44.
10. Klion AD, Law MA, Riemenschneider W, et al. Familial eosinophilia: a benign disorder? Blood 2004;103(11):4050–5.
11. Moore TA, Nutman TB. Eosinophilia in the returning traveler. Infect Dis Clin North Am 1998;12:503–21.
12. Nutman TB. Evaluation and differential diagnosis of marked, persistent eosinophilia. Immunol Allergy Clin North Am 2007;27:529–49.
13. Camus P. Eosinophilic pneumonia (pulmonary infiltrates and eosinophilia). In: Pneumotox Online, the drug-induced respiratory disease Web site. 2012. Available at: http://www.pneumotox.com/pattern/view/4/I.c/eosinophilic-pneumonia-pulmonary-infiltrates-and-eosinophilia/?page=2. Accessed March 14, 2015.
14. Rossert J. Drug-induced acute interstitial nephritis. Kidney Int 2001;60:804–17.
15. Ruffing KA, Hoppes P, Blend D, et al. Eosinophils in the urine revisited. Clin Nephrol 1994;41:163–6.
16. Belongia EA, Hedberg CW, Gleich GJ, et al. An investigation of the cause of the eosinophilia-myalgia syndrome associated with tryptophan use. N Engl J Med 1990;323(6):357–65.
17. Tabuenca JM. Toxic-allergic syndrome caused by ingestion of rapeseed oil denatured with aniline. Lancet 1981;2(8246):567–8.

18. Allen JA, Peterson A, Sufit R, et al. Post-epidemic eosinophilia-myalgia syndrome associated with tryptophan. Arthritis Rheum 2011;63(11):3633–9.
19. Criado PR, Avancini J, Santi CG, et al. Drug reaction with eosinophilia and systemic symptoms (DRESS): a complex interaction of drugs, viruses, and the immune system. Isr Med Assoc J 2012;14:577–82.
20. Oskay T, Karademir A, Erturk OL. Association of anticonvulsant hypersensitivity syndrome with herpesvirus 6, 7. Epilepsy Res 2006;701:27–40.
21. Seishima M, Yamanaka S, Fujisawa T, et al. Reactivation of human herpesvirus (HHV) family members other than HHV-6 in drug induced hypersensitivity syndrome. Br J Dermatol 2006;1552:344–9.
22. Agarwal R. Allergic bronchopulmonary aspergillosis. Chest 2009;135(3):805–26.
23. Tefferi A, Patnaik MM, Pardanani A. Eosinophilia: secondary, clonal and idiopathic. Br J Haematol 2006;133:468–92.
24. Gill GV, Bell DR. *Strongyloides stercoralis* in former Far East prisoners of war. Br Med J 1979;2:572–4.
25. Keiser PB, Nutman TB. *Strongyloides stercoralis* in the immunocompromised population. Clin Microbiol Rev 2004;17(1):208–17.
26. Parasites Home, Strongyloidiasis. Resources for health professionals. Centers for Disease Control and Prevention Web site. Page last updated January 6, 2012. Page last reviewed July 19, 2013. Available at: http://www.cdc.gov/parasites/strongyloides/health_professionals/index.html. Accessed January 20, 2014.
27. Trier JS, Moxey PC, Schimmel EM, et al. Chronic intestinal coccidiosis in man: intestinal morphology and response to treatment. Gastroenterology 1974;66:923–35.
28. Chen X, Zuo Y, Zuo W. Observation on the clinical symptoms and sporocyst excretion in human volunteers experimentally infected with *Sarcocystis hominis*. Zhongguo Ji Sheng Chong Xue Yu Ji Sheng Chong Bing Za Zhi 1999;17:25–7 [in Chinese].
29. Sluzevich JC, Sheth AP, Lucky AW. Persistent eosinophilia as a presenting sign of scabies in patients with disorders of keratinization. Arch Dermatol 2007;143(5):659–75.
30. Klion A. Hypereosinophilic syndrome: current approach to diagnosis and treatment. Annu Rev Med 2009;60:293–306.
31. Kaplan MH, Hall WM, Susin M, et al. Syndrome of severe skin disease, eosinophilia, and dermatopathic lymphadenopathy in patients with HTLV-II complicating human immunodeficiency virus infection. Am J Med 1991;91:300–9.
32. Carvalho EM, Da Fonseca Porto A. Epidemiological and clinical interaction between HTLV-1 and *Strongyloides stercoralis*. Parasite Immunol 2004;26:287–497.
33. Cohen AJ, Steigbigel RT. Eosinophilia in patients infected with human immunodeficiency virus. J Infect Dis 1996;174:615–8.
34. Fearfield LA, Rowe A, Francis N, et al. Itchy folliculitis and human immunodeficiency virus infection: clinicopathological and immunological features, pathogenesis and treatment. Br J Dermatol 1999;141(1):3–11.
35. Harley WB, Blaser MJ. Disseminated coccidioidomycosis associated with extreme eosinophilia. J Infect Dis 1994;18:627–9.
36. Angelis M, Yu M, Takanishi D, et al. Eosinophilia as a marker of adrenal insufficiency in the surgical intensive care unit. J Am Coll Surg 1996;183(6):589–96.
37. Lowe D, Jorizzo J, Hutt MS. Tumour-associated eosinophilia: a review. J Clin Pathol 1981;34:1343–8.
38. Todenhofer R, Wirths S, von Weyhern CH, et al. Severe paraneoplastic hypereosinophilia in metastatic renal cell carcinoma. BMC Urol 2012;12:1–7.

39. Roufosse F, Garaud S, de Leval L. Lymphoproliferative disorders associated with hypereosinophilia. Semin Hematol 2012;49(2):138–48.
40. Greco A, Rizzo MI, De Virgilio A, et al. Churg-Strauss syndrome. Autoimmun Rev 2015;14(4):341–8.
41. Kallenberg CG. Key advances in the clinical approach to ANCA-associated vasculitis. Nat Rev Rheumatol 2014;10:484–93.
42. Maric I, Robyn J, Metcalfe DD, et al. KIT-D816V-associated systemic mastocytosis and FIP1L1-PDGFRA-associated chronic eosinophilic leukemia are distinct entities. J Allergy Clin Immunol 2007;120(3):680–7.
43. Kovalski A, Weller PF. Eosinophilia in mast cell disease. Immunol Allergy Clin North Am 2014;34(2):357–64.
44. Koh H, Kamiishi N, Chiyotani A, et al. Eosinophilic lung disease complicated by Kimura's disease: a case report and literature review. Intern Med 2012;51: 3163–7.
45. Khoury P, Herold J, Alpaugh A, et al. Episodic angioedema with eosinophilia (Gleich's syndrome) is a multilineage cell-cycling disorder. Haematologica 2014;100(3):300–7.
46. Lasalle P, Gosset P, Gruart V, et al. Presence of antibodies against endothelial cells in patients with episodic angioedema and hypereosinophilia. Clin Exp Immunol 1990;82:38–43.
47. Butterfield JH, Leiferman KM, Gleich GJ. Nodules, eosinophilia, rheumatism, dermatitis and swelling (NERDS): a novel eosinophilic disorder. Clin Exp Allergy 1993;23:571–80.
48. Hruz PL, Straumann A. Chapter 44: eosinophil-associated gastrointestinal disorders. In: Rich RR, Fleisher TA, Shaerer WT, et al, editors. Clinical immunology: principles and practice. 4th edition. Elsevier Saunders; 2013. p. 550–7.
49. Rothenberg ME, Mishra A, Brandt EB, et al. Gastrointestinal eosinophils. Immunol Rev 2001;179:139–55.
50. Sampson HA. Food allergy. Part 1: immunopathogenesis and clinical disorders. J Allergy Clin Immunol 1999;103:717–28.
51. Lee J, Dierkhising R, Wu T-T, et al. Eosinophilic gastrointestinal disorders (EGID) with peripheral eosinophilia: a retrospective review at the Mayo Clinic. Dig Dis Sci 2011;56:3254–61.
52. Chusid MJ, Dale CD, West BC, et al. The hypereosinophilic syndrome: analysis of fourteen cases with review of the literature. Medicine (Baltimore) 1975;54: 1–27.
53. Simon H-U, Rothenburg ME, Bochner BS, et al. Refining the definition of hypereosinophilic syndrome. J Allergy Clin Immunol 2010;126:45–9.
54. Roufosse F, Cogan E, Goldman M. Lymphocytic variant hypereosinophilic syndromes. Immunol Allergy Clin North Am 2007;27(3):551–60.
55. Ravoet M, Sibille C, Roufosse F, et al. 6q- is an early and persistent chromosomal aberration in CD3-CD4+ T-cell clones associated with the lymphocytic variant of hypereosinophilic syndrome. Haematologica 2005;90:753–65.
56. Rothenberg ME, Klion AD, Roufosse FE, et al. Treatment of patients with the hypereosinophilic syndrome with mepolizumab. N Engl J Med 2002;358: 1215–28.
57. Vaklavas C, Tefferi A, Butterfield J, et al. Idiopathic eosinophilia with an occult T-cell clone: prevalence and clinical course. Leuk Res 2007;31:691–4.
58. Cools J, DeAngelo DJ, Gotlib J, et al. A novel tyrosine kinase created by the fusion of the PDGFRA and FIP1L1 genes is a therapeutic target of imatinib in idiopathic hypereosinophilic syndrome. N Engl J Med 2003;348:1201–14.

59. Pardnani A, Brockman SR, Paternoster SF, et al. FIP1L1-PDGFRA fusion: prevalence and clinicopathologic correlates in 89 consecutive patients with severe eosinophilia. Blood 2004;104(10):3038–45.
60. Bain BJ. Myeloid and lymphoid neoplasms with eosinophilia and abnormalities of PDGFRA, PDGFRB or FGFR1. Haematologica 2010;95(5):696–8.
61. Lin AY, Nutman TB, Kaslow D, et al. Familial eosinophilia: clinical and laboratory characteristics of a U.S. kindred. Am J Med Genet 1998;76:229–37.
62. Rious JD, Stone VA, Daly MJ, et al. Familial eosinophilia maps to the cytokine gene cluster on human chromosomal region 5q31-q33. Am J Hum Genet 1998; 63:1086–94.
63. Chen Y-Y, Khoury P, Ware JM, et al. Marked and persistent eosinophilia in the absence of clinical manifestations. J Allergy Clin Immunol 2014;133:1195–202.
64. Weller PF, Bubley GJ. The idiopathic hypereosinophilic syndrome. Blood 1994; 83(10):2759–79.
65. Leiferman KM, Gleich GJ, Peters MS. Dermatologic manifestations of the hypereosinophilic syndromes. Immunol Allergy Clin North Am 2007;27(3):415–41.
66. Ogbogu PU, Rosing DR, McDonald KH. Cardiovascular manifestations of hypereosinophilic syndromes. Immunol Allergy Clin North Am 2007;27(3):457–75.
67. Wechsler MM. Pulmonary eosinophilic syndromes. Immunol Allergy Clin North Am 2007;27(3):477–92.
68. Weller PF, Klion A. Approach to the patient with unexplained eosinophilia. In: Mahoney DH, Bochner BS, editors. Waltham (MA): UpToDate; 2014. Available at: http://www.uptodate.com/contents/approach-to-the-patient-with-unexplained-eosinophilia. Accessed January 5, 2015.

Spectrum of Eosinophilic End-Organ Manifestations

Praveen Akuthota, MD[a,b,*], Peter F. Weller, MD[b,c]

KEYWORDS

- Eosinophils pathology • Eosinophils immunology • Humans
- Pulmonary eosinophilia • Eosinophilic esophagitis • Hypereosinophilic syndrome
- Churg-Strauss syndrome • Eosinophilic granulomatous vasculitis

KEY POINTS

- Eosinophilia may affect any organ and cause end-organ damage.
- Mechanisms by which eosinophilia promotes tissue damage include infiltration, fibrosis, thrombosis, and allergic inflammation.
- Patterns of eosinophil-mediated end-organ dysfunction are particularly well characterized for the lungs, heart, and gastrointestinal tract.

INTRODUCTION

The purpose and function of eosinophils in health and disease are complex and cannot be readily crystallized into a single summary statement. This has become increasingly true as myriad potential immunoregulatory behaviors of eosinophils have been uncovered in recent years.[1,2] However, the traditional characterization of eosinophils as end-organ effector cells, causing tissue damage through release of cationic granule proteins, is borne of the observation of a spectrum of eosinophil-associated disorders encompassing practically all organ systems of the body. These disorders may affect one organ alone, such as the eosinophilic pneumonias or eosinophilic esophagitis, or affect multiple organ systems simultaneously, such as the hypereosinophilic

The authors have no financial disclosures or conflicts of interest relevant to the content of this article. Dr P. Akuthota is funded by National Institutes of Health Grant K08HL116429. Dr P.F. Weller is funded by National Institutes of Health grants R37AI020241 and U01AI097073.
[a] Division of Pulmonary, Critical Care, and Sleep Medicine, Beth Israel Deaconess Medical Center, Harvard Medical School, 330 Brookline Avenue, Boston, MA 02215, USA; [b] Division of Allergy and Inflammation, Beth Israel Deaconess Medical Center, Harvard Medical School, 330 Brookline Avenue, Boston, MA 02215, USA; [c] Division of Infectious Diseases, Beth Israel Deaconess Medical Center, Harvard Medical School, 330 Brookline Avenue, Boston, MA 02215, USA
* Corresponding author. 330 Brookline Avenue, E/KSB-23, Boston, MA 02215.
E-mail address: pakuthot@bidmc.harvard.edu

Immunol Allergy Clin N Am 35 (2015) 403–411
http://dx.doi.org/10.1016/j.iac.2015.04.002
0889-8561/15/$ – see front matter © 2015 Elsevier Inc. All rights reserved.

syndromes or eosinophilic granulomatosis with polyangiitis (EGPA, formerly known as Churg-Strauss syndrome).[3–6] This article provides an overview of eosinophilic end-organ manifestations, setting the stage for the organ-specific articles discussed elsewhere in this issue. **Table 1** provides a partial tabulation of organs and organ-systems that may be affected by eosinophilia and potential diagnostic tests and assays that can reflect end-organ dysfunction.

MECHANISMS OF END-ORGAN MANIFESTATIONS

Although the specific mechanisms by which tissue eosinophilia results in end-organ dysfunction require further investigation, some general themes can be constructed based on current knowledge. These themes may be overlapping in specific disease processes but can be useful in parsing the pathologic effects of eosinophils in disease.[7]

The first is that the infiltration of eosinophils in tissue can, in and of itself, be pathologic if it is extensive enough. For example, in the eosinophilic pneumonias, the main finding observed on lung biopsy is often simply extensive infiltration of eosinophils into the lung parenchyma.[3,8,9]

Second, eosinophils may also cause organ damage mediated through associated fibrosis.[10] Several in vitro studies have demonstrated the potential of eosinophils to promote fibroblast activation, proliferation, and extracellular matrix production, likely through their secretion of transforming growth factor (TGF)-β and interleukin (IL)-1β.[11–15] Eosinophil cationic protein, one of the granule-stored proteins of eosinophils, has been observed in vitro to promote fibroblast migration and TGF-β release, potentially implicating granule protein deposition as a mechanism for eosinophil-mediated tissue fibrosis.[16,17] Eosinophil-associated tissue fibrosis is observed in the heart, specifically the endocardium; in hypereosinophilic syndromes; and in the sub-epithelial fibrosis that is characteristic of eosinophilic esophagitis and asthma.[18–20]

Table 1
Detection of eosinophilic end-organ dysfunction

Organ System Affected by Eosinophilia	Selected Studies
Cardiac	Serum troponin Electrocardiogram Echocardiogram Cardiac MRI
Gastrointestinal	Endoscopy with tissue biopsy Serum liver function testing Serum amylase, lipase
Pulmonary	Chest radiograph Chest computed tomography Pulmonary function testing Bronchoscopy with bronchoalveolar lavage Lung biopsy
Neurologic	Head MRI Head computed tomography Nerve conduction studies Nerve biopsy
Skin	Skin biopsy
Renal	Serum creatinine Urine eosinophils Kidney biopsy

Third, allergic mechanisms are a substantial driving force behind a subset of eosinophil-associated diseases and their resulting end-organ manifestations.[21] The T helper-2 cell inflammation that is characteristic of allergic-mediated disease creates an IL-5 rich environment, promoting eosinophil infiltration and survival.[22–24] Additionally, eosinophils have immunoregulatory functions that may promote further inflammation in these tissue environments.[1] Cardinal examples include allergic asthma and atopic dermatitis.[25,26]

Finally, eosinophils have in certain conditions been observed to promote hypercoagulability, which may in turn promote end-organ damage.[20] This effect may be mediated through hypercoagulable and platelet-activating effects of eosinophil granule proteins.[27,28] Such a phenomenon has been reported in the form of thrombotic microangiopathic kidney disease in hypereosinophilic syndromes.[29]

GASTROINTESTINAL

Eosinophils are normally present in all portions of the gastrointestinal tract, with the exception of the esophagus.[30] However, their presence may be pathologic in the gastrointestinal tract when they are present in excess and they are the defining feature of a set of diseases known as the eosinophilic gastrointestinal disorders (EGIDs).[4] These include eosinophilic esophagitis, eosinophilic gastritis and gastroenteritis, and eosinophilic colitis. The degree of end-organ dysfunction in EGID depends on the location and extent of disease. In the esophagus, for example, functional manifestations may include food impaction and general dysphagia, with eosinophilic inflammation and epithelial hyperplasia seen on tissue specimens.[30–32] In progressing distally down the gastrointestinal tract, end-organ manifestations can be characterized by defects in nutrient and calorie absorption, as well as frank protein-losing enteropathy.[30] On endoscopic examination, the examined portions of the gastrointestinal tract are commonly visually abnormal in appearance, emphasizing the functional consequences of tissue eosinophilia.[33]

Eosinophilia involving the gastrointestinal tract may be part of the spectrum of systemic illness in EGPA.[6] The small bowel is most commonly affected and can lead to abdominal pain and gastrointestinal bleeding. In severe cases, bowel ischemia can occur.[6]

Tissue eosinophilia may be seen in the liver and, in particular, be associated with frank hepatitis and hepatic injury in systemic eosinophilia associated with severe drug reactions, known as drug reaction with eosinophilia and systemic symptoms (DRESS) syndrome.[34] In this condition, liver injury can be detected by elevation in serum transaminases.[35] Though rare, eosinophilic infiltration resulting in pancreatitis has been described.[36]

PULMONARY

The lung is perhaps the organ in which tissue eosinophilia intersects most distinctly with organ infiltration to result in a set of specific disease entities. These include allergic asthma, acute and chronic eosinophilic pneumonia, allergic bronchopulmonary aspergillosis, and EGPA, as well as a host of infectious entities that are predominantly parasitic in nature.[3] From a functional perspective, eosinophilic infiltration can be thought of as affecting 2 separate but intimately related compartments, the airways and alveolar spaces (along with accompanying interstitium).

Tissue eosinophilia of the airway wall contributes to the obstructive physiology characteristic of asthma, promoting subepithelial fibrosis and airways hyperresponsiveness.[19] Similar physiology associated with tissue eosinophilia may be found in related disorders that can mimic traditional asthma, principally EGPA and allergic bronchopulmonary aspergillosis. The resulting obstruction is manifest in dyspnea and wheeze that are often experienced by patients and may be quantified by a characteristic pattern on pulmonary function testing.[3]

Eosinophilic infiltration of the alveolar spaces and associated interstitium are characteristic of the eosinophilic pneumonias and may be seen in EGPA as well. Involvement of these areas of lung responsible for gas exchange not only results in dyspnea but also in hypoxemia.[37,38] Gas exchange abnormalities can result in respiratory failure in severe cases with extensive parenchymal involvement.[37,38] In acute eosinophilic pneumonia, diffuse alveolar damage may accompany eosinophilic infiltration on pathologic specimens.[37] In EGPA, eosinophilic vasculitis in the pulmonary interstitium can be observed (though not necessarily), as the name of the disorder implies.[6] Eosinophilic inflammation of the alveolar spaces may be detected by the observation of eosinophils in bronchoalveolar lavage specimens taken during bronchoscopy.[3]

Eosinophilic effusions can also form in the pleural space, affecting lung function through extraparenchymal compression, leading to shortness of breath and impaired gas exchange.[39] Eosinophilic pleural effusions may be idiopathic in nature, although they are also associated with other specific processes, including pathologic drug reactions, malignancy, and parasitic infections.[39]

UPPER AIRWAY AND SINUSES

As a disease entity, chronic rhinosinusitis is strongly associated with tissue eosinophilia.[40] In particular, eosinophilia is associated with rhinosinusitis accompanied by nasal polyposis.[41] Chronic rhinosinusitis can occur independently in atopic individuals or in close association with allergic asthma or EGPA. From an end-organ dysfunction perspective, loss of smell can occur, along with sinus pain and pressure, mucus production, and nasal blockage.[40] Although no specific functional studies are characteristic of eosinophilic infiltration of the sinuses and nasal tissue, eosinophilia may be noted in pathologic specimens obtained in therapeutic surgical procedures.

CARDIOVASCULAR

Eosinophilic inflammation affects the heart in systemic eosinophilic processes such as hypereosinophilic syndromes and EGPA, as well as in concert with helminthic processes and tropical eosinophilia.[20,42,43] End-organ damage to the heart occurs through multiple pathways, including endocardial necrosis, fibrosis, intraluminal thrombosis, and ischemia due to epicardial vascular involvement.[7,20]

In the hypereosinophilic syndromes, endocardial damage occurs initially as necrosis and progresses to endocardial fibrosis.[44,45] Endocardial damage can affect the systolic and diastolic functionality of the heart.[46] When fibrosis affects the chordae tendineae, valvular function can potentially be impaired. The endocardial damage and eosinophilia in hypereosinophilic states also promote intraluminal thrombosis, which has the potential to further impair cardiac function through impairment of filling and flow through the ventricular outflow tract.[20,28] These end-organ cardiac manifestations lead to dyspnea when symptomatic. Although endocardial inflammation is also seen as the primary cardiac pattern in EGPA, small vessel coronary vasculitis and pericarditis may be seen and represent additional patterns of cardiac end-organ dysfunction related to eosinophilia.[42,43]

Echocardiography may detect impairment of cardiac and valvular function and visualize thrombus, whereas cardiac MRI is emerging as a useful modality to detect endocardial fibrosis before functional consequences are readily apparent.[47–49]

Electrocardiogram is nonspecific but is also abnormal with endocardial, pericardial, and ischemic eosinophilic cardiac processes.[50] In eosinophilic disorders, serum troponin is a useful clinical tool to detect any possible active cardiomyocyte cell damage or death.[51]

NEUROLOGIC

The idiopathic hypereosinophilic syndromes and EGPA each have the potential to demonstrate end-organ neurologic manifestations, with the ability to affect both the peripheral and central nervous systems.[52] The peripheral neuropathies that occur with hypereosinophilic syndromes may have motor and sensory components of varied distributions.[44] Direct eosinophil infiltration is often not seen on pathologic examination, making the exact mechanism of end-organ dysfunction somewhat unclear.[52] In EGPA, mononeuritis multiplex is commonly seen and is used as a criterion in diagnostic schema, including the often-cited 1990 American College of Rheumatology criteria.[53] Eosinophilic vasculitis may be seen on nerve biopsy specimens in EGPA.[54]

The central nervous system and cranial nerves can be affected in the hypereosinophilic syndromes. However, as with peripheral neuropathy, pathologic testing does not necessarily reveal eosinophilic infiltration.[52,55] Central nervous system and cranial nerve involvement have also been reported in EGPA.[6,54]

As discussed previously, hypereosinophilia is associated with thrombosis, providing an additional thromboembolic mechanism for end-organ neurologic injury.

SKIN

Dermatologic eosinophilia is varied in nature, can involve all layers of the skin, and can be associated with both local and system disease.[56] Although it is challenging to categorize eosinophilia of the skin into patterns of end-organ damage, highlighting dermatologic disorders that are characterized by eosinophilia can be illustrative (see article by Dagmar Simon elsewhere in this issue). Skin biopsy is the key modality in diagnosis of this diverse group of conditions, including atopic dermatitis, eosinophilic cellulitis (Wells syndrome), eosinophilic fasciitis, eosinophilic panniculitis, bullous pemphigoid, urticaria, and drug reactions.[56–60]

In systemic disorders such as EGPA, skin lesions demonstrating eosinophilic vasculitis can be part of the spectrum of disease.[54] Hypereosinophilic syndromes, particularly lymphocytic variants, can demonstrate urticaria and angioedema or, alternatively, erythematous papules and nodules.[52] Episodic angioedema with eosinophilia, known as Gleich syndrome, represents another distinct entity with its own dermatologic end-organ manifestation.[61]

RENAL AND GENITOURINARY

Eosinophiluria can indicate eosinophilic end-organ disease of the kidney in acute interstitial nephritis related to drug exposure. Common offenders include nonsteroidal antiinflammatory medications and antibiotics.[62] Acute interstitial nephritis may also be seen in systemic infections and inflammatory conditions such as Sjögren syndrome and sarcoidosis.[63,64]

The kidneys can be involved in EGPA, in particular in patients with circulating anti-neutrophil cytoplasmic antibodies.[6,54] End-organ dysfunction of the kidney is reflected in elevated serum creatinine.

Eosinophilic cystitis and eosinophilic prostatitis do not just cause end-organ damage to the bladder and prostate, respectively, but can also lead to renal failure.[65,66]

SUMMARY

This article does not represent an exhaustive list of the potential end-organ manifestations of eosinophilia. Many other entities, such as eosinophilic myositis and localized eosinophilic vasculitis of the skin, belong on the full roster of eosinophilic conditions with end-organ consequences.[67,68] Although eosinophilic disorders encompass a broad range of conditions that are not easily categorized other than the common characteristic of the presence of eosinophils, whether they be present in the blood, in tissues, or in combination, it is clear that eosinophilia can cause significant dysfunction of virtually any organ or organ system.

REFERENCES

1. Akuthota P, Wang HB, Spencer LA, et al. Immunoregulatory roles of eosinophils: a new look at a familiar cell. Clin Exp Allergy 2008;38(8):1254–63.
2. Shamri R, Xenakis JJ, Spencer LA. Eosinophils in innate immunity: an evolving story. Cell Tissue Res 2011;343(1):57–83.
3. Akuthota P, Weller PF. Eosinophilic pneumonias. Clin Microbiol Rev 2012;25(4): 649–60.
4. DeBrosse CW, Rothenberg ME. Allergy and eosinophil-associated gastrointestinal disorders (EGID). Curr Opin Immunol 2008;20(6):703–8.
5. Ogbogu PU, Bochner BS, Butterfield JH, et al. Hypereosinophilic syndrome: a multicenter, retrospective analysis of clinical characteristics and response to therapy. J Allergy Clin Immunol 2009;124(6):1319–25.e3.
6. Vaglio A, Buzio C, Zwerina J. Eosinophilic granulomatosis with polyangiitis (Churg-Strauss): state of the art. Allergy 2013;68(3):261–73.
7. Akuthota P, Weller PF. Eosinophils and disease pathogenesis. Semin Hematol 2012;49(2):113–9.
8. Carrington CB, Addington WW, Goff AM, et al. Chronic eosinophilic pneumonia. N Engl J Med 1969;280(15):787–98.
9. Tazelaar HD, Linz LJ, Colby TV, et al. Acute eosinophilic pneumonia: histopathologic findings in nine patients. Am J Respir Crit Care Med 1997;155(1):296–302.
10. Noguchi H, Kephart GM, Colby TV, et al. Tissue eosinophilia and eosinophil degranulation in syndromes associated with fibrosis. Am J Pathol 1992;140(2): 521–8.
11. Gomes I, Mathur SK, Espenshade BM, et al. Eosinophil-fibroblast interactions induce fibroblast IL-6 secretion and extracellular matrix gene expression: implications in fibrogenesis. J Allergy Clin Immunol 2005;116(4):796–804.
12. Levi-Schaffer F, Garbuzenko E, Rubin A, et al. Human eosinophils regulate human lung- and skin-derived fibroblast properties in vitro: a role for transforming growth factor beta (TGF-beta). Proc Natl Acad Sci U S A 1999;96(17):9660–5.
13. Shock A, Rabe KF, Dent G, et al. Eosinophils adhere to and stimulate replication of lung fibroblasts 'in vitro'. Clin Exp Immunol 1991;86(1):185–90.
14. Wong DT, Elovic A, Matossian K, et al. Eosinophils from patients with blood eosinophilia express transforming growth factor beta 1. Blood 1991;78(10):2702–7.
15. Pincus SH, Ramesh KS, Wyler DJ. Eosinophils stimulate fibroblast DNA synthesis. Blood 1987;70(2):572–4.
16. Zagai U, Lundahl J, Klominek J, et al. Eosinophil cationic protein stimulates migration of human lung fibroblasts in vitro. Scand J Immunol 2009;69(4):381–6.
17. Zagai U, Dadfar E, Lundahl J, et al. Eosinophil cationic protein stimulates TGF-beta1 release by human lung fibroblasts in vitro. Inflammation 2007;30(5): 153–60.

18. Aceves SS, Ackerman SJ. Relationships between eosinophilic inflammation, tissue remodeling, and fibrosis in eosinophilic esophagitis. Immunol Allergy Clin North Am 2009;29(1):197–211, xiii–xiv.
19. Aceves SS, Broide DH. Airway fibrosis and angiogenesis due to eosinophil trafficking in chronic asthma. Curr Mol Med 2008;8(5):350–8.
20. Ogbogu PU, Rosing DR, Horne MK 3rd. Cardiovascular manifestations of hypereosinophilic syndromes. Immunol Allergy Clin North Am 2007;27(3):457–75.
21. Akuthota P, Xenakis JJ, Weller PF. Eosinophils: offenders or general bystanders in allergic airway disease and pulmonary immunity? J Innate Immun 2011;3(2): 113–9.
22. Kita H. Eosinophils: multifaceted biological properties and roles in health and disease. Immunol Rev 2011;242(1):161–77.
23. Warringa RA, Schweizer RC, Maikoe T, et al. Modulation of eosinophil chemotaxis by interleukin-5. Am J Respir Cell Mol Biol 1992;7(6):631–6.
24. Yamaguchi Y, Hayashi Y, Sugama Y, et al. Highly purified murine interleukin 5 (IL-5) stimulates eosinophil function and prolongs in vitro survival. IL-5 as an eosinophil chemotactic factor. J Exp Med 1988;167(5):1737–42.
25. Fajt ML, Wenzel SE. Asthma phenotypes and the use of biologic medications in asthma and allergic disease: The next steps toward personalized care. J Allergy Clin Immunol 2015;135(2):299–310.
26. Simon D, Wardlaw A, Rothenberg ME. Organ-specific eosinophilic disorders of the skin, lung, and gastrointestinal tract. J Allergy Clin Immunol 2010;126(1): 3–13.
27. Rohrbach MS, Wheatley CL, Slifman NR, et al. Activation of platelets by eosinophil granule proteins. J Exp Med 1990;172(4):1271–4.
28. Slungaard A, Vercellotti GM, Tran T, et al. Eosinophil cationic granule proteins impair thrombomodulin function. A potential mechanism for thromboembolism in hypereosinophilic heart disease. J Clin Invest 1993;91(4):1721–30.
29. Liapis H, Ho AK, Brown D, et al. Thrombotic microangiopathy associated with the hypereosinophilic syndrome. Kidney Int 2005;67(5):1806–11.
30. Davis BP, Rothenberg ME. Eosinophils and gastrointestinal disease. In: Lee J, Rosenberg HF, editors. Eosinophils in health and disease. 1st edition. London; Waltham (MA): Elsevier/Academic Press; 2013. p. 484–93.
31. Rothenberg ME, Mishra A, Collins MH, et al. Pathogenesis and clinical features of eosinophilic esophagitis. J Allergy Clin Immunol 2001;108(6):891–4.
32. Orenstein SR, Shalaby TM, Di Lorenzo C, et al. The spectrum of pediatric eosinophilic esophagitis beyond infancy: a clinical series of 30 children. Am J Gastroenterol 2000;95(6):1422–30.
33. Croese J, Fairley SK, Masson JW, et al. Clinical and endoscopic features of eosinophilic esophagitis in adults. Gastrointest Endosc 2003;58(4):516–22.
34. Husain Z, Reddy BY, Schwartz RA. DRESS syndrome: part I. Clinical perspectives. J Am Acad Dermatol 2013;68(5):693.e1–14.
35. Bjornsson E, Olsson R. Outcome and prognostic markers in severe drug-induced liver disease. Hepatology 2005;42(2):481–9.
36. Abraham SC, Leach S, Yeo CJ, et al. Eosinophilic pancreatitis and increased eosinophils in the pancreas. Am J Surg Pathol 2003;27(3):334–42.
37. Janz DR, O'Neal HR Jr, Ely EW. Acute eosinophilic pneumonia: a case report and review of the literature. Crit Care Med 2009;37(4):1470–4.
38. Jederlinic PJ, Sicilian L, Gaensler EA. Chronic eosinophilic pneumonia. A report of 19 cases and a review of the literature. Medicine (Baltimore) 1988;67(3): 154–62.

39. Kalomenidis I, Light RW. Eosinophilic pleural effusions. Curr Opin Pulm Med 2003;9(4):254–60.
40. Schleimer RP, Kato A, Kern R. Eosinophils and chronic rhinosinusitis. In: Lee J, Rosenberg HF, editors. Eosinophils in health and disease. 1st edition. London; Waltham (MA): Elsevier/Academic Press; 2013. p. 508–19.
41. Van Zele T, Claeys S, Gevaert P, et al. Differentiation of chronic sinus diseases by measurement of inflammatory mediators. Allergy 2006;61(11):1280–9.
42. Neumann T, Manger B, Schmid M, et al. Cardiac involvement in Churg-Strauss syndrome: impact of endomyocarditis. Medicine (Baltimore) 2009;88(4):236–43.
43. Dennert RM, van Paassen P, Schalla S, et al. Cardiac involvement in Churg-Strauss syndrome. Arthritis Rheum 2010;62(2):627–34.
44. Weller PF, Bubley GJ. The idiopathic hypereosinophilic syndrome. Blood 1994; 83(10):2759–79.
45. Tai PC, Ackerman SJ, Spry CJ, et al. Deposits of eosinophil granule proteins in cardiac tissues of patients with eosinophilic endomyocardial disease. Lancet 1987;1(8534):643–7.
46. Zientek DM, King DL, Dewan SJ, et al. Hypereosinophilic syndrome with rapid progression of cardiac involvement and early echocardiographic abnormalities. Am Heart J 1995;130(6):1295–8.
47. Shah R, Ananthasubramaniam K. Evaluation of cardiac involvement in hypereosinophilic syndrome: complementary roles of transthoracic, transesophageal, and contrast echocardiography. Echocardiography 2006;23(8):689–91.
48. Syed IS, Martinez MW, Feng DL, et al. Cardiac magnetic resonance imaging of eosinophilic endomyocardial disease. Int J Cardiol 2008;126(3):e50–2.
49. Plastiras SC, Economopoulos N, Kelekis NL, et al. Magnetic resonance imaging of the heart in a patient with hypereosinophilic syndrome. Am J Med 2006;119(2):130–2.
50. Parrillo JE, Borer JS, Henry WL, et al. The cardiovascular manifestations of the hypereosinophilic syndrome. Prospective study of 26 patients, with review of the literature. Am J Med 1979;67(4):572–82.
51. Pitini V, Arrigo C, Azzarello D, et al. Serum concentration of cardiac Troponin T in patients with hypereosinophilic syndrome treated with imatinib is predictive of adverse outcomes. Blood 2003;102(9):3456–7 [author reply: 3457].
52. Sheikh J, Weller PF. Clinical overview of hypereosinophilic syndromes. Immunol Allergy Clin North Am 2007;27(3):333–55.
53. Masi AT, Hunder GG, Lie JT, et al. The American College of Rheumatology 1990 criteria for the classification of Churg-Strauss syndrome (allergic granulomatosis and angiitis). Arthritis Rheum 1990;33(8):1094–100.
54. Comarmond C, Pagnoux C, Khellaf M, et al. Eosinophilic granulomatosis with polyangiitis (Churg-Strauss): clinical characteristics and long-term followup of the 383 patients enrolled in the French Vasculitis Study Group cohort. Arthritis Rheum 2013;65(1):270–81.
55. Moore PM, Harley JB, Fauci AS. Neurologic dysfunction in the idiopathic hypereosinophilic syndrome. Ann Intern Med 1985;102(1):109–14.
56. Simon D, Simon HU. Eosinophils and skin diseases. In: Lee J, Rosenberg HF, editors. Eosinophils in health and disease. 1st edition. London; Waltham (MA): Elsevier/Academic Press; 2013. p. 442–8.
57. Adame J, Cohen PR. Eosinophilic panniculitis: diagnostic considerations and evaluation. J Am Acad Dermatol 1996;34(2 Pt 1):229–34.
58. Caputo R, Marzano AV, Vezzoli P, et al. Wells syndrome in adults and children: a report of 19 cases. Arch Dermatol 2006;142(9):1157–61.

59. Doyle JA, Ginsburg WW. Eosinophilic fasciitis. Med Clin North Am 1989;73(5): 1157–66.
60. Leiferman KM. Eosinophils in atopic dermatitis. J Allergy Clin Immunol 1994;94(6 Pt 2):1310–7.
61. Gleich GJ, Schroeter AL, Marcoux JP, et al. Episodic angioedema associated with eosinophilia. N Engl J Med 1984;310(25):1621–6.
62. Praga M, Gonzalez E. Acute interstitial nephritis. Kidney Int 2010;77(11):956–61.
63. Maripuri S, Grande JP, Osborn TG, et al. Renal involvement in primary Sjögren's syndrome: a clinicopathologic study. Clin J Am Soc Nephrol 2009;4(9):1423–31.
64. Casella FJ, Allon M. The kidney in sarcoidosis. J Am Soc Nephrol 1993;3(9): 1555–62.
65. Kilic S, Erguvan R, Ipek D, et al. Eosinophilic cystitis. A rare inflammatory pathology mimicking bladder neoplasms. Urol Int 2003;71(3):285–9.
66. Liu S, Miller PD, Holmes SA, et al. Eosinophilic prostatitis and prostatic specific antigen. Br J Urol 1992;69(1):61–3.
67. Chen KR, Su WP, Pittelkow MR, et al. Eosinophilic vasculitis syndrome: recurrent cutaneous eosinophilic necrotizing vasculitis. Semin Dermatol 1995;14(2): 106–10.
68. Selva-O'Callaghan A, Trallero-Araguas E, Grau JM. Eosinophilic myositis: an updated review. Autoimmun Rev 2014;13(4–5):375–8.

Eosinophils in Gastrointestinal Disorders

Eosinophilic Gastrointestinal Diseases, Celiac Disease, Inflammatory Bowel Diseases, and Parasitic Infections

Pooja Mehta, MD, Glenn T. Furuta, MD*

KEYWORDS

- Eosinophil • Esophagitis • Eosinophilic esophagitis • Eosinophilic gastritis
- Eosinophilic gastroenteritis • Eosinophilic colitis • Parasitic infection

KEY POINTS

- Eosinophilic gastrointestinal diseases (EGIDs) describe a group of diseases occurring in children and adults and are characterized by symptoms related to gastrointestinal (GI) dysfunction and inflammation consistent with increased intestinal eosinophilia.
- Eosinophilic esophagitis, the most common EGID, presents in children with feeding problems, abdominal pain, and symptoms recalcitrant to acid inhibition, and in adults with food impaction and dysphagia.
- Eosinophilic gastritis, gastroenteritis, and colitis are uncommon and present with abdominal pain, vomiting, diarrhea, and bleeding.
- The association of celiac disease with eosinophils in the small intestinal and esophageal mucosa is increasingly recognized and requires individualized assessment and treatment.
- The association of inflammatory bowel diseases (IBDs) with mucosal eosinophilia and its secreted products is increasing, but the role of eosinophils in the pathogenesis of IBD remains uncertain.
- Intestinal helminth infection can produce a clinical picture indistinguishable from eosinophilic gastroenteritis.

P. Mehta has nothing to disclose. G.T. Furuta is co-founder of EnteroTrack and recipient of NIH grant 1K24DK100303 and the Consortium for Gastrointestinal Eosinophilic Researchers (CEGIR). CEGIR (U54 AI117804) is part of the Rare Diseases Clinical Research Network (RDCRN), an initiative of the Office of Rare Diseases Research (ORDR), NCATS, and is funded through collaboration between NIAID, NIDDK, and NCATS.
Department of Pediatrics, Gastrointestinal Eosinophilic Diseases Program, Section of Pediatric Gastroenterology, Hepatology, and Nutrition, Digestive Health Institute, Children's Hospital Colorado, University of Colorado School of Medicine, 13123 East 16th Ave B290, Aurora, CO 80045, USA
* Corresponding author. University of Colorado School of Medicine, Denver, CO.
E-mail address: glenn.furuta@childrenscolorado.org

Immunol Allergy Clin N Am 35 (2015) 413–437
http://dx.doi.org/10.1016/j.iac.2015.04.003
0889-8561/15/$ – see front matter © 2015 Elsevier Inc. All rights reserved.

immunology.theclinics.com

INTRODUCTION

The gastrointestinal (GI) tract possesses the greatest surface area of any organ in the body and contains the largest number of immune cells and products. Functionally, the gut must maintain critical functions of nutrition absorption and of oral tolerance. How this latter process occurs in such a fine-tuned and regulated fashion remains an area of active investigation.

Over the past few decades, the identification of eosinophils in the GI tract has begun to arouse suspicion that they play a role in GI health and/or disease.[1,2] In contrast to the neutrophil, which is typically absent in the healthy GI tract, eosinophils reside in varying quantities in the mucosa. During disease states, eosinophils increase and have been implicated in the pathogenesis of ongoing inflammatory processes (**Table 1**). These observations are typically limited to enumerating eosinophils in the epithelium or mucosal surface; the exact depth, distribution, and state of activation in these circumstances are still undergoing definition.

This article focuses on 4 diseases in which mucosal eosinophils are clearly associated, eosinophilic gastrointestinal diseases (EGIDs), celiac disease, inflammatory bowel diseases (IBDs), and parasitic infections. Here we will provide an overview of their clinical features and summarize the association of eosinophils with each inflammatory state.

EOSINOPHILIC GASTROINTESTINAL DISEASES
Eosinophilic Esophagitis

Epidemiology
Eosinophilic esophagitis (EoE) has been reported in all continents, except Africa, and consistently has been shown to occur more commonly in male individuals with a 3:1 ratio.[3–6] Because this is an emerging disease, the exact incidence is difficult to predict, but estimates range from 1 to 4 in 10,000 in North America. There does not appear to be a clear predilection toward one ethnicity.

Risk factors
Recent studies and clinical experiences provide some insights into potential risk factors but these are difficult to identify completely because the exact pathogenesis is uncertain. A recent twin study revealed that if a sibling has EoE, there exists a risk of 2.4% of subsequent children developing EoE.[7] A variety of EoE genes provides clues to dysfunction of the epithelial barrier (filaggrin),[8] immune system (thymic stromal lymphopoietin, eotaxin-3)[9–11] and other yet to be identified areas (calpain-14).[12,13]

Pathophysiology
Within the epithelia, the prominence of eosinophils, interleukin (IL)-5–expressing T cells, B cells, and increased mast cells suggests an immunologically mediated Th2-type inflammatory disease.[14] In further support, clinical characterization of children and adults reveals many highly atopic patients posses a Th2-type inflammatory profile. Basic studies in experimental models of EoE reveal that T-cell–deficient mice, but not B-cell–deficient mice, were protected from esophageal inflammation and esophageal inflammation induced by aero-allergens and food allergens, IL-13, and IL-5.[15–20] Together, these clinical and basic studies provide strong support for allergy as a pathogenic etiology for EoE. In contrast, some patients do not exhibit the same degree of atopy and thus may indicate alternative mechanisms and EoE phenotypes.[21]

Pathologic remodeling represents the likely underlying mechanism of problematic EoE complications, such as esophageal stricture and food impaction.[22–25] A number of basic and translational studies suggest a wide variety of mechanisms related to

Table 1
Gastrointestinal diseases associated with eosinophilia

Disease	Clinical Presentation	Laboratory Findings (Possible Findings)	Radiographic Findings (Possible Findings)	Histological Findings	Therapy
Eosinophilic esophagitis (EoE)	Poor growth, feeding difficulties, dysphagia, food impaction	Peripheral eosinophilia	Esophageal mucosal irregularity, narrowing or stricture, Schatzki rings	Mucosal eosinophilia >15 eos/HPF, lamina propria fibrosis	Dietary avoidance of allergens and/or topical steroid
Eosinophilic gastritis (EG)	Abdominal pain, vomiting, hematemesis	Peripheral eosinophilia, anemia	Thickened gastric mucosal folds, ulceration, partial obstruction	Mucosal eosinophilia >30 eos/HPF or twice normal value	Dietary avoidance of allergens, corticosteroids, immunosuppressive agents
Eosinophilic gastroenteritis (EGE)	Abdominal pain, diarrhea, protein-losing enteropathy	Peripheral eosinophilia, anemia, hypoalbuminemia	Small bowel mucosal thickening	Dense mucosal eosinophilia	Dietary avoidance of allergens, corticosteroids, immunosuppressive agents
Eosinophilic colitis	Abdominal pain, diarrhea, hematochezia, tenesmus	Peripheral eosinophilia, anemia, hypoalbuminemia	Colonic mucosal thickening	Mucosal eosinophilia >65 eos/HPF or twice normal value	Dietary avoidance of allergens, corticosteroids, immunosuppressive agents
Celiac disease	Abdominal pain, diarrhea, weight loss, bloating, extraintestinal manifestations	Peripheral eosinophilia	Small bowel mucosal thickening	Duodenal villous blunting, intraepithelial lymphocytes; esophageal eosinophilic infiltrate	Gluten-free diet; if esophageal eosinophilia, consider gluten-free diet plus PPI therapy; if esophageal eosinophilia persists despite treatment, consider treatment for EoE
Inflammatory bowel disease	Abdominal pain, diarrhea, weight loss, bloody stools	Peripheral eosinophilia, anemia, elevated inflammatory markers	Bowel wall thickening, abscesses, stricture formation	Mucosal eosinophilia may be present	Corticosteroids, antibiotics, aminosalicylates, immunomodulators surgery

Abbreviations: eos/HPF, eosinophils per high-power field; PPI, proton pump inhibitor.

altered permeability, fibrosis, epithelial mesenchymal transition, and dysmotility. Phospholamban, transforming growth factor-β, and other inflammatory mediators are involved, but their exact role in the pathogenesis of esophageal dysfunction, dysmotility, and fibrosis is uncertain.[26–30]

Clinical features

The clinical presentation of EoE varies depending on the patient's abilities to report symptoms associated with esophageal dysfunction.[4,31–35] For instance, young children often present with nonspecific symptoms, such as vomiting, abdominal pain, and feeding problems; whereas adolescents and adults report dysphagia, heartburn, retrosternal pain, or recurrent food impactions. Symptoms that are unresponsive to medical or surgical treatments for gastroesophageal reflux disease (GERD) should raise consideration for EoE. Alternatively, patients may develop coping strategies surrounding eating difficulties and it may be necessary to ask additional questions, such as, "Do you avoid foods like meats or breads? Do you need to use liquids, ketchup, or gravy to help your food go down? Are you the last one to leave the table? Do you chew your food for a long time?"[36]

EoE in adolescents and adults presents with symptoms that can be intermittent or regular, severe or subtle. For instance, swallowing disturbances may be only noticeable when food's consistency is dry or textured, a large food bolus is ingested, or when patients eat too quickly. Alternatively, patients may note only rare and isolated instances of food impactions. EoE remains one of the most common causes of food impaction presenting to emergency rooms.[37–41] Retrosternal pain can often be exacerbated by the ingestion of alcohol.[35]

Physical examinations are usually normal except for manifestations of other atopic diseases that can occur in up to 75% of patients. Peripheral eosinophilia may or may not be present. Approximately 70% of patients have elevated total immunoglobulin (Ig) E levels. Esophagrams can be very helpful in examining luminal circumference, as esophageal narrowing may not be detected at the time of endoscopy.[42] Contrast radiography can detect isolated or long-segment esophageal strictures or Schatzki rings. Histopathology is not pathognomonic and other causes of mucosal eosinophilia, such as GERD, should be ruled out before assigning the diagnosis of EoE.[43] The epithelial surface appears highly proliferative, as evidenced by basal cell hyperplasia, and contains not only eosinophils but also other leukocytes, including lymphocytes, mast cells, and basophils.

Association with eosinophilia

EoE is associated with eosinophilia in 2 circumstances. First, some patients may manifest peripheral eosinophilia, but this finding is nonspecific and may be related to associated atopic diseases. Second, the healthy esophageal mucosa, unlike the rest of the GI tract, is completely devoid of eosinophils. In the proper clinical context, the presence of eosinophils in the esophageal mucosa is highly suggestive of the diagnosis of EoE. Other causes of this inflammation need to be ruled out. Enumeration of eosinophils is problematic because of the limited sample size assessed with mucosal biopsies (2–3 mm per biopsy) that leads to uncertainty as to the extent of eosinophilia, state of eosinophil activation, and its impact on associated resident and recruited cells.[43] Future studies defining functional readouts, clinically meaningful outcome metrics, and histologic parameters that focus on histologic features other than eosinophil numbers are needed.

Acute and chronic management

Overview Although research studies continue to focus on both symptoms and histologic responses to treatments, debate still rages among clinicians who wonder whether the focus of EoE treatment should be directed toward only a symptomatic response or if symptomatic and histologic response is necessary. It is the opinion of the authors that there are at least 3 good reasons to treat patients to clinical and histologic remission. First, treatment may enhance the quality of life because dysphagia, with its ongoing risk of food impaction, can have a marked negative and limiting impact on the patient's daily life.[44–46] Second, treatment reduces the risk of severe esophageal injury by preventing long-lasting food impactions, an incident occurring at the time of esophageal contractions or secondary to stricture formation.[47] Third, treatment prevents esophageal damage caused by tissue remodeling due to unbridled eosinophilic inflammation.[48] Clinical experience, as well as a growing body of literature, supports the premise that treatment can impact the natural history, but future long-term studies will provide critical information to answer these treatment questions.

Acute Acute treatment relates to treatment of esophageal foreign body impaction. When this occurs, patients need to have emergent removal of the foreign body, most often a food product. Patients are taken to the operating room and provided airway protection for safe removal of the esophageal foreign body. Following removal, evaluations need to ensue to determine the reason for the impaction, such as ongoing inflammation or isolated or long-segment esophageal narrowing.

Chronic EoE is a chronic disease, so treatment needs to be not only initiated, but also continued. The 3 D's of treatment, drugs, diet, and dilation, have been used with remarkable outcomes.[49]

Drugs

Systemic and topical corticosteroids Although effective in reducing symptoms and resolving mucosal eosinophilia, the chronic use of prednisone is not desired, leading to a number of studies in adults and children using topical swallowed steroids delivered by a metered dose inhaler (MDI).[21,50–55] Steroids administered in this way provide less of a systemic burden, are deposited directly on the esophageal mucosa, and are highly effective in resolving symptoms and mucosal eosinophilia with response rates ranging from 50% to 90%. One prospective pediatric trial comparing swallowed topical fluticasone with oral prednisone, showed similarity in responses and that relapse occurred at same rate when either of these medications was discontinued.[56] The inability of some children to be able to correctly use MDIs to take the steroids led to the development of a viscous product. This product consists of mixing liquid budesonide respules with sucralose, thus creating a mixture termed oral viscous budesonide.[57,58] Because EoE is a chronic disease, it is important to remember that if treatment is stopped, symptoms and inflammation will likely recur; thus, it is the practice of the authors to continue topical steroid treatment with the minimal amount of steroid necessary. Long-term studies are still necessary to identify the best maintenance strategy.

Proton pump inhibitors Proton pump inhibitors (PPIs) play at least 3 potential roles in the care of patients with EoE.[59,60] PPIs are potent drugs in stopping acid production from parietal cells and therefore are useful in ruling out GERD as a cause for esophageal eosinophilia. Second, patients with EoE may have comorbid GERD and need intermittent treatment with PPIs or other acid suppression. Finally, emerging data suggest that PPIs can downregulate epithelial expression of proinflammatory cytokines, such as IL-8 and eotaxin-3, molecules that are known to be critical for leukocyte infiltration.[61,62] These latter findings support a potential role for PPIs in the treatment of EoE.

Biologic agents Humanized anti–IL-5 antibody has been shown to significantly reduce esophageal eosinophilia in adult and pediatric subjects.[63–65] Significant improvement in symptoms has not been consistently shown, and placebo-treated subjects respond in a similar positive fashion. Anti–IL-13 was effective in reducing mucosal eosinophilia in an adult study.[66]

Diet Dietary management of EoE seeks to eliminate the offending food allergen in patients with EoE and takes 1 of 3 forms.[67] Elemental, targeted elimination and 6 food group elimination diets have all been useful in removing allergenic stimuli from contacting the esophageal mucosa and reducing symptoms. Each has significant positive and negative aspects that will be highlighted in the following sections.

Elemental diet Amino acid–based formulas are highly effective (often >96% response) in treating children and adults with EoE, as shown in a limited number of studies.[68,69] Because patients with EoE may have multiple food sensitizations and highly accurate predictive testing for EoE food triggers awaits discovery, an elemental diet can be very useful in inducing a remission. Problematic features of this treatment are adherence to a formula-based diet, cost, and convenience.

Targeted diet A targeted elimination diet based on skin and specific serum IgE (ImmunoCAP) testing for allergenic foods is effective in 53% to 72% of patients.[70–72] Targeted testing is based on the diet history and can be highly beneficial because it is not as restrictive as the elemental diet. Convenience and determining the clinically relevant allergens are potential problems with this approach.

Six food group elimination diet Elimination of the most common allergenic food groups, termed the 6-food elimination diet, is another successful approach to treating EoE, with approximately 74% undergoing remission.[73–78] This is based on empirical removal of the most common food allergen groups (dairy, soy, wheat, egg, nuts, fish). A potential drawback of the 6-food elimination diet is the elimination of a food that may not serve as an offending allergen. There are other potential elimination diets that have shown some efficacy, including the 4-food elimination diet (dairy, wheat, egg, legumes) as well as milk-only elimination.[74,79,80]

Dilation Dilation of isolated or long segments of the narrowed esophagus is often necessary to allow safe passage of food. A number of recent studies have shown the long-lasting benefits of this approach as well as the low incidence of complications, including pain and perforations.[81–88] Dilation does not address the underlying pathophysiology of EoE, as it has no anti-inflammatory effect.

Other considerations The inclusion of subspecialists' expertise in treating patients with EoE can provide significant benefit. A gastroenterologist can provide experience with identifying comorbid GI diseases, such as GERD, and perform endoscopies to assess for mucosal healing and dilations. An allergist can be a vital participant to help identify EoE-related food allergens as well as comorbid allergic diseases such as IgE-mediated food allergies, asthma, atopic dermatitis, rhinitis, and conjunctivitis.[89,90] A dietician can be a key participant in developing a practical plan to eliminate foods and ensure adherence.[91,92] Feeding specialists may be needed to teach new feeding skills or interrupt acquired habits to maximize eating.[36,93,94] Psychosocial expertise may be necessary to help severely affected patients cope with this chronic disease.[45,95]

Differential diagnosis The differential diagnosis for young children with refluxlike symptoms, abdominal pain, or feeding dysfunction includes anatomic malformations and peptic disease. Mucosal eosinophilia can be confused most commonly with GERD. In adults, dysphagia and food impaction can be presentations of esophageal cancer, peptic stricture, achalasia, motility disorders, and GERD.

Prognosis EoE is a chronic disease that requires ongoing treatment, or symptoms and inflammation will return.[48] Complications associated with EoE include esophageal stricture, food impactions, and feeding dysfunction, leading to malnutrition. To date, EoE has not been associated with cancers and does not lead to shortened life span.

Eosinophilic gastritis, gastroenteritis, and colitis

Eosinophilic gastritis (EG), gastroenteritis (EGE), and colitis (EC) are rare diseases characterized by GI symptoms that occur in association with dense mucosal eosinophilia. Other diseases that can be associated with these findings need to be ruled out before the diagnosis of EG, EGE, or EC can be made. These diseases occur in both children and adults, and because they are uncommon, epidemiologic features, risk factors, and pathophysiological mechanisms are not certain.

Clinical features Patients with EG can present with nonspecific symptoms, including vomiting, abdominal pain, or even hematemesis.[96–98] Laboratory analyses can reveal peripheral eosinophilia and anemia but rarely show signs of peripheral inflammation, such as elevated sedimentation rate or C-reactive protein. Radiographic imaging may reveal thickened mucosal folds, ulceration, or partial obstruction.

EGE presents with symptoms consistent with small intestinal dysfunction, such as abdominal pain, diarrhea, and peripheral edema secondary to protein and blood loss.[99] Some patients may develop protein-losing enteropathy or profound anemia requiring albumin or blood transfusions. Upper GI with small bowel follow-through can reveal mucosal thickening, and direct luminal imaging with endoscopy or capsule studies can reveal ulcers, polyps, or normal mucosa.

A wide severity of symptoms has been associated with EC.[100–105] Some reports note diarrhea and lower abdominal pain, whereas others describe hematochezia, tenesmus, and severe rectal pain with a presentation quite similar to that of IBD. Laboratory testing can reveal anemia and hypoalbuminemia but does not always show signs of peripheral inflammation such as elevated sedimentation rate or C-reactive protein.

Association with eosinophilia

The normal numbers of eosinophils vary along the gastrointestinal tract. Except for the esophagus, which has no eosinophils, normal values for eosinophil counts in the rest of the GI tract are less certain. At least 2 studies identified an increasing gradient of eosinophils from the proximal small intestine to the colon.[106,107]

EG, EGE, and EC are associated with dense mucosal eosinophilia. Initial studies classified these EGIDs as mucosal, muscular, and serosal diseases related to not only the site of eosinophilia but also to their clinical presentations.[108,109] For example, muscular disease presented with symptoms of GI obstruction and serosal disease with ascites. With the advent of GI endoscopy, increasing attention has been paid to the mucosal variety.

Presently, histologic features of EGIDs focus strictly the number of mucosal eosinophils. Because eosinophils are normal constituents of the intestinal mucosa, clear definitions of an absolute diagnostic threshold number of eosinophil for EG, EGE, and EC remain under investigation. Thresholds for EG or EC continue to undergo definition; review of the literature and clinical experience suggest that a reasonable threshold value for EG is greater than 25 to 30 eosinophils per high-power field (eos/HPF) and for EC is greater than 65 eos/HPF.[106,107] As with EoE, additional features related to eosinophils, such as location and level of degranulation, as well as features associated with other resident cells (epithelia, fibroblasts, neurons, and others) and infiltrating cells will be critical to increasing understanding disease pathogenesis and providing diagnostic clarity.

Acute and chronic management

Treatment options for EG, EGE, and EC remain quite limited and have focused on the use of corticosteroids, immunosuppressive agents, and diet restriction.[96,103,110,111] No prospective controlled trials have been completed, and recommendations have been based on case series and clinical experiences. Systemic steroid use is often necessary for acute management, and topical steroid use with budesonide (Entocort) or aminosalicylates has been used for chronic management.[100] Clinical experiences suggest that eosinophilia past the esophagus is less likely to respond to removal of dietary allergens. Using the minimal amount of steroids for treatment and monitoring for side effects, such as bone demineralization and adrenal suppression, are important considerations.

Differential diagnosis

EG and EGE should be differentiated from peptic disease, Menetrier disease, vasculitis, and allergic enteropathy. In addition to vasculitis and allergy, EC must be differentiated from IBD.

Natural history

Tertiary centers report the world's largest clinical experiences and descriptions of the natural history of adults with EGIDs.[108,109,112] Over the course of the past 50 years, they found an increase from 1 patient per year from 1950 to 1987 to 3 per year between 1987 and 2007. No significant complications were reported. Clinical experiences suggest that patients with EG and EC may have a waxing and waning course, but no long-term studies are available.

CELIAC DISEASE

Key points for celiac disease are shown in **Box 1**.

Epidemiology

Celiac disease occurs primarily in Non-Hispanic white individuals, with a prevalence of 1 in 133 in the United States and Europe.[113–115] Celiac disease affects both children and adults with female individuals being affected twice as often as male individuals. With better serologic testing, the number of "asymptomatic" patients, either with risk factors listed in the next section who were identified at screening or with an

---

Box 1
Key points for celiac disease

- Celiac disease is an immune-mediated disease in which gluten-containing foods stimulate a reproducible clinical and histologic response.
- Removal of gluten from the diet remains the primary treatment.
- The association with eosinophils in the small intestinal and esophageal mucosa is increasingly recognized and requires individualized assessment and treatment.

abnormal duodenal biopsy done at the time of an endoscopy performed for alternative reasons, is increasing.

Risk Factors

Celiac disease is both associated with environmental factors and carries a strong genetic disposition, especially in those patients with human leukocyte antigen (HLA)-DQ2 and HLA-DQ8.[116] In fact, a recent large multicenter prospective cohort study showed that children homozygous for HLA DR3-DQ2 were at particularly high risk for developing celiac disease.[117] At-risk groups also include first-degree and second-degree relatives of those with celiac disease and patients with autoimmune thyroid disease, Down syndrome, Type 1 diabetes, Williams and Turner syndromes, and IgA deficiency; these patients may have a higher prevalence than the general population. A recent study showed that early introduction of wheat is not a risk factor for developing celiac disease.[118]

Pathophysiology

A multiple-hit model has been proposed as underlying celiac disease. Although 40% of the Western world is susceptible based on HLA typing, only 1% develops disease. Once the disease has been initiated, enzymatically digested gluten fragments bind to predisposing HLA molecules and trigger a T-cell response and mucosal damage. Tissue transglutaminase is released and modifies gluten peptides, allowing the peptides to bind to HLA molecules with higher affinity, further perpetuating inflammation.[119] Inflammation is characterized by findings ranging from lymphocytic inflammation of the lamina propria with increased intraepithelial lymphocytes to total villous blunting.

Clinical Features

Clinically, celiac disease can present at any age but is most often recognized in young children soon after the introduction of wheat-containing foods into their diet. Symptoms, including diarrhea, steatorrhea, weight loss, and bloating, are related to villous damage with resultant malabsorption. Laboratory findings include anemia, hypoalbuminemia, and elevated transaminases.[120] Other patients may have non-GI–related symptoms, such as short stature, neurologic symptoms (ataxia, epilepsy, depression, and neuropathy), dermatitis herpetiformis, and dental enamel defects.

In patients with suspected celiac disease, celiac disease–specific antibodies should be measured. Most commonly, IgA class antitissue transglutaminase type 2 (TG2) antibodies are initially obtained in conjunction with total serum IgA level. If screening testing is positive, diagnosis should be confirmed with the procurement of a mucosal biopsy.[116] A gluten-free diet should not be initiated until the diagnostic process is complete. Clinical experience suggests a mucosal biopsy may not be necessary to establish a diagnosis, but this has not become the standard of care in the United States yet.

Association with Eosinophilia

An eosinophilic infiltrate also has been described in the duodenal mucosa of patients with active celiac disease.[121] In a case series of 150 newly diagnosed patients, biopsy specimens showed anywhere between 3 and 50 eos/HPF. Mucosal eosinophilia was associated with advanced histologic staging of the disease, suggesting that eosinophils may play a role in mucosal damage.[122]

Recently, a link between esophageal eosinophilia and celiac disease has been noted. Although celiac disease and EoE are separate gastrointestinal disorders, several studies have postulated a coexistence of esophageal eosinophilia in patients with celiac disease. In a study of 1000 randomly selected adults from the general population, there was no increased risk of celiac disease in persons with esophageal eosinophilia.[123] In a second study, the prevalence of esophageal eosinophilia was measured in a retrospective analysis of 120 children with celiac disease compared with healthy controls. This study found no differences in the incidence of esophageal eosinophilia between the two.[124] These results imply that esophageal eosinophilia in patients with celiac disease may be incidental rather than causal. Reports of improvement of esophageal eosinophilia on a gluten-free diet have been mixed, with some studies showing resolution and others show no improvement.[125–128] Based on these limited data, we suggest that patients with celiac disease and esophageal eosinophilia first undergo treatment with a PPI and a gluten-free diet. Depending on clinical symptoms and response to treatment, additional dietary elimination or topical corticosteroids for treatment of EoE can be considered. Thus, esophageal eosinophilia may be a representation of immunologic dysregulation underlying celiac disease or may occur independently as a manifestation of EoE. Future studies determining the fate of eosinophilic inflammation after celiac treatment will begin to tease out mechanisms of this finding.

Acute and Chronic Management

Treatment for celiac disease is based on complete elimination of gluten from the diet.[129] To guide care, a recent National Institutes of Health panel suggested the mnemonic, *CELIAC* representing, *C*onsultation with a skilled dietitian, *E*ducation about the disease, *L*ifelong adherence to a gluten-free diet, *I*dentification and treatment of nutritional deficiencies, *A*ccess to an advocacy group, *C*ontinuous long-term follow-up by a multidisciplinary team (http://celiac.nih.gov/materials.aspx). Dieticians are central to the management of patients with celiac disease to ensure that the diet is gluten-free and nutritionally replete.

INFLAMMATORY BOWEL DISEASES

Key points for IBDs are shown in **Box 2**.

Epidemiology

IBD often presents in the second or third decade; however, childhood presentation can occur. Ulcerative colitis (UC) incidence is 2 to 19 per 100,000, and Crohn disease (CrD) incidence is 3 to 20 per 100,000. UC tends to occur more commonly in male individuals; whereas, CrD occurs more often in female individuals. A first-degree relative with IBD is found in 10% to 25% of patients.

Box 2
Key points for inflammatory bowel diseases

- Inflammatory bowel diseases (IBD) consist of at least 2 immune-mediated chronic inflammatory diseases of the gastrointestinal tract: Crohn disease and ulcerative colitis.

- Treatments for IBDs include corticosteroids for acute exacerbations, and 5-aminosalicylates, immunosuppressives and biologics directed against tumor necrosis factor-α for maintenance management.

- The association of IBDs with mucosal eosinophilia and its secreted products is increasing, but the role of eosinophils in the pathogenesis of IBD remains uncertain.

Risk Factors

A number of factors seem to pose increased risk for developing IBD, but these vary between UC and CrD.[130] For instance, smoking is associated with an increased risk of CrD but may be protective in UC. Dietary factors may contribute to the development of IBD with processed, fried, and sugary foods being associated with the development of IBDs, whereas long-term intake of dietary fiber is protective.

Pathophysiology

The intestinal tract is composed of a complex and ingenious architecture that blends together soluble elements, extracellular matrices, and a wide array of cells to create an effective barrier separating luminal contents from the rest of the body. Functional elements, such as secretion of trefoil peptides and cryptdins and rhythmic peristalsis, aid in protecting the epithelial barrier from penetration and binding of noxious particles and microbes. In addition, the innate and adaptive immune system arm the underlying mucosa with nonspecific and acquired elements to process antigenic materials that are encountered. When any of these elements is ineffective, the potential for inflammation ensues.

In the case of IBD, the etiology remains unknown, but it is thought that environmental factors as well as genetic predisposition lead to gastrointestinal immune dysregulation.[131–133] To date, more than 160 genetic loci are associated with human IBDs.[134] When grouping these loci and gene products, a pattern of expression related to mucosal homeostasis, inflammation, and healing can help to visualize the potential underlying defects observed in these diseases. For instance, dysregulation of homeostasis can take the form of altered intestinal permeability, increased antigen uptake, and change in patterns of tolerance. Although inflammation is necessary to limit the exposure of the immunomicromilieu to exogenous antigens, when uncontrolled, clinical manifestations of IBD may arise. For instance, a large body of research is investigating not only the specific microbiome associated with the mucosa affected by IBD, but also how these microbial patterns are sensed.[135] Healing defects may not allow for proper resolution of mucosal injury and inflammation and perpetuate IBD. The role of exogenous factors, such as diet, is an active area of investigation as mentioned earlier, with certain nutritional components being protective, such as vitamin D and high fiber, and others, in excess, being permissive, such as total or polyunsaturated fats and sugary foods.

Clinical Features

Most patients with CrD have abdominal pain, diarrhea, and weight loss.[136] Although grossly bloody stool can be seen with colonic disease, it is unusual with isolated small bowel disease. Other features of CrD, including growth retardation, nausea and vomiting, perirectal disease, or extraintestinal manifestations, occur in up to 25% of patients.[137] UC presents with diarrhea, rectal bleeding, and abdominal pain.[132] Diagnosis is confirmed by histologic characteristics of chronic inflammatory changes, including cryptitis in UC and transmural infiltration of lymphocytes and granuloma formation in CrD.

Association with Eosinophilia

Eosinophils have been implicated in the pathogenesis of IBD; however, their relationship to these diseases remains unclear.[2,138,139] At least 2 different postulates have been developed. The most commonly held belief, based on clinical observations and mouse models, is that eosinophils accumulate in the mucosa where they synthesize and release inflammatory mediators that lead to tissue damage.[139–151] A less common thought is that eosinophils may serve an innate protective role that heals or prevents inflammation. This is based on the clinical finding that mucosal eosinophilia precedes the onset of IBD and mouse data supporting a role for eosinophils in healing epithelial barrier function.[152] Future studies determining the underlying role of eosinophils in the pathogenesis of IBD will permit clinical studies examining the utility of measuring eosinophils as biomarkers.

Mucosal eosinophilia

Early studies describing mucosal biopsies of patients with IBD revealed mucosal eosinophilia compared with healthy controls. Unlike the esophagus, eosinophils are resident cells of the small and large intestines; the normal number of eosinophils is not well-defined, making interpretation of pathologic intestinal eosinophilia difficult.[2] Clinical implications of mucosal eosinophils in IBD are unknown, especially because mucosal eosinophilia is increased in IBD compared with irritable bowel syndrome. One study found that the severity of eosinophilic inflammation in patients with UC was the most significant predictor of lack of response to therapy.[153]

Eosinophil products and inflammatory bowel disease

Eosinophils secrete eosinophil granule proteins (EGP), such as ECP, EPO, EDN, and MBP, and increased EGP levels of these products in tissues and stool effluent provide circumstantial support for a role in IBD. Early electron microscopic studies of colonic resection specimens from patients with CrD identified numerous eosinophils, extracellular eosinophil MBP granule deposition, and cytotoxic tissue changes.[154,155] At least one study revealed not only increased mucosal eosinophilia, but also IL-5, in resected colon of patients with CrD, a finding that was associated with endoscopic recurrence.[156] A number of studies have analyzed the concentrations of EGPs in stool and correlated increased EGP concentrations with severity of disease. Granule proteins may indicate relapse as suggested in a study demonstrating that ECP and EPX fecal levels increased when intestinal inflammation increased.[157] Finally, declining stool EGP levels may indicate disease remission. For instance, fecal EPX levels in patients with UC decreased after corticosteroid treatment.[158]

These last studies raise the possibility that eosinophils may be beneficial in IBD. To address this, we induced colitis in wild-type and eosinophil-deficient PHIL mice.[152] When colitis was induced in PHIL mice, they developed more severe colitis than their eosinophil-competent controls. These mice also had greater numbers of neutrophils and increased levels of chemokines that attract neutrophils. Further dissection of the mechanism revealed that PHIL mice were lacking in the barrier protective molecule, protectin D1. Rescue of PHIL with protectin reduced the severity of colitis. In contrast to these findings, at least 2 other studies have shown a deleterious role for eosinophils in mouse colitis.[159,160]

Acute and Chronic Management

The acute management of the severely ill patient with IBD consists of bowel rest, intravenous fluids, and nutrition, and immunosuppression with corticosteroids, but after the diagnosis, most patients can be cared for as outpatients.[161] Medications are focused on reducing inflammation and maintaining remission.[151] Immunosuppressives used include 6-mercaptopurine, azathioprine, and biologics including anti–tumor necrosis factor (TNF) antibodies.[162] Additional medications include 5-aminosalicylates that can be administered as topical agents, swallowed or in enema form, depending on the site of the inflammation. In some circumstances, antibiotics may be helpful, and recent works have begun to investigate the role of the microbiome in IBD thera-peutics.[163] Care must be taken to ensure adequate nutrition to supply calories, pro-teins, and micronutrients, especially to the growing child.[164] Surgery may be indicated in some patients with recalcitrant disease, obstruction, or uncontrollable hemorrhage.

Differential Diagnosis

The differential diagnosis for patients with abdominal pain, bloody diarrhea, and ane-mia includes infections, immunodeficiency, eosinophilic colitis, and vasculitis. The diagnosis of IBD is based on exclusion of these entities and the findings of chronic inflammation on mucosal biopsies and, in the case of CrD, granulomas.

Prognosis

Patients with IBD experience a course of exacerbations and remissions. If a patient with CrD is in remission for 1 year, there is an 80% chance of remaining in remission for subsequent years. Patients with CrD may have an increased risk of cancer, and those taking a combination of anti-TNF medications and azathioprine may be at increased risk of hepatosplenic T-cell lymphoma.[165] Two-thirds of patients with UC will have 1 relapse in the 10 years after diagnosis. Up to one-third of patients will require surgery or colectomy for complications. There is an increased risk of cancer that begins 10 years after the onset of symptoms.

PARASITIC INFECTIONS

Key points for parasitic infections are shown in **Box 3**.

Introduction

Blood eosinophilia is a common finding in tropical developing countries and is strongly associated with the presence of parasitic disease, particularly intestinal helminth infection.[164] In travelers returning from the tropics, there is a significant chance of hel-minth infection in the setting of eosinophilia.[165] Even in patients who are asymptom-atic, eosinophilia can be associated with intestinal parasitic infections.[166] Despite the association of eosinophilia with parasitic infection, patients may have eosinophilia in the absence of infection and vice versa.[164,165] In fact, in a large study looking at 14,298 returning travelers, fewer than 50% of patients with helminth infections had blood eosinophilia.[165] Sustained peripheral eosinophilia is usually associated with par-asites that invade tissues, as this leads to contact with immune effector cells. Conversely, infections that are entirely intraluminal, such as tapeworm infection, are unlikely to cause peripheral eosinophilia.[167]

Although intestinal parasites are relatively common in some developing countries, they are an uncommon cause of GI disease in developed countries. In a large

---

Box 3
Key points for parasitic infections

- Intestinal parasites are an uncommon cause of gastrointestinal disease in developed countries.
- Patients may have eosinophilia in the absence of parasitic infections and vice versa.
- Intestinal helminth infection can produce a clinical picture indistinguishable from eosinophilic gastroenteritis.

systematic review and meta-analysis assessing GI pathogens in developed and developing countries, parasites were the least common cause of GI illness after viral and bacterial causes, respectively, and of the parasitic causes of GI disease, *Giardia intestinalis*, and *Cryptosporidium* species (neither of which are associated with eosinophilia) were the most common.[166] Nevertheless, it is important to consider helminth infection in the differential diagnosis of a patient presenting with blood or tissue eosinophilia and gastrointestinal symptoms, because therapy is typically curative and differs substantially from that for other causes of GI disorders. *Strongyloides stercoralis* is of particular importance because administration of corticosteroids, which may be used to treat EGID, can lead to the development of potentially fatal hyperinfection syndrome.

Although some parasitic infections, such as trichinosis, can cause acute GI symptoms associated with eosinophilia, these symptoms are transient and associated with other clinical manifestations. Consequently, patients rarely present to gastroenterologists. In contrast, patients with chronic intestinal parasitic infection, such as that caused by hookworm or *Strongyloides*, may present with nonspecific GI complaints with or without peripheral eosinophilia. Moreover, as in EGID, endoscopic biopsies may reveal tissue eosinophilia (**Table 2**). Although a comprehensive discussion of parasitic causes of EGIDs is beyond the scope of this article (and is reviewed by O'Connell and Nutman, elsewhere in this issue), hookworm infection and strongyloidiasis provide 2 illustrative examples.

Hookworm Infection

Ancylostoma duodenale and *Necator americanus*, commonly referred to as "hookworms," are estimated to infect up to 740 million people worldwide.[167] Although newer studies are lacking, prevalence in the United States was estimated to be 19.6% in 1982, particularly in the southern United States, including Appalachia.[172] Hookworms are found in soil and generally penetrate human skin and migrate to the lungs. Hookworm larvae are then swallowed with bronchial secretions and eventually mature worms attach to the wall of the small intestine. A pruritic skin rash is sometimes noticeable at site of penetration into skin. Chronic infections are generally asymptomatic unless there is a large intestinal worm burden. Although this can cause a gastroenteritislike syndrome, most concerning are an associated anemia from production of an anticoagulant substance and protein-losing enteropathy.[173] Laboratory evaluation can reveal eosinophilia and a moderate increase in IgE levels.[174,175] Diagnosis is made by microscopic visualization of hookworm eggs or larvae in feces. First-line treatment is albendazole.

Strongyloidiasis

Strongyloides stercoralis is endemic worldwide, including the United States and Europe, with an estimated global prevalence of up to 100 million people. Outbreaks of strongyloidiasis have been reported in the southeastern part of the United States, particularly Kentucky, Tennessee, and Florida.[172–175] Transmission occurs when larvae from infected soil penetrate the skin. Because of its unique autoinfective life cycle, the parasite can persist for decades in an infected host,[176] whereas some individuals with strongyloidiasis complain of abdominal pain, diarrhea, urticaria, or rash, many are asymptomatic.[173] Immunosuppression (typically with corticosteroids) causes potentially fatal acceleration of the autoinfective cycle (hyperinfection syndrome) and/or dissemination of infection. Peripheral and small bowel eosinophilia are commonly seen and can mimic EGID.[177] Diagnosis can be difficult in immunocompetent hosts because larvae are excreted only intermittently and in small numbers,

Table 2
Selected parasitic diseases associated with gastrointestinal manifestations and eosinophilia

Parasite	Clinical Presentation	Peripheral Blood Eosinophil Count	Tissue Eosinophilia	Diagnosis	Treatment
Hookworm (Ancylostoma duodenale and Necator americanus)	Skin rash on inoculation, asymptomatic to mild GI disease, anemia and protein-losing enteropathy with large burden	Elevated	GI	Direct visualization of eggs or larvae on microscopy	Albendazole
Trichinella spiralis	Diarrhea may be seen early in infection before the development of myalgia and other symptoms	Elevated	Muscle	Serology, muscle biopsy	Albendazole, steroids
Strongyloides stercoralis	Abdominal pain, diarrhea, rash, or asymptomatic in chronic infection	Elevated	GI	Multiple modalities, including stool and serology	Ivermectin, albendazole
Cystisospora belli	Diarrhea	Elevated	GI[168]	Stool examination for cysts	Trimethoprim sulfamethoxazole
Anisakis	Abdominal pain, allergic gastroenteritis	Elevated	GI[169–171]	Endoscopic visualization of worm	Removal of worm

Abbreviation: GI, gastrointestinal.

and commercial serologic tests vary in sensitivity and specificity and do not distinguish active from past infection.[178] Recommended treatment is with ivermectin (200 µg/kg daily for 1–2 days) or albendazole (400 mg daily for 3 days and followup at 2 weeks to confirm cure).

Diagnostic Approach

In patients with unknown eosinophilia, parasitic infection should be considered. The approach to these patients will depend on their travel history, other medical conditions, and clinical signs and symptoms. Eosinophilia should first be confirmed by obtaining an absolute eosinophil count. If history and physical examination do not elucidate a cause of eosinophilia and parasitic infection is still considered a potential etiology, 3 separate stool samples and appropriate serology should be obtained.[169]

FUTURE CONSIDERATIONS AND SUMMARY

The diversity of circumstances in which mucosal eosinophils are found in the gut provides a wealth of scientific intrigue and clinical confusion. An increasing body of research focuses on mucosal eosinophilia that is captured by biopsy forceps at the time of endoscopy, but this limited sampling may lead to underestimating the impact of eosinophils that are dispersed throughout the mucosa as well as deeper in the muscular layers. Although there are clinical circumstances when it is highly likely that eosinophils participate in the pathogenesis of a disease, such as EoE, other situations are less certain. The finding of eosinophils in association with other diseases, such as celiac and IBD, raises questions as to whether their role is one of harm or healing. Future studies that help characterize eosinophils in the GI tract, understand its functional role, and determine its viability as a therapeutic target and biomarker will provide much insight into GI health and disease.

REFERENCES

1. Furuta GT, Atkins FD, Lee NA, et al. Changing roles of eosinophils in health and disease. Ann Allergy Asthma Immunol 2014;113(1):3–8.
2. Yantiss RK. Eosinophils in the GI tract: how many is too many and what do they mean? Mod Pathol 2015;28(Suppl 1):S7–21.
3. Attwood S, Smyrk T, Demeester T, et al. Esophageal eosinophilia with dysphagia. A distinct clinicopathologic syndrome. Dig Dis Sci 1993;38:109–16.
4. Straumann A, Spichtin HP, Bernoulli R, et al. Idiopathic eosinophilic esophagitis: a frequently overlooked disease with typical clinical aspects and discrete endoscopic findings. Schweiz Med Wochenschr 1994;124(33):1419–29 [in German].
5. Dellon ES, Gonsalves N, Hirano I, et al. ACG clinical guideline: evidenced based approach to the diagnosis and management of esophageal eosinophilia and eosinophilic esophagitis (EoE). Am J Gastroenterol 2013;108(5):679–92 [quiz: 693].
6. Liacouras CA, Furuta GT, Hirano I, et al. Eosinophilic esophagitis: updated consensus recommendations for children and adults. J Allergy Clin Immunol 2011;128(1):3–20.e6 [quiz: 21–2].
7. Alexander ES, Martin LJ, Collins MH, et al. Twin and family studies reveal strong environmental and weaker genetic cues explaining heritability of eosinophilic esophagitis. J Allergy Clin Immunol 2014;134(5):1084–92.e1.
8. Matoso A, Mukkada VA, Lu S, et al. Expression microarray analysis identifies novel epithelial-derived protein markers in eosinophilic esophagitis. Mod Pathol 2013;26(5):665–76.

9. Rothenberg ME, Spergel JM, Sherrill JD, et al. Common variants at 5q22 associate with pediatric eosinophilic esophagitis. Nat Genet 2010;42(4):289–91.
10. Sherrill JD, Gao PS, Stucke EM, et al. Variants of thymic stromal lymphopoietin and its receptor associate with eosinophilic esophagitis. J Allergy Clin Immunol 2010;126(1):160–5.e3.
11. Blanchard C, Durual S, Estienne M, et al. Eotaxin-3/CCL26 gene expression in intestinal epithelial cells is up-regulated by interleukin-4 and interleukin-13 via the signal transducer and activator of transcription 6. Int J Biochem Cell Biol 2005;37(12):2559–73.
12. Kottyan LC, Davis BP, Sherrill JD, et al. Genome-wide association analysis of eosinophilic esophagitis provides insight into the tissue specificity of this allergic disease. Nat Genet 2014;46(8):895–900.
13. Sleiman PM, Wang ML, Cianferoni A, et al. GWAS identifies four novel eosinophilic esophagitis loci. Nat Commun 2014;5:5593.
14. Sherrill JD, Rothenberg ME. Genetic and epigenetic underpinnings of eosinophilic esophagitis. Gastroenterol Clin North Am 2014;43(2):269–80.
15. Mishra A, Schlotman J, Wang M, et al. Critical role for adaptive T cell immunity in experimental eosinophilic esophagitis in mice. J Leukoc Biol 2007;81(4):916–24.
16. Mishra A, Rothenberg ME. Intratracheal IL-13 induces eosinophilic esophagitis by an IL-5, eotaxin-1, and STAT6-dependent mechanism. Gastroenterology 2003;125(5):1419–27.
17. Mishra A, Hogan SP, Brandt EB, et al. IL-5 promotes eosinophil trafficking to the esophagus. J Immunol 2002;168(5):2464–9.
18. Mishra A, Hogan SP, Brandt EB, et al. An etiological role for aeroallergens and eosinophils in experimental esophagitis. J Clin Invest 2001;107(1):83–90.
19. Mishra A, Hogan SP, Lee JJ, et al. Fundamental signals that regulate eosinophil homing to the gastrointestinal tract. J Clin Invest 1999;103(12):1719–27.
20. Cho JY, Doshi A, Rosenthal P, et al. Smad3 deficient mice have reduced esophageal fibrosis and angiogenesis in a mouse model of egg induced eosinophilic esophagitis. J Pediatr Gastroenterol Nutr 2014;59(1):10–6.
21. Butz BK, Wen T, Gleich GJ, et al. Efficacy, dose reduction, and resistance to high-dose fluticasone in patients with eosinophilic esophagitis. Gastroenterology 2014;147(2):324–33.e5.
22. Lucendo AJ. Cellular and molecular immunological mechanisms in eosinophilic esophagitis: an updated overview of their clinical implications. Expert Rev Gastroenterol Hepatol 2014;8(6):669–85.
23. Hirano I, Aceves SS. Clinical implications and pathogenesis of esophageal remodeling in eosinophilic esophagitis. Gastroenterol Clin North Am 2014;43(2):297–316.
24. Aceves SS. Remodeling and fibrosis in chronic eosinophil inflammation. Dig Dis 2014;32(1–2):15–21.
25. Cheng E, Souza RF, Spechler SJ. Tissue remodeling in eosinophilic esophagitis. Am J Physiol Gastrointest Liver Physiol 2012;303(11):G1175–87.
26. Cho JY, Rosenthal P, Miller M, et al. Targeting AMCase reduces esophageal eosinophilic inflammation and remodeling in a mouse model of egg induced eosinophilic esophagitis. Int Immunopharmacol 2014;18(1):35–42.
27. Beppu LY, Anilkumar AA, Newbury RO, et al. TGF-beta1-induced phospholamban expression alters esophageal smooth muscle cell contraction in patients with eosinophilic esophagitis. J Allergy Clin Immunol 2014;134(5):1100–7.e4.
28. Abdulnour-Nakhoul SM, Al-Tawil Y, Gyftopoulos AA, et al. Alterations in junctional proteins, inflammatory mediators and extracellular matrix molecules in eosinophilic esophagitis. Clin Immunol 2013;148(2):265–78.

29. Kagalwalla AF, Akhtar N, Woodruff SA, et al. Eosinophilic esophagitis: epithelial mesenchymal transition contributes to esophageal remodeling and reverses with treatment. J Allergy Clin Immunol 2012;129(5):1387–96.e7.

30. Mishra A, Wang M, Pemmaraju VR, et al. Esophageal remodeling develops as a consequence of tissue specific IL-5-induced eosinophilia. Gastroenterology 2008;134(1):204–14.

31. Fox VL, Nurko S, Furuta GT. Eosinophilic esophagitis: it's not just kid's stuff. Gastrointest Endosc 2002;56(2):260–70.

32. Liacouras CA. Eosinophilic esophagitis in children and adults. J Pediatr Gastroenterol Nutr 2003;37(Suppl 1):S23–8.

33. Liacouras CA, Spergel JM, Ruchelli E, et al. Eosinophilic esophagitis: a 10-year experience in 381 children. Clin Gastroenterol Hepatol 2005;3(12):1198–206.

34. Putnam PE. Eosinophilic esophagitis in children: clinical manifestations. Gastroenterol Clin North Am 2008;37(2):369–81.

35. Straumann A, Aceves SS, Blanchard C, et al. Pediatric and adult eosinophilic esophagitis: similarities and differences. Allergy 2012;67(4):477–90.

36. Mukkada VA, Haas A, Maune NC, et al. Feeding dysfunction in children with eosinophilic gastrointestinal diseases. Pediatrics 2010;126(3):e672–7.

37. Desai TK, Stecevic V, Chang CH, et al. Association of eosinophilic inflammation with esophageal food impaction in adults. Gastrointest Endosc 2005;61(7):795–801.

38. Nonevski IT, Downs-Kelly E, Falk GW. Eosinophilic esophagitis: an increasingly recognized cause of dysphagia, food impaction, and refractory heartburn. Cleve Clin J Med 2008;75(9):623–6, 629–33.

39. Straumann A, Bussmann C, Zuber M, et al. Eosinophilic esophagitis: analysis of food impaction and perforation in 251 adolescent and adult patients. Clin Gastroenterol Hepatol 2008;6(5):598–600.

40. Hurtado CW, Furuta GT, Kramer RE. Etiology of esophageal food impactions in children. J Pediatr Gastroenterol Nutr 2011;52(1):43–6.

41. El-Matary W, El-Hakim H, Popel J. Eosinophilic esophagitis in children needing emergency endoscopy for foreign body and food bolus impaction. Pediatr Emerg Care 2012;28(7):611–3.

42. Gentile N, Katzka D, Ravi K, et al. Oesophageal narrowing is common and frequently under-appreciated at endoscopy in patients with oesophageal eosinophilia. Aliment Pharmacol Ther 2014;40(11–12):1333–40.

43. Collins MH. Histopathology of eosinophilic esophagitis. Dig Dis 2014;32(1–2):68–73.

44. Franciosi JP, Hommel KA, DeBrosse CW, et al. Quality of life in paediatric eosinophilic oesophagitis: what is important to patients? Child Care Health Dev 2012;38(4):477–83.

45. Klinnert MD, Silveira L, Harris R, et al. Health-related quality of life over time in children with eosinophilic esophagitis and their families. J Pediatr Gastroenterol Nutr 2014;59(3):308–16.

46. Lucendo AJ, Sanchez-Cazalilla M, Molina-Infante J, et al. Transcultural adaptation and validation of the "Adult Eosinophilic Esophagitis Quality of Life Questionnaire" into Spanish. Rev Esp Enferm Dig 2014;106(6):386–94.

47. Schoepfer AM, Safroneeva E, Bussmann C, et al. Delay in diagnosis of eosinophilic esophagitis increases risk for stricture formation, in a time-dependent manner. Gastroenterology 2013;145(6):1230–6.e1–2.

48. Menard-Katcher P, Marks KL, Liacouras CA, et al. The natural history of eosinophilic oesophagitis in the transition from childhood to adulthood. Aliment Pharmacol Ther 2013;37(1):114–21.

49. Straumann A. Treatment of eosinophilic esophagitis: diet, drugs, or dilation? Gastroenterology 2012;142(7):1409–11.

50. Schroeder S, Fleischer DM, Masterson JC, et al. Successful treatment of eosinophilic esophagitis with ciclesonide. J Allergy Clin Immunol 2012;129(5): 1419–21.

51. Straumann A, Conus S, Degen L, et al. Budesonide is effective in adolescent and adult patients with active eosinophilic esophagitis. Gastroenterology 2010;139(5):1526–37, 1537.e1.

52. Arora AS, Perrault J, Smyrk TC. Topical corticosteroid treatment of dysphagia due to eosinophilic esophagitis in adults. Mayo Clin Proc 2003;78(7):830–5.

53. Teitelbaum J, Fox V, Twarog F, et al. Eosinophilic esophagitis in children: immunopathological analysis and response to fluticasone propionate. Gastroenterology 2002;122:1216–25.

54. Faubion WA Jr, Perrault J, Burgart LJ, et al. Treatment of eosinophilic esophagitis with inhaled corticosteroids. J Pediatr Gastroenterol Nutr 1998;27(1):90–3.

55. Konikoff MR, Noel RJ, Blanchard C, et al. A randomized, double-blind, placebo-controlled trial of fluticasone propionate for pediatric eosinophilic esophagitis. Gastroenterology 2006;131(5):1381–91.

56. Schaefer ET, Fitzgerald JF, Molleston JP, et al. Comparison of oral prednisone and topical fluticasone in the treatment of eosinophilic esophagitis: a randomized trial in children. Clin Gastroenterol Hepatol 2008;6(2):165–73.

57. Dohil R, Newbury R, Fox L, et al. Oral viscous budesonide is effective in children with eosinophilic esophagitis in a randomized, placebo-controlled trial. Gastroenterology 2010;139(2):418–29.

58. Aceves SS, Bastian JF, Newbury RO, et al. Oral viscous budesonide: a potential new therapy for eosinophilic esophagitis in children. Am J Gastroenterol 2007; 102(10):2271–9 [quiz: 2280].

59. Kedika RR, Souza RF, Spechler SJ. Potential anti-inflammatory effects of proton pump inhibitors: a review and discussion of the clinical implications. Dig Dis Sci 2009;54(11):2312–7.

60. Spechler SJ, Genta RM, Souza RF. Thoughts on the complex relationship between gastroesophageal reflux disease and eosinophilic esophagitis. Am J Gastroenterol 2007;102(6):1301–6.

61. Cheng E, Zhang X, Huo X, et al. Omeprazole blocks eotaxin-3 expression by oesophageal squamous cells from patients with eosinophilic oesophagitis and GORD. Gut 2013;62(6):824–32.

62. Zhang X, Cheng E, Huo X, et al. Omeprazole blocks STAT6 binding to the eotaxin-3 promoter in eosinophilic esophagitis cells. PLoS One 2012;7(11): e50037.

63. Otani IM, Anilkumar AA, Newbury RO, et al. Anti-IL-5 therapy reduces mast cell and IL-9 cell numbers in pediatric patients with eosinophilic esophagitis. J Allergy Clin Immunol 2013;131(6):1576–82.

64. Spergel JM, Rothenberg ME, Collins MH, et al. Reslizumab in children and adolescents with eosinophilic esophagitis: results of a double-blind, randomized, placebo-controlled trial. J Allergy Clin Immunol 2012;129(2):456–63, 463.e1–3.

65. Assa'ad AH, Gupta SK, Collins MH, et al. An antibody against IL-5 reduces numbers of esophageal intraepithelial eosinophils in children with eosinophilic esophagitis. Gastroenterology 2011;141(5):1593–604.

66. Rothenberg ME, Wen T, Greenberg A, et al. Intravenous anti-IL-13 mAb QAX576 for the treatment of eosinophilic esophagitis. J Allergy Clin Immunol 2015; 135(2):500–7.

67. Arias A, Gonzalez-Cervera J, Tenias JM, et al. Efficacy of dietary interventions for inducing histologic remission in patients with eosinophilic esophagitis: a systematic review and meta-analysis. Gastroenterology 2014;146(7):1639–48.
68. Peterson KA, Byrne KR, Vinson LA, et al. Elemental diet induces histologic response in adult eosinophilic esophagitis. Am J Gastroenterol 2013;108(5):759–66.
69. Kelly KJ, Lazenby AJ, Rowe PC, et al. Eosinophilic esophagitis attributed to gastroesophageal reflux: improvement with an amino acid-based formula. Gastroenterology 1995;109(5):1503–12.
70. Greenhawt M, Rubenstein JH. A tailored vs empiric diet–which is best for eosinophilic esophagitis? Gastroenterology 2013;144(7):1560–1.
71. Spergel JM, Brown-Whitehorn TF, Cianferoni A, et al. Identification of causative foods in children with eosinophilic esophagitis treated with an elimination diet. J Allergy Clin Immunol 2012;130(2):461–7.e5.
72. Henderson CJ, Abonia JP, King EC, et al. Comparative dietary therapy effectiveness in remission of pediatric eosinophilic esophagitis. J Allergy Clin Immunol 2012;129(6):1570–8.
73. Rodriguez-Sanchez J, Gomez Torrijos E, Lopez Viedma B, et al. Efficacy of IgE-targeted vs empiric six-food elimination diets for adult eosinophilic oesophagitis. Allergy 2014;69(7):936–42.
74. Molina-Infante J, Arias A, Barrio J, et al. Four-food group elimination diet for adult eosinophilic esophagitis: a prospective multicenter study. J Allergy Clin Immunol 2014;134(5):1093–9.e1.
75. Gonsalves N, Kagalwalla AF. Dietary treatment of eosinophilic esophagitis. Gastroenterol Clin North Am 2014;43(2):375–83.
76. Lucendo AJ, Arias A, Gonzalez-Cervera J, et al. Empiric 6-food elimination diet induced and maintained prolonged remission in patients with adult eosinophilic esophagitis: a prospective study on the food cause of the disease. J Allergy Clin Immunol 2013;131(3):797–804.
77. Lucendo AJ, Arias A, Gonzalez-Cervera J, et al. Tolerance of a cow's milk-based hydrolyzed formula in patients with eosinophilic esophagitis triggered by milk. Allergy 2013;68(8):1065–72.
78. Kagalwalla AF, Sentongo TA, Ritz S, et al. Effect of six-food elimination diet on clinical and histologic outcomes in eosinophilic esophagitis. Clin Gastroenterol Hepatol 2006;4(9):1097–102.
79. Kagalwalla AF, Amsden K, Shah A, et al. Cow's milk elimination: a novel dietary approach to treat eosinophilic esophagitis. J Pediatr Gastroenterol Nutr 2012;55(6):711–6.
80. Kruszewski PG, Russo JM, Franciosi JP, et al. Prospective, comparative effectiveness trial of cow's milk elimination and swallowed fluticasone for pediatric eosinophilic esophagitis. Dis Esophagus 2015. [Epub ahead of print].
81. Ukleja A, Shiroky J, Agarwal A, et al. Esophageal dilations in eosinophilic esophagitis: a single center experience. World J Gastroenterol 2014;20(28):9549–55.
82. Schoepfer A. Treatment of eosinophilic esophagitis by dilation. Dig Dis 2014;32(1–2):130–3.
83. Lipka S, Keshishian J, Boyce HW, et al. The natural history of steroid-naive eosinophilic esophagitis in adults treated with endoscopic dilation and proton pump inhibitor therapy over a mean duration of nearly 14 years. Gastrointest Endosc 2014;80(4):592–8.
84. Ally MR, Dias J, Veerappan GR, et al. Safety of dilation in adults with eosinophilic esophagitis. Dis Esophagus 2013;26(3):241–5.

85. Schoepfer AM, Gonsalves N, Bussmann C, et al. Esophageal dilation in eosinophilic esophagitis: effectiveness, safety, and impact on the underlying inflammation. Am J Gastroenterol 2010;105(5):1062–70.
86. Hirano I. Dilation in eosinophilic esophagitis: to do or not to do? Gastrointest Endosc 2010;71(4):713–4.
87. Dellon ES, Gibbs WB, Rubinas TC, et al. Esophageal dilation in eosinophilic esophagitis: safety and predictors of clinical response and complications. Gastrointest Endosc 2010;71(4):706–12.
88. Bohm M, Richter JE, Kelsen S, et al. Esophageal dilation: simple and effective treatment for adults with eosinophilic esophagitis and esophageal rings and narrowing. Dis Esophagus 2010;23(5):377–85.
89. Chehade M, Aceves SS, Furuta GT, et al. Food allergy and eosinophilic esophagitis: what do we do? The journal of allergy and clinical immunology. In Pract 2015;3(1):25–32.
90. Aceves SS. Food allergy testing in eosinophilic esophagitis: what the gastroenterologist needs to know. Clin Gastroenterol Hepatol 2014;12(8):1216–23.
91. Papadopoulou A, Koletzko S, Heuschkel R, et al. Management guidelines of eosinophilic esophagitis in childhood. J Pediatr Gastroenterol Nutr 2014;58(1):107–18.
92. Henry ML, Atkins D, Fleischer D, et al. Factors contributing to adherence to dietary treatment of eosinophilic gastrointestinal diseases. J Pediatr Gastroenterol Nutr 2012;54(3):430–2.
93. Menard-Katcher C, Henry M, Furuta GT, et al. Significance of feeding dysfunction in eosinophilic esophagitis. World J Gastroenterol 2014;20(31):11019–22.
94. Pentiuk SP, Miller CK, Kaul A. Eosinophilic esophagitis in infants and toddlers. Dysphagia 2007;22(1):44–8.
95. Klinnert MD. Psychological impact of eosinophilic esophagitis on children and families. Immunol Allergy Clin North Am 2009;29(1):99–107, x.
96. Ko HM, Morotti RA, Yershov O, et al. Eosinophilic gastritis in children: clinicopathological correlation, disease course, and response to therapy. Am J Gastroenterol 2014;109(8):1277–85.
97. Caldwell JM, Collins MH, Stucke EM, et al. Histologic eosinophilic gastritis is a systemic disorder associated with blood and extragastric eosinophilia, TH2 immunity, and a unique gastric transcriptome. J Allergy Clin Immunol 2014;134(5): 1114–24.
98. Lwin T, Melton SD, Genta RM. Eosinophilic gastritis: histopathological characterization and quantification of the normal gastric eosinophil content. Mod Pathol 2011;24(4):556–63.
99. Prussin C. Eosinophilic gastroenteritis and related eosinophilic disorders. Gastroenterol Clin North Am 2014;43(2):317–27.
100. Alfadda AA, Shaffer EA, Urbanski SJ, et al. Eosinophilic colitis is a sporadic self-limited disease of middle-aged people: a population-based study. Colorectal Dis 2014;16(2):123–9.
101. Fernandez Salazar LI, Borrego Pintado H, Velayos Jimenez B, et al. Differential diagnosis and management of histologic eosinophilic colitis. J Crohns Colitis 2013;7(1):e20–1.
102. Brandon JL, Schroeder S, Furuta GT, et al. CT imaging features of eosinophilic colitis in children. Pediatr Radiol 2013;43(6):697–702.
103. Alfadda AA, Storr MA, Shaffer EA. Eosinophilic colitis: epidemiology, clinical features, and current management. Therap Adv Gastroenterol 2011;4(5):301–9.
104. Collins MH. Histopathologic features of eosinophilic esophagitis and eosinophilic gastrointestinal diseases. Gastroenterol Clin North Am 2014;43(2):257–68.

105. Gaertner WB, Macdonald JE, Kwaan MR, et al. Eosinophilic colitis: University of Minnesota experience and literature review. Gastroenterol Res Pract 2011;2011: 857508.
106. DeBrosse CW, Case JW, Putnam PE, et al. Quantity and distribution of eosinophils in the gastrointestinal tract of children. Pediatr Dev Pathol 2006;9(3):210–8.
107. Lowichik A, Welnberg A. A quantitative evaluation of mucosal eosinophils in the pediatric gastrointestinal tract. Mod Pathol 1996;9:110–4.
108. Talley NJ, Shorter RG, Phillips SF, et al. Eosinophilic gastroenteritis: a clinicopathological study of patients with disease of the mucosa, muscle layer, and subserosal tissues. Gut 1990;31(1):54–8.
109. Cello JP. Eosinophilic gastroenteritis—a complex disease entity. Am J Med 1979;67:1097–104.
110. Fleischer DM, Atkins D. Evaluation of the patient with suspected eosinophilic gastrointestinal disease. Immunol Allergy Clin North Am 2009;29(1):53–63, ix.
111. Yan BM, Shaffer EA. Primary eosinophilic disorders of the gastrointestinal tract. Gut 2009;58(5):721–32.
112. Chang JY, Choung RS, Lee RM, et al. A shift in the clinical spectrum of eosinophilic gastroenteritis toward the mucosal disease type. Clin Gastroenterol Hepatol 2010;8(8):669–75 [quiz: e688].
113. Liu E, Lee HS, Agardh D. Risk of celiac disease according to HLA haplotype and country. N Engl J Med 2014;371(11):1074.
114. Soon IS, Butzner JD, Kaplan GG, et al. Incidence and prevalence of eosinophilic esophagitis in children. J Pediatr Gastroenterol Nutr 2013;57(1):72–80.
115. Catassi C, Kryszak D, Bhatti B, et al. Natural history of celiac disease autoimmunity in a USA cohort followed since 1974. Ann Med 2010;42(7):530–8.
116. Husby S, Koletzko S, Korponay-Szabo IR, et al. European Society for Pediatric Gastroenterology, Hepatology, and Nutrition guidelines for the diagnosis of coeliac disease. J Pediatr Gastroenterol Nutr 2012;54(1):136–60.
117. Liu E, Lee HS, Aronsson CA, et al. Risk of pediatric celiac disease according to HLA haplotype and country. N Engl J Med 2014;371(1):42–9.
118. Aronsson CA, Lee HS, Liu E, et al. Age at gluten introduction and risk of celiac disease. Pediatrics 2015;135(2):239–45.
119. Koning F. Pathophysiology of celiac disease. J Pediatr Gastroenterol Nutr 2014; 59(Suppl 1):S1–4.
120. Rubio-Tapia A, Hill ID, Kelly CP, et al, American College of Gastroenterology. ACG clinical guidelines: diagnosis and management of celiac disease. Am J Gastroenterol 2013;108(5):656–76 [quiz: 677].
121. Colombel JF, Torpier G, Janin A, et al. Activated eosinophils in adult coeliac disease: evidence for a local release of major basic protein. Gut 1992;33(9): 1190–4.
122. Brown IS, Smith J, Rosty C. Gastrointestinal pathology in celiac disease: a case series of 150 consecutive newly diagnosed patients. Am J Clin Pathol 2012; 138(1):42–9.
123. Ludvigsson JF, Aro P, Walker MM, et al. Celiac disease, eosinophilic esophagitis and gastroesophageal reflux disease, an adult population-based study. Scand J Gastroenterol 2013;48(7):808–14.
124. Ahmed OI, Qasem SA, Abdulsattar JA, et al. Esophageal eosinophilia in pediatric patients with celiac disease; is it a causal or an incidental association? J Pediatr Gastroenterol Nutr 2014;60(4):493–7.
125. Verzegnassi F, Bua J, De Angelis P, et al. Eosinophilic oesophagitis and coeliac disease: is it just a casual association? Gut 2007;56(7):1029–30.

126. Quaglietta L, Coccorullo P, Miele E, et al. Eosinophilic oesophagitis and coeliac disease: is there an association? Aliment Pharmacol Ther 2007;26(3):487–93.
127. Leslie C, Mews C, Charles A, et al. Celiac disease and eosinophilic esophagitis: a true association. J Pediatr Gastroenterol Nutr 2010;50(4):397–9.
128. Ooi CY, Day AS, Jackson R, et al. Eosinophilic esophagitis in children with celiac disease. J Gastroenterol Hepatol 2008;23(7 Pt 1):1144–8.
129. Fasano A, Catassi C. Clinical practice. Celiac disease. N Engl J Med 2012; 367(25):2419–26.
130. Burisch J, Munkholm P. Inflammatory bowel disease epidemiology. Curr Opin Gastroenterol 2013;29(4):357–62.
131. Loftus EV Jr. Clinical epidemiology of inflammatory bowel disease: incidence, prevalence, and environmental influences. Gastroenterology 2004;126(6):1504–17.
132. Danese S, Fiocchi C. Ulcerative colitis. N Engl J Med 2011;365(18):1713–25.
133. Graham DB, Xavier RJ. From genetics of inflammatory bowel disease towards mechanistic insights. Trends Immunol 2013;34(8):371–8.
134. Ellinghaus D, Bethune J, Petersen BS, et al. The genetics of Crohn's disease and ulcerative colitis–status quo and beyond. Scand J Gastroenterol 2015; 50(1):13–23.
135. Kostic AD, Xavier RJ, Gevers D. The microbiome in inflammatory bowel disease: current status and the future ahead. Gastroenterology 2014;146(6):1489–99.
136. Baumgart DC, Sandborn WJ. Inflammatory bowel disease: clinical aspects and established and evolving therapies. Lancet 2007;369(9573):1641–57.
137. Isene R, Bernklev T, Hoie O, et al. Extraintestinal manifestations in Crohn's disease and ulcerative colitis: results from a prospective, population-based European inception cohort. Scand J Gastroenterol 2015;50(3):300–5.
138. Katsanos KH, Zinovieva E, Lambri E, et al. Eosinophilic-Crohn overlap colitis and review of the literature. J Crohns Colitis 2011;5(3):256–61.
139. Woodruff SA, Masterson JC, Fillon S, et al. Role of eosinophils in inflammatory bowel and gastrointestinal diseases. J Pediatr Gastroenterol Nutr 2011;52(6): 650–61.
140. Choy MY, Walker-Smith JA, Williams CB, et al. Activated eosinophils in chronic inflammatory bowel disease. Lancet 1990;336(8707):126–7.
141. Bischoff SC, Wedemeyer J, Herrmann A, et al. Quantitative assessment of intestinal eosinophils and mast cells in inflammatory bowel disease. Histopathology 1996;28(1):1–13.
142. Bischoff SC, Grabowsky J, Manns MP. Quantification of inflammatory mediators in stool samples of patients with inflammatory bowel disorders and controls. Dig Dis Sci 1997;42(2):394–403.
143. Troncone R, Caputo N, Esposito V, et al. Increased concentrations of eosinophilic cationic protein in whole-gut lavage fluid from children with inflammatory bowel disease. J Pediatr Gastroenterol Nutr 1999;28(2):164–8.
144. Stevceva L, Pavli P, Husband A, et al. Eosinophilia is attenuated in experimental colitis induced in IL-5 deficient mice. Genes Immun 2000;1(3):213–8.
145. Chen W, Paulus B, Shu D, et al. Increased serum levels of eotaxin in patients with inflammatory bowel disease. Scand J Gastroenterol 2001;36(5):515–20.
146. Carvalho AT, Elia CC, de Souza HS, et al. Immunohistochemical study of intestinal eosinophils in inflammatory bowel disease. J Clin Gastroenterol 2003;36(2): 120–5.
147. Furuta GT, Nieuwenhuis EE, Karhausen J, et al. Eosinophils alter colonic epithelial barrier function: role for major basic protein. Am J Physiol Gastrointest Liver Physiol 2005;289(5):G890–7.

148. Uzunismail H, Hatemi I, Dogusoy G, et al. Dense eosinophilic infiltration of the mucosa preceding ulcerative colitis and mimicking eosinophilic colitis: report of two cases. Turk J Gastroenterol 2006;17(1):53–7.

149. Wedemeyer J, Vosskuhl K. Role of gastrointestinal eosinophils in inflammatory bowel disease and intestinal tumours. Best Pract Res Clin Gastroenterol 2008; 22(3):537–49.

150. Masterson JC, McNamee EN, Jedlicka P, et al. CCR3 blockade attenuates eosinophilic ileitis and associated remodeling. Am J Pathol 2011;179(5): 2302–14.

151. Wedrychowicz A, Tomasik P, Pieczarkowski S, et al. Clinical value of serum eosinophilic cationic protein assessment in children with inflammatory bowel disease. Arch Med Sci 2014;10(6):1142–6.

152. Masterson JC, McNamee EN, Fillon SA, et al. Eosinophil-mediated signalling attenuates inflammatory responses in experimental colitis. Gut 2014. [Epub ahead of print].

153. Zezos P, Patsiaoura K, Nakos A, et al. Severe eosinophilic infiltration in colonic biopsies predicts patients with ulcerative colitis not responding to medical therapy. Colorectal Dis 2014;16(12):O420–30.

154. Dvorak AM, Osage JE, Monahan RA, et al. Crohn's disease: transmission electron microscopic studies. III. Target tissues. Proliferation of and injury to smooth muscle and the autonomic nervous system. Hum Pathol 1980;11(6):620–34.

155. Dvorak AM. Ultrastructural evidence for release of major basic protein-containing crystalline cores of eosinophil granules in vivo: cytotoxic potential in Crohn's disease. J Immunol 1980;125(1):460–2.

156. Dubucquoi S, Janin A, Klein O, et al. Activated eosinophils and interleukin 5 expression in early recurrence of Crohn's disease. Gut 1995;37(2):242–6.

157. Saitoh O, Kojima K, Sugi K, et al. Fecal eosinophil granule-derived proteins reflect disease activity in inflammatory bowel disease. Am J Gastroenterol 1999;94(12):3513–20.

158. Peterson CG, Sangfelt P, Wagner M, et al. Fecal levels of leukocyte markers reflect disease activity in patients with ulcerative colitis. Scand J Clin Lab Invest 2007;67(8):810–20.

159. Maltby S, Wohlfarth C, Gold M, et al. CD34 is required for infiltration of eosinophils into the colon and pathology associated with DSS-induced ulcerative colitis. Am J Pathol 2010;177(3):1244–54.

160. Ahrens R, Waddell A, Seidu L, et al. Intestinal macrophage/epithelial cell-derived CCL11/eotaxin-1 mediates eosinophil recruitment and function in pediatric ulcerative colitis. J Immunol 2008;181(10):7390–9.

161. Leiman DA, Lichtenstein GR. Therapy of inflammatory bowel disease: what to expect in the next decade. Curr Opin Gastroenterol 2014;30(4):385–90.

162. Rutgeerts P, Vermeire S, Van Assche G. Biological therapies for inflammatory bowel diseases. Gastroenterology 2009;136(4):1182–97.

163. Hansen JJ, Sartor RB. Therapeutic manipulation of the microbiome in IBD: current results and future approaches. Curr Treat Options Gastroenterol 2015; 13(1):105–20.

164. Lee D, Albenberg L, Compher C, et al. Diet in the pathogenesis and treatment of inflammatory bowel diseases. Gastroenterology 2015;148(6):1087–106.

165. Lichtenstein GR, Rutgeerts P, Sandborn WJ, et al. A pooled analysis of infections, malignancy, and mortality in infliximab- and immunomodulator-treated adult patients with inflammatory bowel disease. Am J Gastroenterol 2012; 107(7):1051–63.

166. Fletcher S, Van Hal S, Andresen D, et al. Gastrointestinal pathogen distribution in symptomatic children in Sydney, Australia. J Epidemiol Glob Health 2013; 3(1):11–21.
167. McCarty TR, Turkeltaub JA, Hotez PJ. Global progress towards eliminating gastrointestinal helminth infections. Curr Opin Gastroenterol 2014;30(1):18–24.
168. Kim MJ, Kim WH, Jung HC, et al. *Isospora belli* infection with chronic diarrhea in an alcoholic patient. Korean J Parasitol 2013;51(2):207–12.
169. Esteve C, Resano A, Diaz-Tejeiro P, et al. Eosinophilic gastritis due to *Anisakis*: a case report. Allergol Immunopathol (Madr) 2000;28(1):21–3.
170. Kim SG, Jo YJ, Park YS, et al. Four cases of gastric submucosal mass suspected as anisakiasis. Korean J Parasitol 2006;44(1):81–6.
171. Montalto M, Miele L, Marcheggiano A, et al. *Anisakis* infestation: a case of acute abdomen mimicking Crohn's disease and eosinophilic gastroenteritis. Dig Liver Dis 2005;37(1):62–4.
172. Centers for Disease Control and Prevention. Notes from the field: strongyloides infection among patients at a long-term care facility–Florida, 2010-2012. MMWR Morb Mortal Wkly Rep 2013;62(42):844.
173. Berk SL, Verghese A, Alvarez S, et al. Clinical and epidemiologic features of strongyloidiasis. A prospective study in rural Tennessee. Arch Intern Med 1987;147(7):1257–61.
174. Centers for Disease Control and Prevention. Notes from the field: strongyloidiasis in a rural setting–Southeastern Kentucky, 2013. MMWR Morb Mortal Wkly Rep 2013;62(42):843.
175. Russell ES, Gray EB, Marshall RE, et al. Prevalence of *Strongyloides stercoralis* antibodies among a rural Appalachian population–Kentucky, 2013. Am J Trop Med Hyg 2014;91(5):1000–1.
176. Pelletier LL Jr, Baker CB, Gam AA, et al. Diagnosis and evaluation of treatment of chronic strongyloidiasis in ex-prisoners of war. J Infect Dis 1988;157(3): 573–6.
177. Thompson BF, Fry LC, Wells CD, et al. The spectrum of GI strongyloidiasis: an endoscopic-pathologic study. Gastrointest Endosc 2004;59(7):906–10.
178. Requena-Mendez A, Chiodini P, Bisoffi Z, et al. The laboratory diagnosis and follow up of strongyloidiasis: a systematic review. PLoS Negl Trop Dis 2013; 7(1):e2002.

Eosinophilia in Hematologic Disorders

Lorenzo Falchi, MD, Srdan Verstovsek, MD, PhD*

KEYWORDS

- Eosinophilia • PDGFRA • PDGFRB • Chronic eosinophilic leukemia
- Hypereosinophilic syndrome • Imatinib

KEY POINTS

- Eosinophilia can subtend a broad differential diagnosis of acute or chronic, benign or malignant disorders.
- Suspecting an eosinophilia-associated myeloid neoplasm is important for prompt initiation of effective therapy.
- Molecular characterization of eosinophilia-associated myeloid neoplasms is critical for selecting the most appropriate targeted therapy.

INTRODUCTION

The upper limit of normal for eosinophils in the peripheral blood is 3% to 5%, corresponding to an absolute eosinophil count (AEC) of 350 to 500/mm³.[1] The severity of eosinophilia has been arbitrarily divided into mild (AEC 500–1500/mm³), moderate (AEC 1500–5000/mm³), and severe (AEC >5000/mm³),[1,2] although the practical significance of this stratification is unclear.

Many different conditions can underlie a finding of eosinophilia. A first broad distinction should be made between reactive and clonal eosinophilia. The first condition is characterized by the proliferation of polyclonal, mature eosinophils and can be sustained by benign or malignant disorders. In the second, eosinophils represent the primary malignant clone, and precursors can be found in the peripheral blood or bone marrow. As an additional category, idiopathic hypereosinophilic syndrome (HES) is a diagnosis of exclusion in patients with sustained eosinophilia and evidence of end-organ damage. It is important to identify the correct type of eosinophilia in a timely manner because a delay in referral and treatment can have profoundly detrimental

The authors have nothing to disclose.
Department of Leukemia, The University of Texas MD Anderson Cancer Center, 1515 Holcombe Boulevard, Houston, TX 77030, USA
* Corresponding author. 1515 Holcombe Boulevard, Unit 428, Houston, TX 77030.
E-mail address: sverstov@mdanderson.org

Immunol Allergy Clin N Am 35 (2015) 439–452
http://dx.doi.org/10.1016/j.iac.2015.04.004   **immunology.theclinics.com**

consequences on patient outcomes. This review discusses the diagnostic approach to eosinophilia from the hematologist's perspective, including elements of suspicion, diagnostic tests, and current treatment approaches for eosinophilia-associated myeloid neoplasms (MN-eos).

REACTIVE EOSINOPHILIA

Reactive eosinophilia is typically caused by increased levels of interleukin (IL)-5. Concomitant elevation in IL-4 and IL-13 can lead to associated hypergammaglobulinemia E (hyper-IgE).[3] In Western countries, reactive eosinophilia is most commonly caused by allergic conditions, whereby increases in IL-5 are mediated by T-helper 2 cells. A detailed clinical history and prick or radioallergosorbent tests usually allow prompt diagnosis and appropriate treatment.[4] In developing countries, the main cause of eosinophilia is invasive parasitic infections (most commonly helminths). A thorough travel history is crucial to elicit clinical suspicion and subsequent testing.[5] Other medical conditions that can present or associate with eosinophilia include a variety of pulmonary, dermatologic, or gastrointestinal disorders,[6] adrenal insufficiency,[7,8] and more rare entities such as hyper-IgE syndrome[9] or Wiscott-Aldrich syndrome.[10] A systematic review of these disorders is offered elsewhere in this issue.

REACTIVE EOSINOPHILIA OF HEMATOLOGIC AND ONCOLOGIC INTEREST

Cancer cells are capable of secreting granulocyte-/monocyte-colony stimulating factor, IL-3, and IL-5, which stimulate the proliferation of polyclonal eosinophils.[11,12] Paraneoplastic eosinophilia occurs in a variety of solid malignancies including, but not limited to, head and neck, lung, gastrointestinal, ovarian, and cervical cancer. Its frequency is 0.5% to 7%.[13] Eosinophilia is usually associated with advanced-stage disease and its prognostic value seems to vary (favorable, unfavorable, or neutral) among tumor types. However, the available data on the clinical significance of tumor-associated tissue eosinophilia are limited and heterogeneous.[14]

Hodgkin lymphoma, especially the mixed cellularity or nodular sclerosis types, can present with peripheral blood or, less frequently, tissue or marrow eosinophilia. Eosinophils are recruited directly by Reed-Sternberg cells. Acute B-cell lymphoblastic leukemia (B-ALL) associated with t(5;14) can also present with eosinophilia. The t(5;14) juxtaposes the IL-3 gene (on chromosome 5) and the immunoglobulin heavy chain (IgH) gene locus (on chromosome 14), resulting in enhanced IL-3 transcription and consequent eosinophilia. Around 10% of cases of adult T-cell leukemia/lymphoma are associated with reactive, IL-5-mediated peripheral blood eosinophilia, and 2% to 20% of patients with non-Hodgkin lymphoma (mostly of T-cell origin) present with elevated AEC (eosinophilia in lymphoproliferative disorders is reviewed in Ref.[15]).

LYMPHOCYTE VARIANT HYPEREOSINOPHILIC SYNDROME

In lymphocytic variant (LV) HES, peripheral blood eosinophilia is sustained by clonal T-helper 2 cells,[16] which may display different phenotypes, such as CD3−/CD4+, CD3+/CD4−/CD8−, and CD3+/CD4+/CD8−. Increased serum IgE levels can also be present. Diagnosis of LV HES, which is not a World Health Organization (WHO)-defined entity, is not standardized. Demonstration of a clonally rearranged T-cell receptor, direct observation of cytokine production by cultured T cells, or a finding of elevated TARC (a T-helper 2 cytokine) may be helpful in supporting the diagnosis. Up to one-fourth of patients with LV HES ultimately develop an overt T-cell malignancy.[17]

EOSINOPHILIC MYELOID DISORDERS
Epidemiology

Analyses of the Surveillance, Epidemiology, and End Results (SEER) database from 2001 to 2005 estimate the incidence rate of MN-eos at 0.036 per 100,000 people per year.[18] The incidence of recurrent genetic abnormalities in patients with HES has been reported to range from 10% to 20%[19,20] HES is most commonly diagnosed between the ages of 20 and 50 years with a male to female ratio of 1.47,[18] although most patients with MN-eos are male.[19,20]

Classification

There are 3 major types of MN-eos (**Box 1**). The 2008 WHO classification of myeloid neoplasms has recognized the pathogenetic, diagnostic, and therapeutic importance of recurrent genetic abnormalities in patients with primary eosinophilia by creating the category "Myeloid and lymphoid neoplasms with eosinophilia and abnormalities of platelet-derived growth factor receptor alpha (*PDGFRA*), platelet-derived growth factor receptor beta (*PDGFRB*), or fibroblast growth factor receptor 1 (*FGFR1*)."[21] A second WHO-defined MN-eos is chronic eosinophilic leukemia not otherwise specified (CEL-NOS), included among the myeloproliferative neoplasms (MPN). This definition is operational and requires: (1) absence of the Philadelphia chromosome or rearrangements of *PDGFRA*, *PDGFRB*, and *FGFR1*, and the exclusion of established myeloid neoplasms associated with eosinophilia; (2) demonstration of increased marrow blasts; and (3) evidence of clonality of the eosinophil population.[22] A diagnosis of idiopathic HES is one of exclusion, requiring the exclusion of all the aforementioned primary and secondary causes of eosinophilia and the demonstration of an AEC greater than 1500/mm^3 sustained for longer than 6 months with concomitant tissue damage.[22] Given the potential risk of end-organ damage when therapy is delayed, especially in patients with marked peripheral blood or tissue eosinophilia, a consensus definition of hypereosinophilia (HE) includes: AEC greater than 1500/mm^3 on 2 occasions 4 weeks or more apart, and/or tissue HE (defined as >20% marrow eosinophils, extensive eosinophil infiltration in the pathologist's opinion, or marked deposition of eosinophil granule proteins). A diagnosis of HES is made when there is concomitant end-organ damage that is attributable solely to eosinophilic infiltration.[23]

Diagnostic Workup

Manifestations of eosinophilia are heterogeneous. Patients can be paucisymptomatic or experience a rapidly fatal course, mainly attributable to advanced cardiomyopathy or transformation into acute leukemia. Virtually any organ can be infiltrated by eosinophils. In addition to peripheral blood work and bone marrow examination (where indicated), the diagnostic workup of patients presenting with eosinophilia should include, at a minimum, chest radiograph, pulmonary function tests, echocardiogram, and measurement of troponin levels. Further testing should be guided by the individual patient's symptoms. Selected clinical features of eosinophilia, including warning signs that should raise suspicion of eosinophilia related to a hematologic disorder, are summarized in **Table 1**.

When clonal eosinophilia is suspected, peripheral blood smear and bone marrow sampling for morphology, conventional cytogenetics, and immunohistochemistry should be performed to ascertain whether an underlying WHO-defined myeloid disorder, such as systemic mastocytosis (SM), chronic myelogenous leukemia (CML), acute myeloid leukemia (AML), myelodysplastic syndrome (MDS), or MDS/MPN overlap entities (ie, chronic myelomonocytic leukemia [CMML]), is present. Common marrow

Box 1
Classification and diagnostic criteria of primary hypereosinophilic disorders

Myeloid and Lymphoid Neoplasms with Eosinophilia and Abnormalities of PDGFRA, PDGFRB, or FGFR1

PDGFRA rearrangements:

  A Ph-negative MPN OR AML OR B/T-lymphoblastic leukemia/lymphoma

  Prominent eosinophilia

  Presence of *FIP1L1-PDGFRA* fusion gene

PDGFRB rearrangements:

  Ph-negative MPN

  Prominent eosinophilia[a]

  Presence of t(5;12)(q31-q33;p12) or variant OR *ETV6-PDGFRB* fusion gene OR other *PDGFRB* rearrangement

FGFR1 rearrangements:

  A Ph-negative MPN OR AML OR B/T-lymphoblastic leukemia/lymphoma

  Prominent eosinophilia[a]

  Presence of t(8;13)(p11;q12) OR variant and presence of FGFR1 rearrangement in myeloid cells and/or lymphoblasts

CEL-NOS

  AEC greater than 1500/μL

  Blast cell count less than 20% and no other diagnostic criteria of AML

  Blast cells greater than 2% in peripheral blood or greater than 5% in the bone marrow OR clonal cytogenetic or molecular abnormality

  Absence of Ph- or BCR-ABL-positive or -negative MPN or MDS/MPN overlap disorder

  Absence of *PDFGRA, PDGFRB,* or *FGFR1* rearrangements

Idiopathic HES

  AEC greater than 1500/μL (sustained for >6 months)

  Evidence of organ damage[b]

  Exclusion of the following conditions:

  1. Reactive eosinophilia

  2. LV HES

  3. CEL-NOS

  4. WHO-defined MN-eos (ie, AML, MDS, MPN, MDS/MPN overlapping disorders)

  5. MN-eos with rearrangements of *PDGFRA, PDGFRB,* or *FGFR1*

Abbreviations: AEC, absolute eosinophil count; AML, acute myeloid leukemia; CEL-NOS, chronic eosinophilic leukemia not otherwise specified; LV HES, lymphocyte variant hypereosinophilic syndrome; MDS, myelodysplastic syndrome; MN-eos, eosinophilia-associated myeloid neoplasm; MPN, myeloproliferative neoplasm; Ph, Philadelphia chromosome.
  [a] Neutrophilia or monocytosis can be present.
  [b] If no organ damage is present, a diagnosis of idiopathic hypereosinophilia is made.
  Data from Bain BJ, Gilliland DG, Horny HP, et al. Chronic eosinophilic leukaemia, not otherwise specified. In: Swerdlow S, Harris NL, Stein H, et al, editors. World Health Organization classification of tumours. Pathology and genetics of tumours of haematopoietic and lymphoid tissues. Lyon (France): IARC Press; 2008. p. 51–3; and Bain BJ, Gilliland DG, Horny HP, et al. Myeloid and lymphoid neoplasms with eosinophilia and abnormalities of PDGFRA, PDGFRB, orFGFR1. In: Swerdlow S, Harris NL, Stein H, et al, editors. World Health Organization classification of tumours. Pathology and genetics of tumours of haematopoietic and lymphoid tissues. Lyon (France): IARC Press; 2008. p. 68–73.

Table 1
Selected clinical manifestations of sustained eosinophilia

Organ/System	Manifestations	Findings
Nonhematologic		
General	Fatigue	—
	Fever	—
Dermatologic	Pruritus	Urticaria
	Angioedema	Erythematous papules
Cardiac	Signs/symptoms of heart failure	Inflammatory/infiltrative cardiomyopathy
	—	Endomyocardial fibrosis, including valvulopathy
	Signs/symptoms of systemic embolization	Mural platelet thrombi
Pulmonary	Cough, rhinitis	—
	Shortness of breath	Pleural effusion
	—	Pulmonary infiltrates
Gastrointestinal	Diarrhea, with or without blood	Eosinophilic colitis
	Dysphagia/regurgitation	Eosinophilic esophagitis/ esophageal eosinophilia
	Vomiting/dyspepsia/ malabsorption	Eosinophilic gastroenteritis
Neurologic	Dysesthesia	Polyneuropathy
	Loss of vision	Optic neuritis
Musculoskeletal	Myalgias	Eosinophilic myositis/fasciitis
Hematologic		
Peripheral blood	—	Leukocytosis[a]
	—	Eosinophilia[a]
	—	Neutrophilia
	—	Basophilia[b]
	—	Left shift[b]
	—	Circulating blasts[b]
	—	Uni- or multilineage dysplasia[b]
	Pallor	Anemia[a]
	Bruisability/thrombosis	Thrombocytopenia/ thrombocytosis[a]
Reticuloendothelial	Abdominal pain	Hepato-/splenomegaly[b]
	—	Hepatic/splenic infarct[b]
	Lymph node swelling	Superficial and/or deep adenopathy[b]

[a] If severe, upfront bone marrow examination should be performed.
[b] Upfront bone marrow examination must be performed.

findings in patients with MN-eos include hypercellularity, prominent eosinophilia with or without dysplasia, increased blasts, marrow fibrosis, and Charcot-Leyden crystals. Conventional cytogenetics can provide important diagnostic information. Indeed, rearrangements of genes commonly involved in the pathogenesis of MN-eos often have a cytogenetic counterpart (ie, rearrangements of *PDGFRA*, *PDGFRB*, and *FGFR1* are associated with abnormalities of chromosomes 4q12, 5q31-33, and 8p11-13, respectively).[21]

For practical purposes, however, screening of primary eosinophilia is typically performed by reverse transcriptase–polymerase chain reaction (RT-PCR) of peripheral blood or interphase/metaphase fluorescent in situ hybridization (FISH) to detect the *FIP1L1-PDGFRA* fusion gene. FISH probes are used to detect the cytogenetically occult 800-kb deletion on chromosome 4q12 that generates *FIP1L1-PDGFRA*.[24] Deletion of the *CHIC2* gene, which is found in this region, is used as a surrogate marker for the *FIP1L1-PDGFRA* fusion gene in FISH.[25] Finally, the *FIP1L1-PDGFRA* has been described in cases of eosinophilia-associated AML and T-cell lymphoblastic lymphoma.[26]

When *FIP1L1-PDGFRA* cannot be identified in a patient otherwise suspected to have primary eosinophilia, a search for other recurrent molecular abnormalities should be initiated. *PDGFRB* rearrangements have been identified in cases of CMML, atypical CML, and juvenile myelomonocytic leukemia. Although rare, this molecular finding is of critical importance given the responsiveness of PDGFRB-driven disorders to imatinib mesylate (IM) (see later discussion). More than 20 fusion-gene partners of *PDGFRB* have been described.[21,27] MN-eos sustained by fusion genes involving *FGFR1* (formerly known as 8p11 myeloproliferative syndrome) are very rare. Since the discovery of the *ZNF198-FGFR1* fusion gene 17 years ago,[28] more than 10 fusion partners of *FGFR1* have been identified.[27] These disorders can present as MPN, with or without peripheral or tissue eosinophilia, AML, or T-cell lymphoblastic lymphoma. At present, MN-eos that are triple-negative (ie, lacking *PDGFRA*, *PDGFRB*, and *FGFR1* rearrangements) are diagnosed as CEL-NOS, idiopathic HES, or idiopathic HE (if there is no organ damage).

Treatment

Patients with no symptoms or evidence of organ damage are generally observed without intervention. However, the clinical aggressiveness of CEL-NOS and HES and the availability of effective targeted therapy for molecularly defined entities have persuaded many clinicians to manage these patients proactively rather than conservatively. A treatment algorithm is presented in **Fig. 1**. In patients with eosinophilia-associated WHO-defined myeloid or lymphoid malignancy, treatment should follow disease-specific guidelines.

Molecularly defined eosinophilia-associated myeloid neoplasms

IM is a multikinase inhibitor that blocks the activity of the BCR-ABL oncoprotein in CML, thereby inhibiting the proliferation and survival of the leukemic cells.[29] Treatment of CML with IM has elicited unprecedented high rates of deep cytogenetic and molecular responses and, ultimately, dramatically improved patient outcomes.[30] Based on such tremendous success, IM was empirically tested in patients with MN-eos.

The first studies of IM (100–400 mg/d) in patients with HES were reported about a decade ago as case reports or small series. Most patients treated achieved early complete hematologic responses (CHR), usually defined as resolution of clinical symptoms and normalization of blood counts.[31–33] The subsequent identification of FIP1L1-PDGFRA as a therapeutic target of IM[24] enabled the selection of HES patients suitable for targeted therapy, leading to the reclassification of these MN-eos as WHO-defined entities.[21] Moreover, the availability of a molecular marker improved the assessment and monitoring of response to IM. Several studies have shown that most patients with FIP1L1-PDGFRA-positive disease treated with IM experience complete molecular remission, defined as no detectable fusion transcript by RT-PCR (**Table 2**). Results of these studies suggest that IM effectively suppresses the *FIP1L1-PDGFRA* clone. However, discontinuation of IM often results in disease reappearance and clinical relapse. In one study, 5 patients with molecularly undetectable disease had molecular relapse on IM dose deescalation, but were able to regain molecular remission after

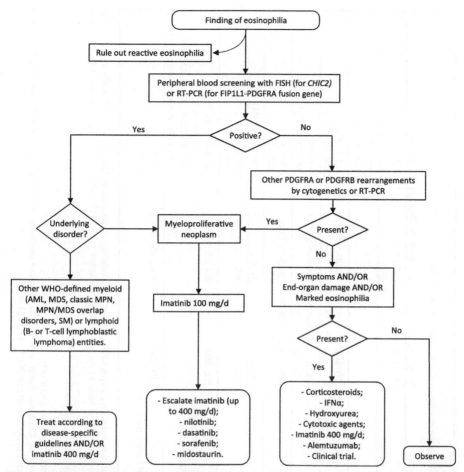

Fig. 1. Suggested treatment algorithm for patients with primary eosinophilia (MN-eos). IFN, interferon.

resuming treatment.[34] In another study, 6 of 11 patients who discontinued IM relapsed while 5 maintained their molecular remission after 9 to 88 months.[35] Although a few patients may maintain their remission after discontinuation, whether IM can eradicate the disease remains unclear at this time. Therefore, treatment discontinuation is currently considered experimental. Of note, because end-organ damage cannot be reversed with treatment in most cases, prompt initiation of IM is critical once a target molecular lesion is identified.

Primary or acquired resistance to IM has only occasionally been reported in patients with *FIP1L1-PDGFRA*–positive disease. The T674I point mutation within the adenosine triphosphate–binding domain of PDGFRA is the most common mechanism of acquired resistance to IM in *PDGFRA-FIP1L1*–positive disease. Its pharmacodynamic consequences are similar to those caused by T315I in CML, which renders BCR-ABL resistant to IM and other tyrosine kinase inhibitors (TKIs).[24] T674I mutated clones are sensitive to nilotinib, sorafenib, and midostaurin in vitro. However, preliminary clinical experience with these agents has been disappointing.[36] The D842V mutation has been found in patients whose disease progressed after treatment with nilotinib or

Table 2
Published studies of MN-eos with *PDGFRA* or *PDGFRB* rearrangements treated with imatinib mesylate

Study	No. of Patients	Gene Rearrangement	Dose (mg/d)	Duration of Therapy	Response
Klion et al,[56] 2004	6	*FIP1L1-PDGFRA*	100–400	1–12 mo	CHR 100% CMR 5/6 (83%)
Metzgeroth et al,[57] 2008	16	*FIP1L1-PDGFRA*	—	12 mo	CHR 100% CMR 14/16 (87%)
Helbig et al,[58] 2008	6	*FIP1L1-PDGFRA*	100–400[a]	Median 30 mo	CHR 100% CMR 5/6 (83%)
Legrand et al,[35] 2013[b]	44	*FIP1L1-PDGFRA*	Mean, 165 induction/ 58 maintenance	Median 52 mo	CHR 100% CMR 43/44 (95%)
Baccarani et al,[59] 2007	27	*FIP1L1-PDGFRA*	100 escalated to 400	Median 1 mo	CHR 100% CMR 100%
Jovanovic et al,[60] 2007[b]	11	*FIP1L1-PDGFRA*	100–400	12 mo	CMR 9/11 (82%)
Arefi et al,[61] 2012[b]	8	*FIP1L1-PDGFRA*	100	NR	CHR 100% MR[9] 100%
David et al,[62] 2007[c]	20	10 *ETV6-PDGFRB* 7 various *PDGFRB* fusion partners 3 unknown *PDGFRB* fusion partners	200–800	0.1–60 mo	CHR 16/20 (80%) CCyR 15/20 (75%) CMR: 4/8 (50%) *ETV6-PDGFRB*, 1/8 (12%) other rearrangements
Cheah et al,[63] 2007[d]	26	18 *ETV6-PDGFRB* 8 various *PDGFRB* fusion partners	100–400	Median, 10.2 y	OR 96% CCyR 52% CMR 32%

Abbreviations: CCyR, complete cytogenetic remission, defined as normal karyotype; CHR, complete hematologic response, defined as resolution of symptoms and normalization of blood counts; CMR, complete molecular response defined, as no detectable transcript by RT-PCR; MR, molecular response; OR, objective response.

[a] Patients were transitioned to once-weekly dosing after achieving remission.
[b] Multicenter retrospective study.
[c] Multicenter, prospective study + review and update of data from the literature.
[d] Multicenter retrospective study, including data from David M, Cross NC, Burgstaller S, et al. Durable responses to imatinib in patients with PDGFRB fusion gene-positive and BCR-ABL–negative chronic myeloproliferative disorders. Blood 2007;109(1):61–4.

sorafenib, and is not sensitive in vitro to second-generation TKIs. The low frequency of TKI resistance in *FIP1L1-PDGFRA*–positive disease might be explained by the limited repertoire of mutations that can affect the PDGFRA kinase domain.[37] Allogeneic hematopoietic stem cell transplantation has been performed successfully in patients with HES,[38] and should be considered a priority in cases of TKI-resistant *PDGFRA-FIP1L1*–positive disease.

IM has also been used successfully in MN-eos patients with a variety of other rearrangements involving *PDGFRA* or *PDGFRB* (more than half of whom harbor *ETV6-PDGFRB* fusion gene, see **Table 2**).

Eosinophilia-associated *FGFR1*-positive disease is the least common subtype of MN-eos. The clinical course is aggressive with frequent evolution into AML within 1 to 2 years. These disorders can present with or, more commonly, without peripheral blood or tissue eosinophilia. Eosinophilia-associated manifestations are also uncommon. Histopathology is usually consistent with T-cell lymphoblastic leukemia/lymphoma or a myeloid/T-cell phenotype.[21] Treatment is directed at the lymphoma and usually involves intensive chemotherapy followed by allogeneic transplantation whenever possible. Data on the efficacy of multiple TKIs, including IM, ponatinib,[39] dovitinib,[40] and midostaurin[41] in vitro are promising, but experience in the clinical setting is limited.

IM and other TKIs have been generally well tolerated in patients with MN-eos, with a toxicity profile largely overlapping that observed in CML patients. However, because some patients have experienced cardiogenic shock after receiving IM,[42] prophylactic steroids are recommended for the first 7 to 10 days of treatment in patients with known cardiac comorbidities, elevated baseline serum troponin levels attributable to eosinophil cardiac infiltration, or both.

Recurrent rearrangements of genes other than *PDGFRA*, *PDGFRB*, or *FGFR1* have been identified in patients with MN-eos. The most important ones involve *JAK2* and *FLT3*, each of which are fused with several different partners. Of 4 patients with *JAK2*-positive MN-eos treated with the JAK1/2 inhibitor ruxolitinib, all have been reported to achieve a hematologic and cytogenetic response.[43,44] Another extremely rare condition, *ETV6-FLT3*–positive MN-eos, has been reported in 5 cases.[45–48] Three patients received an FLT3 inhibitor[46,48] and achieved clinical and cytogenetic responses. Because these 2 entities have a clinical-hematologic phenotype similar to that of WHO-defined MN-eos and are driven by targetable molecular lesions, their recognition in the WHO framework seems appropriate.

Idiopathic hypereosinophilic syndrome and chronic eosinophilic leukemia not otherwise specified

Systemic corticosteroids exert quick and effective eosinophil-lytic activity and remain the first-line treatment of patients with primary eosinophilia without a defined molecular lesion. However, treatment duration is limited by numerous side effects. Among patients treated with 30 to 40 mg of prednisone daily, with subsequent tapering to a maintenance dose, objective response rates range from 65% to 85%.[49,50] Disease progression while on prednisone doses greater than 10 mg daily warrants the addition of a second agent. Hydroxyurea has been used alone or together with corticosteroids in previously untreated or steroid-refractory HES patients with response rates of approximately 70%.[51] For patients who fail to respond to corticosteroids and hydroxyurea, interferon (IFN)-α represents a viable option.[52] Reported response rates are approximately 50% and increase to 75% with the addition of prednisone. The optimal induction and maintenance doses are not defined.[49] IFN-α therapy is burdened with side effects (eg, flu-like syndrome, fatigue, cytopenia, mood disorders, hypothyroidism) in a significant proportion of patients. The pegylated formulation of IFN-α may decrease the incidence and severity of these complications while preserving efficacy.[53] Other treatment options for patients who did not respond to or were intolerant of the aforementioned agents include vincristine, cyclophosphamide, etoposide, and cladribine, alone or in combination with cytarabine, and cyclosporin A.[36] The "molecularly blind" use of IM in this patient population has limited efficacy, and the few responses observed are conceivably explained by the presence of occult molecular targets.

Novel monoclonal antibodies (MoAb) that target the pathophysiology of eosinophilia have been used in patients whose disease cannot be controlled with conventional approaches. Mepolizumab, a MoAb against IL-5, was compared as a steroid-sparing agent with placebo in a randomized trial.[54] Significantly more patients in the mepolizumab arm achieved doses of prednisone less than 10 mg daily for longer than 8 weeks. Some patients were able to avoid prednisone for at least 3 months. Alemtuzumab, an anti-CD52 MoAb, induced CHR in most patients.[55] However, the response duration is short and patients typically require a maintenance regimen. Moreover, because alemtuzumab is profoundly immune suppressive, close monitoring and anti-infectious prophylaxis are recommended during and after treatment. A more extensive review of MoAbs for the treatment of HES is offered elsewhere in this issue.

SUMMARY

A finding of eosinophilia, isolated or in conjunction with other clinical manifestations, opens a broad differential diagnosis for clinicians, as it can subtend many different disorders be they acute or chronic, benign or malignant. In the context of myeloid neoplasms that present or are associated with eosinophilia, an equally large number of different conditions must be considered in the diagnostic approach. For molecularly defined MN-eos, targeted agents such as IM represent definitive therapy for most patients. By contrast, the relatively vast armamentarium used to treat CEL-NOS or HES has yielded insufficient results. As our knowledge of the pathogenesis of MN-eos expands and new targeted molecules become available, more cases currently labeled as CEL-NOS/HES will likely be reclassified as WHO-defined entities. Thus, in the future it will be important to devise MN-eos–specific molecular diagnostic panels that encompass core genetic driving lesions, thus providing clinicians with reliable and timely guidance for patient management.

REFERENCES

1. Rothenberg ME. Eosinophilia. N Engl J Med 1998;338(22):1592–600.
2. Tefferi A, Patnaik MM, Pardanani A. Eosinophilia: secondary, clonal and idiopathic. Br J Haematol 2006;133(5):468–92.
3. Valent P, Gleich GJ, Reiter A, et al. Pathogenesis and classification of eosinophil disorders: a review of recent developments in the field. Expert Rev Hematol 2012; 5(2):157–76.
4. Lombardi C, Passalacqua G. Eosinophilia and diseases: clinical review of 1862 cases. Arch Intern Med 2003;163:1371–3.
5. Siddiqui AA, Berk SL. Diagnosis of *Strongyloides stercoralis* infection. Clin Infect Dis 2001;33:1040–7.
6. Simon D, Wardlaw A, Rothenberg ME. Organ-specific eosinophilic disorders of the skin, lung, and gastrointestinal tract. J Allergy Clin Immunol 2010;126(1): 3–13 [quiz: 14–5].
7. Spry C. Eosinophilia in Addison's disease. Yale J Biol Med 1976;49(4):411–3.

8. Beishuizen A, Vermes I, Hylkema BS, et al. Relative eosinophilia and functional adrenal insufficiency in critically ill patients. Lancet 1999;353(9165): 1675–6.
9. Sowerwine KJ, Holland SM, Freeman AF. Hyper-IgE syndrome update. Ann N Y Acad Sci 2012;1250:25–32.
10. Ochs HD, Thrasher AJ. The Wiskott-Aldrich syndrome. J Allergy Clin Immunol 2006;117(4):725–38 [quiz: 739].
11. Pandit R, Scholnik A, Wulfekuhler L, et al. Non-small-cell lung cancer associated with excessive eosinophilia and secretion of interleukin-5 as a paraneoplastic syndrome. Am J Hematol 2007;82(3):234–7.
12. Stefanini M, Claustro JC, Motos RA, et al. Blood and bone marrow eosinophilia in malignant tumors. Role and nature of blood and tissue eosinophil colony-stimulating factor(s) in two patients. Cancer 1991;68(3):543–8.
13. Isaacson NH, Rapoport P. Eosinophilia in malignant tumors: its significance. Ann Intern Med 1946;25(6):893–902.
14. Jain M, Kasetty S, Khan S, et al. Tissue eosinophilia in head and neck squamous neoplasia: an update. Exp Oncol 2014;36(3):157–61.
15. Roufosse F, Garaud S, de Leval L. Lymphoproliferative disorders associated with hypereosinophilia. Semin Hematol 2012;49(2):138–48.
16. Simon HU, Plotz SG, Dummer R, et al. Abnormal clones of T cells producing interleukin-5 in idiopathic eosinophilia. N Engl J Med 1999;341:1112–20.
17. Roufosse F, Cogan E, Goldman M. Lymphocytic variant hypereosinophilic syndromes. Immunol Allergy Clin North Am 2007;27(3):389–413.
18. Crane MM, Chang CM, Kobayashi MG, et al. Incidence of myeloproliferative hypereosinophilic syndrome in the United States and an estimate of all hypereosinophilic syndrome incidence. J Allergy Clin Immunol 2010;126(1):179–81.
19. Pardanani A, Brockman SR, Paternoster SF, et al. FIP1L1-PDGFRA fusion: prevalence and clinicopathologic correlates in 89 consecutive patients with moderate to severe eosinophilia. Blood 2004;104(10):3038–45.
20. Pardanani A, Ketterling RP, Li CY, et al. FIP1L1-PDGFRA in eosinophilic disorders: prevalence in routine clinical practice, long-term experience with imatinib therapy, and a critical review of the literature. Leuk Res 2006;30(8):965–70.
21. Bain BJ, Gilliland DG, Horny H-P, et al. Myeloid and lymphoid neoplasms with eosinophilia and abnormalities of PDGFRA, PDGFRB, or FGFR1. In: Swerdlow S, Harris NL, Stein H, et al, editors. World Health Organization classification of tumours. Pathology and genetics of tumours of haematopoietic and lymphoid tissues. Lyon (France): IARC Press; 2008. p. 68–73.
22. Bain BJ, Gilliland DG, Horny HP, et al. Chronic eosinophilic leukemia, not otherwise specified. In: Swerdlow SH, Campo E, Harris NL, et al, editors. WHO classification of tumours of the haematopoietic and lymphoid tissues. Lyon (France): IARC Press; 2008. p. 51–3.
23. Valent P, Klion AD, Horny HP, et al. Contemporary consensus proposal on criteria and classification of eosinophilic disorders and related syndromes. J Allergy Clin Immunol 2012;130(3):607–12.e9.
24. Cools J, Deangelo DJ, Gotlib J, et al. A tyrosine kinase created by fusion of the PDGFRA and FIP1L1 genes as a therapeutic target of imatinib in idiopathic hypereosinophilic syndrome. N Engl J Med 2003;348:1201–14.
25. Pardanani A, Ketterling RP, Brockman SR, et al. CHIC2 deletion, a surrogate for FIP1L1-PDGFRA fusion, occurs in systemic mastocytosis associated with eosinophilia and predicts response to imatinib mesylate therapy. Blood 2003;102(9): 3093–6.

26. Metzgeroth G, Walz C, Score J, et al. Recurrent finding of the FIP1L1-PDGFRA fusion gene in eosinophilia-associated acute myeloid leukemia and lymphoblastic T-cell lymphoma. Leukemia 2007;21(6):1183–8.

27. Gotlib J, Cools J. Five years since the discovery of FIP1L1-PDGFRA: what we have learned about the fusion and other molecularly defined eosinophilias. Leukemia 2008;22(11):1999–2010.

28. Xiao S, Nalabolu SR, Aster JC, et al. FGFR1 is fused with a novel zinc-finger gene, ZNF198, in the t(8;13) leukaemia/lymphoma syndrome. Nat Genet 1998;18:84–7.

29. Druker BJ, Tamura S, Fau - Buchdunger E, et al. Effects of a selective inhibitor of the Abl tyrosine kinase on the growth of Bcr-Abl positive cells. Nat Med 1996;2(5):561–6.

30. Druker BJ, Guilhot F, O'Brien SG, et al. Five-year follow-up of patients receiving imatinib for chronic myeloid leukemia. N Engl J Med 2006;355:2408–17.

31. Schaller JL, Burkland GA. Case report: rapid and complete control of idiopathic hypereosinophilia with imatinib mesylate. MedGenMed 2001;3(5):9.

32. Gleich GJ, Leiferman KM, Pardanani A, et al. Treatment of hypereosinophilic syndrome with imatinib mesylate. Lancet 2002;359(9317):1577–8.

33. Cortes J, Ault P, Koller C, et al. Efficacy of imatinib mesylate in the treatment of idiopathic hypereosinophilic syndrome. Blood 2003;101(12):4714–6.

34. Klion AD, Robyn J, Maric I, et al. Relapse following discontinuation of imatinib mesylate therapy for FIP1L1/PDGFRA-positive chronic eosinophilic leukemia: implications for optimal dosing. Blood 2007;110(10):3552–6.

35. Legrand F, Renneville A, Macintyre E, et al. The spectrum of FIP1L1-PDGFRA-associated chronic eosinophilic leukemia: new insights based on a survey of 44 cases. Medicine 2013;92(5):e1–9.

36. Gotlib J. World Health Organization-defined eosinophilic disorders: 2014 update on diagnosis, risk stratification, and management. Am J Hematol 2014;89(3):325–37.

37. von Bubnoff N, Gorantla SP, Engh RA, et al. The low frequency of clinical resistance to PDGFR inhibitors in myeloid neoplasms with abnormalities of PDGFRA might be related to the limited repertoire of possible PDGFRA kinase domain mutations in vitro. Oncogene 2011;30(8):933–43.

38. Halaburda K, Prejzner W, Szatkowski D, et al. Allogeneic bone marrow transplantation for hypereosinophilic syndrome: long-term follow-up with eradication of FIP1L1-PDGFRA fusion transcript. Bone Marrow Transplant 2006;38(4):319–20.

39. Lierman E, Smits S, Cools J, et al. Ponatinib is active against imatinib-resistant mutants of FIP1L1-PDGFRA and KIT, and against FGFR1-derived fusion kinases. Leukemia 2012;26(7):1693–5.

40. Wasag B, Lierman E, Meeus P, et al. The kinase inhibitor TKI258 is active against the novel CUX1-FGFR1 fusion detected in a patient with T-lymphoblastic leukemia/lymphoma and t(7;8)(q22;p11). Haematologica 2011;96(6):922–6.

41. Chen J, Deangelo DJ, Kutok JL, et al. PKC412 inhibits the zinc finger 198-fibroblast growth factor receptor 1 fusion tyrosine kinase and is active in treatment of stem cell myeloproliferative disorder. Proc Natl Acad Sci U S A 2004;101(40):14479–84.

42. Pitini V, Arrigo C, Azzarello D, et al. Serum concentration of cardiac troponin T in patients with hypereosinophilic syndrome treated with imatinib is predictive of adverse outcomes. Blood 2003;102(9):3456–7.

43. Schwaab J, Knut M, Haferlach C, et al. Limited duration of complete remission on ruxolitinib in myeloid neoplasms with PCM1-JAK2 and BCR-JAK2 fusion genes. Ann Hematol 2015;94(2):233–8.

44. Bain BJ, Ahmad S. Should myeloid and lymphoid neoplasms with PCM1-JAK2 and other rearrangements of JAK2 be recognized as specific entities? Br J Haematol 2014;166(6):809–17.
45. Vu HA, Xinh PT, Masuda M, et al. FLT3 is fused to ETV6 in a myeloproliferative disorder with hypereosinophilia and a t(12;13)(p13;q12) translocation. Leukemia 2006;20(8):1414–21.
46. Walz C, Erben P, Ritter M, et al. Response of ETV6-FLT3-positive myeloid/lymphoid neoplasm with eosinophilia to inhibitors of FMS-like tyrosine kinase 3. Blood 2011;118(8):2239–42.
47. Chonabayashi K, Hishizawa M, Matsui M, et al. Successful allogeneic stem cell transplantation with long-term remission of ETV6/FLT3-positive myeloid/lymphoid neoplasm with eosinophilia. Ann Hematol 2014;93(3):535–7.
48. Falchi L, Mehrotra M, Newberry KJ, et al. ETV6-FLT3 fusion gene-positive, eosinophilia-associated myeloproliferative neoplasm successfully treated with sorafenib and allogeneic stem cell transplant. Leukemia 2014;28(10):2090–2.
49. Ogbogu PU, Bochner BS, Butterfield JH, et al. Hypereosinophilic syndrome: a multicenter, retrospective analysis of clinical characteristics and response to therapy. J Allergy Clin Immunol 2009;124(6):1319–25.e3.
50. Helbig G, Wisniewska-Piaty K, Francuz T, et al. Diversity of clinical manifestations and response to corticosteroids for idiopathic hypereosinophilic syndrome: retrospective study in 33 patients. Leuk Lymphoma 2013;54(4):807–11.
51. Fauci AS, Harley JB, Roberts WC, et al. The idiopathic hypereosinophilic syndrome: clinical, pathophysiologic, and therapeutic considerations. Ann Intern Med 1982;97:78–92.
52. Butterfield JH. Interferon treatment for hypereosinophilic syndromes and systemic mastocytosis. Acta Haematol 2005;114(1):26–40.
53. Jabbour E, Kantarjian H, Cortes J, et al. PEG-IFN-alpha-2b therapy in BCR-ABL-negative myeloproliferative disorders: final result of a phase 2 study. Cancer 2007;110(9):2012–8.
54. Rothenberg ME, Klion AD, Roufosse FE, et al. Treatment of patients with the hypereosinophilic syndrome with mepolizumab. N Engl J Med 2008;358(12):1215–28.
55. Verstovsek S, Tefferi A, Kantarjian H, et al. Alemtuzumab therapy for hypereosinophilic syndrome and chronic eosinophilic leukemia. Clin Cancer Res 2009;15(1):368–73.
56. Klion AD, Robyn J, Akin C, et al. Molecular remission and reversal of myelofibrosis in response to imatinib mesylate treatment in patients with the myeloproliferative variant of hypereosinophilic syndrome. Blood 2004;103(2):473–8.
57. Metzgeroth G, Walz C, Erben P, et al. Safety and efficacy of imatinib in chronic eosinophilic leukaemia and hypereosinophilic syndrome: a phase-II study. Br J Haematol 2008;143(5):707–15.
58. Helbig G, Stella-Holowiecka B, Majewski M, et al. A single weekly dose of imatinib is sufficient to induce and maintain remission of chronic eosinophilic leukaemia in FIP1L1-PDGFRA-expressing patients. Br J Haematol 2008;141(2):200–4.
59. Baccarani M, Cilloni D, Rondoni M, et al. The efficacy of imatinib mesylate in patients with FIP1L1-PDGFR -positive hypereosinophilic syndrome. Results of a multicenter prospective study. Haematologica 2007;92(9):1173–9.
60. Jovanovic JV, Score J, Waghorn K, et al. Low-dose imatinib mesylate leads to rapid induction of major molecular responses and achievement of complete molecular remission in FIP1L1-PDGFRA-positive chronic eosinophilic leukemia. Blood 2007;109:4635–40.

61. Arefi M, Garcia JL, Briz MM, et al. Response to imatinib mesylate in patients with hypereosinophilic syndrome. Int J Hematol 2012;96(3):320–6.
62. David M, Cross NC, Burgstaller S, et al. Durable responses to imatinib in patients with PDGFRB fusion gene-positive and BCR-ABL-negative chronic myeloproliferative disorders. Blood 2007;109(1):61–4.
63. Cheah CY, Burbury K, Apperley JF, et al. Patients with myeloid malignancies bearing PDGFRB fusion genes achieve durable long-term remissions with imatinib. Blood 2014;123(23):3574–7.

Eosinophilia in Rheumatologic/Vascular Disorders

Hiromichi Tamaki, MD[a], Soumya Chatterjee, MD, MS, FRCP[a],
Carol A. Langford, MD, MHS[b],*

KEYWORDS

- Eosinophilic granulomatosis with polyangiitis (Churg-Strauss)
- Diffuse fasciitis with eosinophilia • Eosinophilic fasciitis
- Immunoglobulin G4-related disease • Eosinophilic myositis
- Eosinophilia-myalgia syndrome

KEY POINTS

- Rheumatologic and vascular conditions associated with peripheral or tissue eosinophilia are rare and can manifest with single-organ or systemic disease.
- The pathophysiology of rheumatologic and vascular conditions associated with peripheral or tissue eosinophilia remains largely unknown.
- A limited number of randomized controlled therapeutic trials have been performed in rheumatologic and vascular conditions associated with peripheral or tissue eosinophilia so that treatment is largely based on open-label and cohort studies.

INTRODUCTION

Eosinophilia in blood or tissue can be seen in many rheumatologic and vascular conditions (**Box 1**). Although this occurs as an uncommon but described feature in several diseases, for some entities eosinophilia seems to have a significant clinical and pathophysiologic role. When eosinophilia is seen in rheumatic or vascular conditions where this is not generally considered to be an integral part of the clinical picture, care should be taken to consider other causes of eosinophilia. These other causes can particularly include medications; allergic diseases; infections, especially parasitic

H. Tamaki and S. Chatterjee have nothing to disclose. C.A. Langford reports GlaxoSmithKline NCT02020889 research funds for conducting a clinical trial.
[a] Department of Rheumatic and Immunologic Diseases, Cleveland Clinic, 9500 Euclid Avenue, A50, Cleveland, OH 44195, USA; [b] Department of Rheumatic and Immunologic Diseases, Center for Vasculitis Care and Research, Cleveland Clinic, 9500 Euclid Avenue, A50, Cleveland, OH 44195, USA
* Corresponding author.
E-mail address: langfoc@ccf.org

Immunol Allergy Clin N Am 35 (2015) 453–476
http://dx.doi.org/10.1016/j.iac.2015.05.001
0889-8561/15/$ – see front matter © 2015 Elsevier Inc. All rights reserved.

immunology.theclinics.com

Box 1
Rheumatologic or vascular conditions associated with tissue and blood eosinophilia

Common

EGPA (Churg-Strauss)

IgG4-related disease

DFE

Eosinophilia myalgia syndrome

EM

Less common

GPA (Wegener)

Polymyositis

Dermatomyositis

Inclusion body myositis

Rheumatoid arthritis

Systemic sclerosis

Sjögren syndrome

Systemic lupus erythematosus

Behçet disease

---

diseases; hematologic conditions; or the possibility of an alternative diagnosis. This article examines 5 rheumatologic and vascular conditions wherein peripheral blood or tissue eosinophilia is a prominent feature: eosinophilic granulomatosis with polyangiitis (Churg-Strauss) (EGPA), immunoglobulin G4 (IgG4)-related disease (IgG4RD), diffuse fasciitis with eosinophilia (DFE), eosinophilia-myalgia syndrome (EMS), and eosinophilic myositis (EM).

EOSINOPHILIC GRANULOMATOSIS WITH POLYANGIITIS (CHURG-STRAUSS)

EGPA is a form of primary systemic vasculitis defined by the presence of eosinophil-rich and necrotizing granulomatous inflammation often involving the respiratory tract, necrotizing vasculitis of the small to medium vessels, and an association with asthma and eosinophilia.[1] EGPA carries a wide spectrum of clinical manifestations and can be life-threatening. Although EGPA is considered within the family of antineutrophil cytoplasmic antibody (ANCA) -associated vasculitides, ANCA are found in a minority of patients and cannot confirm or exclude the diagnosis.

Epidemiology

Epidemiologic studies in EGPA have been difficult to perform. The incidence of EGPA has varied between 0 and 3.7 per million person-years with a prevalence of 2 to 22.3 million inhabitants.[2,3] In studies of patients with asthma, the incidence of EGPA was reported to be 34.6 to 67 per million person-years.[4,5] The mean age of diagnosis of EGPA is between 40 and 50 years with an equal occurrence in men and women.

Risk Factors

Two studies found an association between HLA and EGPA. HLA-DRB1*04 and HLA-DRB1*7 seemed to enhance disease risk, whereas HLA-DRB1*03 and HLA-DRB1*13 conferred protection.[6,7] Single-nucleotide polymorphisms tagging the promoter haplotypes of IL10 gene (IL10–3575, IL10–1082, and IL10–592) were associated with EGPA, especially with ANCA-negative EGPA.[8]

The role of leukotriene receptor antagonists (LTRA) as a risk factor for the development of EGPA remains controversial. Following up on case reports, larger studies suggested an association between EGPA and LTRA.[9,10] From a review of the US Food and Drug Administration (FDA) Adverse Event Reporting System database, LTRA were listed as suspect medications in 90% of the 181 reported cases of possible drug-induced EGPA.[11] Beyond a direct cause-effect relationship, one hypothesis has been that EGPA become unmasked when LTRA use allows asthmatic patients to taper glucocorticoids. It remains unclear to date whether LTRA have a direct role in the development of EGPA or if LTRA are a confounding factor in patients experiencing worsening asthma before the onset of other EGPA features.

Pathophysiology

The pathogenesis of EGPA is unknown, although eosinophils are thought to play a central role. Eosinophil cationic protein has been found in serum and tissues of patients with active EGPA and is thought to cause tissue damage.[12,13] Interleukin (IL)-5 production is increased in patients with EGPA and is involved in the maturation and survival of eosinophils.[14,15] Other Th2 cytokines, such as IL-4 and IL-13, have also been found to be increased in EGPA,[15,16] leading to the hypothesis that this may be a Th2-driven disease. However, the histologic features of EGPA cannot be entirely explained by Th2 responses, and Th1 responses are thought to contribute to granuloma formation In EGPA.[16] Other studies have demonstrated an increase in Th17 cells[17] and reductions in T-regulatory cells.[17,18]

Clinical Features and Diagnostic Investigation

In 1984, Lanham and colleagues[19] described 3 phases of EGPA: a prodromal phase with allergic features, an eosinophilic phase characterized by peripheral and tissue eosinophilia, and a vasculitic phase with small to medium vessel vasculitis. Although recognition of these phases is conceptually helpful, they do not occur in all patients or always occur in sequence.

Long-standing sinonasal symptoms with allergic rhinitis and nasal polyps are common. Asthma is seen in more than 90% of patients[19–22] and usually precedes the diagnosis of EGPA by 4 to 9 years. The asthma of EGPA typically begins in adulthood or becomes markedly worse in those with childhood onset. Parenchymal lung disease occurs in 37% to 63% and can manifest as fleeting peripheral pulmonary infiltrates or alveolar hemorrhage. Vasculitic features most commonly involve the peripheral nerve (motor or sensory mononeuritis multiplex) or skin (purpura, nodules, ulcerating lesions, livedo reticularis). Renal involvement is seen in 13% to 58% of patients. Although glomerulonephritis occurs less commonly than that in granulomatosis with polyangiitis (GPA) and microscopic polyangiitis (MPA), it has an identical histologic appearance in being a segmental, necrotizing, crescentic glomerulonephritis with few to no immune complexes (pauci-immune glomerulonephritis). Gastrointestinal disease in EGPA can be related to eosinophilic infiltration or vasculitis. Cardiac involvement (cardiomyopathy from myocarditis, pericarditis, endocarditis, valvulitis, coronary vasculitis) is important to recognize because it is the main cause of patient mortality and occurs in 12% to 58% of patients. An echocardiogram should be performed in all EGPA patients at the time of diagnosis and cardiac MRI may be useful in detecting cardiac involvement when this is suspected (**Fig. 1**). Patients with cardiac

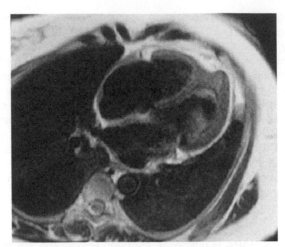

Fig. 1. Cardiac MRI demonstrating complications from heart involvement in EGPA (Churg-Strauss). This patient has endomyocardial fibrosis at the left ventricular apex with a large apical thrombus.

involvement tend to have a higher number of eosinophils and a negative ANCA,[22,23] whereas more patients with a glomerulonephritis had a positive ANCA.[24,25]

Diagnosing EGPA can be challenging because of the diversity of clinical features, the potential for these to be seen in other settings, and the frequent use of glucocorticoids for asthma, which will blunt peripheral eosinophilia. Central to the diagnosis of EGPA is the identification of vasculitic manifestations although this can be difficult to prove histologically. ANCA, which is more commonly myeloperoxidase ANCA, is seen in less than 40% of patients with EGPA and do not play a meaningful diagnostic role.

Differential Diagnosis

The 2 major categories within the differential diagnoses for EGPA are other eosinophilic disorders and diseases associated with small- to medium-vessel vasculitis (**Box 2**). The clinical manifestations of aspirin exacerbated respiratory disease (AERD) are asthma, chronic sinusitis, nasal polyps, and reaction to cyclooxygenase-inhibiting nonsteroidal anti-inflammatory drugs (NSAIDs). Lung infiltrates or other systemic manifestations seen in EGPA are uncommon in AERD. Patients with chronic eosinophilic pneumonia exhibit pulmonary symptoms but do not have granuloma characteristic for EGPA in the lung histopathology and lack vasculitic features. Allergic bronchopulmonary aspergillosis causes asthma, lung infiltrates, rhinitis, sinusitis, and eosinophilia but does not affect other organ systems.

Hypereosinophilic syndrome (HES) is often the main diagnosis being differentiated from EGPA. It is defined by a combination of hypereosinophilia and organ damage or dysfunction attributable to hypereosinophilia, provided that other possible causes of organ damage are excluded.[26] The challenge in differentiating EGPA from HES lies in the similarity of organ involvement because of tissue infiltration of eosinophils in both conditions.[27] The presence of vasculitis is a key differentiating factor between HES and EGPA but can be difficult to confirm, and asthma is uncommon in HES. Certain types of HES are associated with cytogenic abnormalities on bone marrow biopsy that are not seen in EGPA.

Box 2
Differential diagnosis for eosinophilic granulomatosis with polyangiitis (Churg-Strauss)
Eosinophilic disorders
Hypereosinophilic syndrome
AERD
Eosinophilic pneumonia
Allergic bronchopulmonary aspergillosis
Gleich syndrome (episodic angioedema and eosinophilia)
Parasitic diseases
Hypersensitivity syndromes
Vasculitis
GPA (Wegener)
MPA
Cryoglobulinemic vasculitis
IgA vasculitis (Henoch-Schönlein)
Polyarteritis nodosa

The main vasculitic diseases that can have a similar appearance to EGPA are GPA and MPA, which can also affect the lungs, kidneys, skin, and peripheral nerve. However, asthma and peripheral eosinophilia are uncommon in GPA or MPA. Although sinus and lung disease can occur in both GPA and EGPA, GPA is associated with a far greater degree of tissue necrosis, which is not seen in EGPA.

Management

Treatment of EGPA is determined by the disease manifestations and their severity. Glucocorticoids are the foundation of treatment of EGPA, and for those patients with nonsevere EGPA, prednisone alone can be sufficient.[28] Asthma in particular is typically glucocorticoid responsive and also is the main factor that limits glucocorticoid tapering. Use of an additional immunosuppressive agent beyond glucocorticoids is based on the degree of disease severity. The 5-factor score (FFS) is a severity scoring system derived from patients with MPA, polyarteritis nodosa, and EGPA consisting of proteinuria greater than 1 g/L, creatinine greater than 1.58 mg/dL, cardiomyopathy, central nervous system disease, and gastrointestinal involvement.[29,30] In one study of 64 patients, those with an FFS greater than or equal to 2 had an improved outcome when treated with cyclophosphamide,[31] supporting that EGPA patients with organ- or life-threatening involvement should be treated with combined therapy. Cardiac involvement in particular should be treated with prednisone and cyclophosphamide given its risk of mortality and improvement in cardiac function with this treatment.

The treatment of severe EGPA has been extrapolated from that used in GPA and MPA. Although several EGPA studies have used intravenous cyclophosphamide, superiority over that of daily cyclophosphamide in EGPA has not been proven.[32] The authors' approach in severe EGPA is to combine prednisone with daily cyclophosphamide, given for 3 to 6 months, after which time cyclophosphamide is stopped and switched to a less toxic maintenance agent, usually consisting of either azathioprine or methotrexate.[33] Although there have been no controlled trials examining the use of these agents in EGPA, azathioprine or methotrexate combined with prednisone has also been used for less severe features, where the disease remains active or where there is an inability to taper prednisone to acceptable levels. Although this can provide benefit in those with vasculitic features, it has been less effective in those with predominantly sinus disease and asthma, although individual patient responses can be seen.

Experience with biologic agents in EGPA remains limited. The largest report of 41 patients with EGPA treated with rituximab showed improvement in 83% of patients.[34] Mepolizumab, an anti-IL-5 antibody, has been used for EGPA in a small number of patients with promising results.[35,36]

Prognosis

The prognosis of EGPA has improved greatly.[37] Long-term outcomes in 2 treatment studies revealed a survival rate and disease-free survival rate of 98%/74% at 1 year, 94%/61% at 3 years, 92%/54% at 5 years, and 90%/51% at 7 years, respectively.[33] Another study of 383 patients with EGPA reported a 5-year survival of 89% and 10-year survival of 79%.[22]

IMMUNOGLOBULIN G4-RELATED DISEASE

IgG4RD is a relatively newly defined systemic fibrotic inflammatory condition, which can involve multiple organ systems. Many manifestations of IgG4RD, such as autoimmune pancreatitis (AIP),[38] retroperitoneal fibrosis, Riedel thyroiditis, Küttner tumor, and Mikulicz disease (MD), were previously recognized as separate diseases but are now considered within the spectrum of IgG4RD. Histopathologic findings, including lymphoplasmacytic infiltrate with a high percentage of IgG4-positive plasma cells, storiform fibrosis, obliterative phlebitis, and mild to moderate tissue eosinophilia and elevated IgG4 levels, have aided in the recognition and diagnosis of IgG4RD.[39–42]

Epidemiology

The epidemiology of IgG4RD is yet to be investigated. A nationwide survey on the epidemiology of AIP in Japan revealed a prevalence of 2.2 per 100,000 and an incidence of 0.9 per 100,000 person-years.[43] In this study, the male-to-female ratio was 3.7:1 with disease occurring at a mean age of 63 years.

Risk Factors

Genetic risk factors for AIP have been explored in the Japanese population, where a possible link with HLA DRB1*0405-DQB1*0401 was suggested as well as an association with Fc receptor-like 3, KCNA3, and CTLA4 polymorphisms.[44–47]

Pathophysiology

The pathogenesis of IgG4RD is unknown. IgG4 is considered noninflammatory, and it is currently unclear whether IgG4 plays a role in IgG4RD pathophysiology. Although eosinophils are often found on tissue biopsies in IgG4RD, current evidence does not support a pathogenic role. The expression of Th2 cytokines and regulatory cytokines were upregulated in affected tissues from patients with AIP as well as labial salivary gland specimens of MD.[48] Th2 is known to promote fibrosis by stimulating fibroblasts,[49] and one hypothesis is that Th2 predominance is the central pathway of fibrotic organ damage in IgG4RD. However, Th1 predominance was also reported in 10 patients with IgG4-related sialadenitis,[50] and the numbers of regulatory T cells were also increased in peripheral blood from patients with AIP.

Clinical Features and Diagnostic Investigation

The range of clinical manifestations of IgG4RD continues to be actively described with features reported in almost every organ system where this can manifest as single-organ or multiorgan disease (**Box 3**).[39,42]

Elevated serum IgG4 levels alone are not diagnostic because increased levels can be seen with patients with pancreatic cancer, and a normal serum IgG4 level does not rule out IgG4RD.[51,52] In one study, the sensitivity of elevated serum IgG4 level greater than 135 mg/dL for the diagnosis of either definite or probable IgG4RD was 90%, whereas the specificity was 60%. If a higher cutoff of 270 mg/dL was used, the sensitivity was 35% and specificity was 91%.[53]

The diagnosis of IgG4RD is based on its clinical features together with compatible histopathology, if feasible. Specific pathologic criteria for each organ have been proposed.[40,54]

Differential Diagnosis

In patients with IgG4RD affecting a single organ, the differential diagnosis is tailored toward that specific site. Many systemic diseases can mimic the presentation of multiorgan IgG4RD.

For features such as aortitis and retroperitoneal fibrosis (**Fig. 2**), whereby access to tissue is difficult, evaluating for characteristic features of other diseases within the differential is important (**Box 4**). Takayasu arteritis is a granulomatous large-vessel vasculitis involving the aorta and its primary branches, which predominantly affects women 20 to 40 years of age. Giant cell arteritis is a granulomatous large- to medium-vessel vasculitis that has a predilection for branches of the carotid artery often presenting with cranial features and polymyalgia rheumatic, which predominantly affects people older than the age of 50. Erdheim-Chester disease (ECD) is a very rare multisystemic disease caused by the non-Langerhans form of histiocytosis that can manifest with circumferential periaortic sheathing of the thoracic or abdominal aorta. ECD is highly suggested by long bone uptake on bone scintigraphy and hairy kidney on abdominal CT scan.[55] The possibility of infectious aortitis needs to be carefully evaluated because atypical pathogens such as *Mycobacterium tuberculosis, Treponema pallidum*, or *Coxiella burnetti* can have a subacute course similar to IgG4RD. Lymphoma can present with retroperitoneal disease, and tissue biopsy should be considered wherever this is feasible in settings where lymphoma remains strongly in the differential.

Management

Glucocorticoids are the first-line treatment of IgGRD based on cohort studies. Cyclophosphamide, azathioprine, methotrexate, mycophenolate mofetil, and cyclosporine have been used for IgG4RD; however, the experience is limited.[56,57] Small series including an open-label prospective trial have found rituximab to be effective in patients with refractory IgG4RD.[58,59]

Prognosis

The prognosis of IgG4RD has not been well described. A multicenter analysis revealed 99% of patients with type 1 AIP treated with glucocorticoids achieved remission compared with 55% of those managed conservatively. More than one-third of these patients had at least one relapse with 67% of relapses occurring after glucocorticoid

Box 3
Clinical manifestations of immunoglobulin G4–related disease

Head, eyes, ears, nose, throat, and neck

Chronic sclerosing dacryoadenitis

Orbital pseudotumor

Orbital myositis

Dacryoadenitis

Submandibular and parotid gland enlargement

Scleritis

Nasolacrimal duct obstruction

Chronic sclerosing sialadenitis

Eosinophilic angiocentric fibrosis

Rhinitis

Nasal polyps

Chronic sinusitis

Otitis media with effusions

Eosinophilic otitis media

Sensorineural hearing loss

Inflammation of pharynx, hypopharynx

Tracheal inflammation

Vocal cord inflammation

Thyroid

Riedel thyroiditis

Fibrosing Hashimoto thyroiditis

Cardiovascular

Aortitis

Periaortitis

Constrictive pericarditis

Lungs and mediastinum

Inflammatory nodule

Thickening of the bronchovascular bundle

Interstitial pneumonitis

Sclerosing pleuritis

Fibrosing mediastinitis

Lymph nodes

Lymphadenopathy

Breast

Inflammatory pseudotumor

Sclerosing mastitis

Kidney/genitourinary

Tubulointerstitial nephritis

Membranous nephropathy

Low-density renal parenchymal lesions

Chronic sclerosing pyelitis

Prostatitis

Orchitis

Paratesticular pseudotumor

Abdomen

Type I AIP

Sclerosing cholangitis

Sclerosing mesenteritis

IgG4 hepatopathy

Liver inflammatory pseudotumor

Colonic pseudotumor

Retroperitoneal fibrosis

Central nervous system

Hypertrophic pachymeningitis

Hypophysitis

Hypopituitarism

Peripheral nervous system

Perineural inflammation

Skin

Skin nodules, papules

Psoriasis-like lesions

Erythematous maculopapular rashes

Systemic and other features

Fever

Weight loss

Multifocal fibrosclerosis

Data from Brito-Zerón P, Ramos-Casals M, Bosch X, et al. The clinical spectrum of IgG4-related disease. Autoimmun Rev 2014;13(12):1203–10; and Kamisawa T, Zen Y, Pillai S, et al. IgG4-related disease. Lancet 2014;385(9976):1460–71.

discontinuation.[57] Outcome may also be affected by a possible association between IgG4RD and malignancy.[60,61]

DIFFUSE FASCIITIS WITH EOSINOPHILIA

DFE is an uncommon disorder characterized by thickened skin, peripheral eosinophilia, and hypergammaglobulinemia. Tissue eosinophilia is not essential for the diagnosis; hence, the preferred terminology is *diffuse fasciitis with eosinophilia* as opposed to *eosinophilic fasciitis*. The first 2 cases were described by Dr Shulman in 1974, such that DFE has also been called Shulman disease.[62]

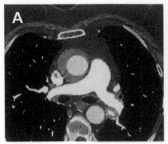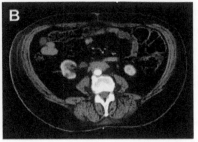

Fig. 2. Computed tomography showing periaortitis in a patient with IgG4-related disease. (*A*) Circumferential tissue thickening around the ascending aorta. (*B*) Heterogeneous region of soft tissue thickening just anterior to the infrarenal aorta.

Epidemiology

DFE is a very rare disorder and its epidemiology is unknown. A retrospective analysis of 52 cases revealed a slight female predominance (56%).[63] The mean age in this study was 40 to 50 years, although this has varied widely in other series.

Risk Factors

Multiple risk factors have been anecdotally linked to DFE, including physical stress, trauma, medications,[64–70] chemicals,[71] and infections.[72–74] In one study of 52 cases

---

Box 4
Differential diagnosis for aortitis and retroperitoneal fibrosis manifestations of immunoglobulin G4–related disease

Aortitis

Primary vasculitic diseases

- Giant cell arteritis
- Takayasu arteritis
- Cogan syndrome
- Behçet disease

ECD

Sarcoidosis

Ankylosing spondylitis

Relapsing polychondritis

Infectious aortitis

Retroperitoneal fibrosis

Idiopathic retroperitoneal fibrosis

Lymphoma

Sarcoma

Tuberculosis

Retroperitoneal fibromatosis (desmoid tumors)

Methysergide-induced retroperitoneal fibrosis

of DFE, 5 patients (9%) had hematologic disorders including 2 patients with thrombo-cytopenia, one with myelomonocytic leukemia, one with chronic lymphocytic leuke-mia, and one with evolving myeloproliferative disorder.[63] Associations with other hematological disorders have been reported anecdotally.[75–87]

Pathophysiology

The pathophysiology of DFE remains to be elucidated, but limited data suggest immune dysregulation. The inflammatory cells in tissue histopathology[88] consist of eo-sinophils, CD8+ lymphocytes, and macrophages, which have been thought to cause tissue damage in DFE.[89] T cells in DFE stimulated by T-cell activator phytohemagglu-tinin produce more Th2 cytokines as well as Th1 cytokines compared with healthy controls.[90] The serum and tissue levels of tissue inhibitor of metalloproteinase-1 was elevated in DFE,[91] which was implicated as a potent stimulator of systemic sclerosis (SSc) fibroblasts.

Clinical Features and Diagnostic Investigation

DFE is characterized by acute or subacute symmetric swelling, erythema, and stiff-ness of the distal extremities sometimes with pitting edema. These early changes evolve into woody induration, and eventually DFE patients exhibit a characteristic appearance of skin puckering (peau d'orange appearance) and depressed veins (groove sign) (**Fig. 3**).[92,93] The level of inflammation and fibrosis is deep in the subcutis. Hence, the epidermis is normal on examination, but there is a deeper level of indura-tion (subcutaneous rather than dermal as seen in SSc). DFE predominantly involves the extremities and can cause joint contractures and tendon retractions. In one report of 52 patients, all patients had extremity involvement, with other affected areas, including the abdomen (23%), chest (17%), back (6%), buttocks (6%), and face/neck (6%).[63] Polyarthritis can be seen in up to 40% of patients[63] and carpal tunnel syndrome in up to 23% of patients.[63]

The diagnosis of DFE is based on clinical features and histopathology on a full-thickness biopsy of an affected area (including skin, subcutaneous fat, and fascia). A punch biopsy is not adequate because it will miss the fascia, the main site of path-ologic abnormality in DFE (**Fig. 4**). Pinal-Fernandez and colleagues[93] proposed diag-nostic criteria of DFE requiring the presence of both major criteria, or one major criterion plus 2 minor criteria, following the exclusion of SSc. Major criteria include (1) swelling, induration, and thickening of the skin and subcutaneous tissue that is symmetric or nonsymmetric, diffuse (extremities, trunk, and abdomen), or localized (extremities); (2) fascial thickening with accumulation of lymphocytes and

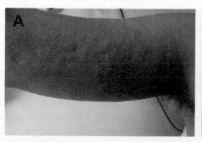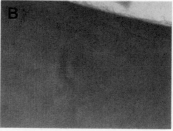

Fig. 3. Clinical findings in a patient with DFE. (*A*) Peau d'orange of the upper extremity. (*B*) Groove sign representing depressed veins.

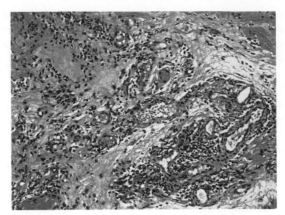

Fig. 4. Histologic section shows a prominent chronic inflammatory cell infiltrate primarily involving the deep fascia. There is no evidence of necrotizing vasculitis or granulomatous inflammation. These findings are consistent with chronic fasciitis as is seen in DFE (Hematoxylin and eosin, ×200).

macrophages with or without eosinophilic infiltration (determined by full-thickness wedge biopsy of clinically affected skin). Minor criteria include (1) eosinophilia greater than 0.5×10^9/L; (2) hypergammaglobulinemia greater than 1.5 g/L; (3) muscle weakness or elevated aldolase levels; (4) groove sign or peau d'orange; (5) hyperintense fascia on MRI T2-weighted images.

Differential Diagnosis

The major differential diagnoses of DFE include SSc and its mimics. In a retrospective study of 52 patients with DFE, only one patient had Raynaud phenomenon,[63] whereas more than 90% of patients with SSc have Raynaud phenomenon. Fingers, feet, and face are typically not affected in DFE compared with SSc. Nailfold capillaries are usually normal in DFE, whereas abnormal nailfold capillaries tend to be seen in SSc.[94] Visceral involvement is uncommon in DFE, whereas SSc can affect the pulmonary, cardiovascular, gastrointestinal, and renal systems. Antinuclear antibodies (ANA) can be found in 85% to 90% of patients with SSc, but in a study of 52 DFE patients, only 3 (6%) were positive for ANA.[63] Other entities including chronic graft-versus-host disease, nephrogenic systemic fibrosis, scleromyxedema, and scleredema can be differentiated from DFE based on clinical features and skin biopsy.[95]

The differential diagnoses for skin thickening with eosinophilia include EMS and toxic oil syndrome. Pneumonitis or neuropathy can be seen in EMS.[96,97] Toxic oil syndrome was associated with adulterated rapeseed oil in an endemic outbreak in Spain during the 1980s. Clinical manifestations include dyspnea, myalgia, arthralgia, and neuropathy with eosinophilia and elevation of serum creatine kinase.[97,98]

Management

The treatment approach to DFE has been based on case reports and cohort series. Spontaneous recovery has been noted, but most reported patients were treated with immunosuppressive agents. In a series of 52 patients, 34 were initially treated with prednisone 40 to 60 mg daily, which resulted in complete resolution in 15%, partial response (>25% improvement) in 59%, and poor response in 27%. In 5 patients who received no treatment, resolution occurred in 40%, more than 50% improvement in 40%, and no improvement in 20%.[63] In a retrospective study of 34 patients with DFE where the mean initial dose of prednisone was 0.77 mg/kg, 44% received an additional immunosuppressive agent due to an inadequate clinical response (methotrexate 86%, azathioprine 14%).[99] Overall, 69% of patients achieved a complete remission, with 19% experiencing remission with disability, and 12% having treatment failure. Fifteen patients (47%) were treated with methylprednisolone pulses before prednisone and were found to require a second immunosuppressive less frequently (20% vs 65%, $P = .02$) and more readily achieve complete remission (87% vs 53%, $P = .06$).[99] Cyclosporine, cyclophosphamide, hydroxychloroquine, and sulfasalazine have been used in small case series. There has been only anecdotal experience with infliximab,[100–102] etanercept,[103] and rituximab.[104]

Prognosis

The prognosis of patients with DFE is not well documented. From a retrospective study, predictors for poor outcomes included diagnosis delay greater than 6 months and absence of methylprednisolone pulses at treatment initiation.[99]

EOSINOPHILIA-MYALGIA SYNDROME

EMS first emerged as a disease entity in 1989 with a new epidemic in the United States of a multisystem disease characterized by severe muscle pain and profound eosinophilia.[105] Case control studies in Minnesota, Oregon, and New Mexico determined an association between antecedent tryptophan consumption and EMS.[106,107]

Epidemiology

In 1989, more than 1500 cases of EMS related to tryptophan occurred in the United States that resulted in 36 deaths by 1991.[108] After the FDA banned the sale of products containing tryptophan, the incidence of EMS declined rapidly. An isolated case associated with L-tryptophan was reported in 2005.[109]

Risk Factors

Tryptophan was identified as a causative agent for EMS in epidemiologic studies.[106,107] Further investigation revealed a strong association with the consumption of L-tryptophan produced by one company.[110,111] More than 60 minor impurities were detected in this company's products, 6 of which were reported to be associated with EMS.[112] Lewis rats treated with one of these impurities, 1,1'-ethylidenebis (tryptophan) (EBT) or case-associated L-tryptophan, developed myofascial thickening similar to human EMS, but Lewis rats treated with L-tryptophan without EBT also showed mild myofascial thickening.[113] Another impurity, 3-(phenylamino) alanine, shares chemical properties with 3-(M-phenylamino)-1,2-propanediol, which was implicated as a causative agent of toxic oil syndrome in Spain in 1981.[114]

Pathophysiology

The pathophysiology of EMS remains unclear. The cellular immune response and cytokines/growth factors, such as IL-2, IL-4, IL-5, interferon-γ, granulocyte-macrophage colony-stimulating factor, and transforming growth factor-β, have been implicated in the pathophysiology of EMS.[115]

Clinical Features and Diagnostic Investigation

The cardinal features of EMS are severe muscle pain and peripheral eosinophilia. Criteria established by the US Centers for Disease Control and Prevention include eosinophil count greater than or equal to 1.0×10^9 cells/L, generalized myalgia severe enough to interfere with normal daily activities, and no infectious or neoplastic condition that could account for these findings. Cough or dyspnea can be seen in up to 60% of patients and chest radiograph abnormality was seen in approximately 20% of the cases. Neuropathy can be seen in up to 30% of patients and was more common in those with a fatal outcome. Other common manifestations include fever (35%), rash (60%), arthralgia (70%), peripheral edema (60%), and thickened skin (35%).[108]

The diagnosis of EMS is based on a compatible clinical presentation, peripheral blood eosinophilia, and histopathology, which reveals perimyositis with inflammatory cells predominantly consisting of mononuclear cells and eosinophils.[116]

Differential Diagnosis

The differential diagnosis of EMS is similar to that of DFE as listed previously. The clinical differences between DFE and EMS can be subtle or none and they are mainly differentiated by prior exposure to tryptophan that occurs in EMS.[117–119] Severe myalgias, neuropathy, respiratory symptoms, and cognitive impairment are not seen in DFE.

Management

Treatment of EMS beyond discontinuation of the offending substance is not well established. Glucocorticoids or other immunosuppressive agents have been used.

Prognosis

A report of 205 patients with EMS with 18- to 24-month follow-up after disease onset showed improvement in myalgias (67%), respiratory symptoms (74%), muscle weakness (60%), arthralgias (66%), fever (88%), swelling (80%), and paresthesia (51%). Prednisone was used in most patients with full improvement by physician's evaluation in 19% of patients and partial improvement in 60%.[120]

EOSINOPHILIC MYOSITIS

EM is a very rare disease and contains a diverse group of disorders. EM includes 3 major subtypes: eosinophilic polymyositis (EP), eosinophilic perimyositis (EPM), and focal eosinophilic myositis (FEM). These disorders have only been reported in case reports or small case series.

Epidemiology

No population-based epidemiologic data are available. In one review of 20 men and 11 women, the mean age was 47 years, consisting of 13 patients with EPM, 7 with EP, 10 with FEM, and 1 patient with cyclic EM (unclassified).[121]

Risk Factors

No major risk factors for EM have been identified because of its rarity. Heavy alcohol use was suggested as a trigger for FEM in case reports[122,123] as well as trauma.[124]

Pathophysiology

The pathophysiology of EM is unknown because of its rarity. It is generally thought that eosinophils and cytotoxic proteins released by eosinophils as well as cytotoxic T cells elicit muscular injury.[125] Muscle biopsy specimens from 3 patients with EP revealed elevated IL-5 messenger RNA levels, suggesting that local expression of IL-5 led to an accumulation of eosinophils in the muscle.[126]

Clinical Features and Diagnostic Investigation

Diagnostic criteria for FEM, EPM, and EM have been proposed[127] (**Box 5**). These criteria are based on the main clinical, laboratory, and histologic features that have been described in these diseases.[121–129]

Box 5
Proposed diagnostic criteria for focal eosinophilic myositis, eosinophilic polymyositis, and eosinophilic perimyositis

Proposed diagnostic criteria for focal eosinophilic myositis

Deep vein thrombosis, cellulitis, and parasitic infections must be excluded to apply these criteria.

To fulfill the criteria, 2 major criteria or one major criterion and all minor criteria are required.

Major criteria:

1. Pain and calf swelling (other muscles can be affected)

2. Deep mononuclear cell infiltration (eosinophilic or not), with muscle fiber invasion and necrosis on muscle biopsy

Minor criteria:

1. Elevated serum levels of creatine kinase and aldolase (2- to 10-fold)

2. MRI or electromyographic evidence of focal myositis

3. Absence of systemic illness

4. Eosinophilia greater than 0.5×10^9/L

Proposed diagnostic criteria for eosinophilic polymyositis

To fulfill the criteria, presence of both major criteria or one major criterion and 2 minor criteria are required.

Exclusion: Hypereosinophilic syndrome, T-cell clonality, dermatomyositis, vasculitis (EGPA [Churg-Strauss]), drugs, limb girdle muscle disease (Becker muscular dystrophy, calpainopathy, and sarcoglycanopathy), and parasitic infections must be excluded.

Major criteria:

1. Proximal weakness exists, affecting limb-girdle muscles, sometimes severe.

2. Widespread deep infiltration of eosinophils into muscle, with eosinophilic cuffing on histology study. Myonecrosis and endomysial inflammation usually present. In the absence of eosinophil infiltration, major basic protein deposition should be demonstrated by specific immunostaining.

Minor criteria:

1. Elevated serum levels of creatine kinase and aldolase (usually high, >10 upper limit of normal)

2. Eosinophilia greater than 0.5×10^9/L

3. Systemic illness with frequent cardiac involvement

4. Corticosteroids are needed

Proposed diagnostic criteria for eosinophilic perimyositis

Toxic oil syndrome, myalgia-eosinophilia, exposure to other inorganic or organic substances should be excluded.

Presence of both major criteria and major criterion number 2 plus 2 minor criteria are required for the diagnosis.

Major criteria:

1. Myalgia, proximal mild weakness

2. Eosinophilic infiltrate confined to fascia and superficial perimysium, absence of myofiber necrosis

Minor criteria:

1. Absence of systemic manifestations

2. Normal creatinine kinase, aldolase levels slightly elevated (less than 2- to 3-fold of upper limit of normal).

3. Eosinophilia greater than 0.5×10^9/L

Adapted from Selva-O'Callaghan A, Trallero-Araguas E, Grau JM. Eosinophilic myositis: an updated review. Autoimmun Rev 2014;13(4–5):375–8.

Management

No treatment trials have been conducted in EM because of its rarity and lack of consensus criteria such that treatment is based on case reports. FEM can improve spontaneously, but rapid response to glucocorticoids has been reported. Some patients with FEM were treated with NSAIDs. EPM usually responds to glucocorticoids but often long-term treatment is necessary. EP typically spontaneously resolves but glucocorticoids or NSAIDs have been used with success, although relapses were noted.[121,124,128,130]

Differential Diagnosis

Evaluation for secondary causes of EM is necessary to explore potential parasitic infestations, such as trichinosis, cysticercosis, sarcocystis, or toxoplasmosis,[131–135] or a systemic eosinophilic disorder that can cause EM. HES can mimic EPM, especially in the setting of myocardial involvement. However, in a retrospective multicenter study of 188 patients with HES, only one had myositis and 9 had myalgias as the initial presentation.[27] In a retrospective study of 383 patients with EGPA, 39% had myalgias at diagnosis[22]; however, true myositis is rare.[136] Recently, cases of EM associated with muscular dystrophies have been reported.[137–144] Major differential diagnoses of FEM include deep vein thrombosis, inflammatory pseudotumor, and parasitic infestations. Differential diagnoses of EP include EMS or toxic oil syndrome.

Prognosis

Prognosis of this diverse disease group is unknown.

SUMMARY

The rheumatologic and vascular disorders associated with eosinophilia represent an uncommon but important group of disease entities. Despite their rarity, increasing knowledge has been accumulated in recent years and novel therapies are being explored, particularly in those diseases whereby the consensus for their classification/diagnostic criteria have been established and wherein collaborative work has been performed. Establishment of disease definitions is necessary in some of rheumatologic and vascular disorders associated with eosinophilia to promote more accurate and detailed description of the diseases and to meet unmet needs; this is critically important given that multicenter collaboration will play an essential role to further investigate these rare disease entities.

REFERENCES

1. Jennette JC, Falk RJ, Bacon PA, et al. 2012 revised International Chapel Hill Consensus Conference Nomenclature of Vasculitides. Arthritis Rheum 2013; 65(1):1–11.
2. Gibelin A, Maldini C, Mahr A. Epidemiology and etiology of Wegener granulomatosis, microscopic polyangiitis, Churg-Strauss syndrome and Goodpasture syndrome: vasculitides with frequent lung involvement. Semin Respir Crit Care Med 2011;32(3):264–73.
3. Sada KE, Amano K, Uehara R, et al. A nationwide survey on the epidemiology and clinical features of eosinophilic granulomatosis with polyangiitis (Churg-Strauss) in Japan. Mod Rheumatol 2014;24(4):640–4.
4. Loughlin JE, Cole JA, Rothman KJ, et al. Prevalence of serious eosinophilia and incidence of Churg-Strauss syndrome in a cohort of asthma patients. Ann Allergy Asthma Immunol 2002;88(3):319–25.
5. Harrold LR, Andrade SE, Go AS, et al. Incidence of Churg-Strauss syndrome in asthma drug users: a population-based perspective. J Rheumatol 2005;32(6): 1076–80.
6. Vaglio A, Martorana D, Maggiore U, et al. HLA-DRB4 as a genetic risk factor for Churg-Strauss syndrome. Arthritis Rheum 2007;56(9):3159–66.
7. Wieczorek S, Hellmich B, Gross WL, et al. Associations of Churg-Strauss syndrome with the HLA-DRB1 locus, and relationship to the genetics of antineutrophil cytoplasmic antibody-associated vasculitides: comment on the article by Vaglio et al. Arthritis Rheum 2008;58(1):329–30.
8. Wieczorek S, Hellmich B, Arning L, et al. Functionally relevant variations of the interleukin-10 gene associated with antineutrophil cytoplasmic antibody-negative Churg-Strauss syndrome, but not with Wegener's granulomatosis. Arthritis Rheum 2008;58(6):1839–48.
9. Hauser T, Mahr A, Metzler C, et al. The leucotriene receptor antagonist montelukast and the risk of Churg-Strauss syndrome: a case-crossover study. Thorax 2008;63(8):677–82.
10. Nathani N, Little MA, Kunst H, et al. Churg-Strauss syndrome and leukotriene antagonist use: a respiratory perspective. Thorax 2008;63(10):883–8.
11. Bibby S, Healy B, Steele R, et al. Association between leukotriene receptor antagonist therapy and Churg-Strauss syndrome: an analysis of the FDA AERS database. Thorax 2010;65(2):132–8.
12. Tai PC, Holt ME, Denny P, et al. Deposition of eosinophil cationic protein in granulomas in allergic granulomatosis and vasculitis: the Churg-Strauss syndrome. Br Med J (Clin Res Ed) 1984;289(6442):400–2.
13. Hurst S, Chizzolini C, Dayer JM, et al. Usefulness of serum eosinophil cationic protein (ECP) in predicting relapse of Churg and Strauss vasculitis. Clin Exp Rheumatol 2000;18(6):784–5.
14. Tsukadaira A, Okubo Y, Kitano K, et al. Eosinophil active cytokines and surface analysis of eosinophils in Churg-Strauss syndrome. Allergy Asthma Proc 1999; 20(1):39–44.

15. Kurosawa M, Nakagami R, Morioka J, et al. Interleukins in Churg-Strauss syndrome. Allergy 2000;55(8):785–7.
16. Kiene M, Csernok E, Muller A, et al. Elevated interleukin-4 and interleukin-13 production by T cell lines from patients with Churg-Strauss syndrome. Arthritis Rheum 2001;44(2):469–73.
17. Jakiela B, Sanak M, Szczeklik W, et al. Both Th2 and Th17 responses are involved in the pathogenesis of Churg-Strauss syndrome. Clin Exp Rheumatol 2011;29(1 Suppl 64):S23–34.
18. Saito H, Tsurikisawa N, Tsuburai T, et al. The proportion of regulatory T cells in the peripheral blood reflects the relapse or remission status of patients with Churg-Strauss syndrome. Int Arch Allergy Immunol 2011;155(Suppl 1):46–52.
19. Lanham JG, Elkon KB, Pusey CD, et al. Systemic vasculitis with asthma and eosinophilia: a clinical approach to the Churg-Strauss syndrome. Medicine (Baltimore) 1984;63(2):65–81.
20. Guillevin L, Cohen P, Gayraud M, et al. Churg-Strauss syndrome. Clinical study and long-term follow-up of 96 patients. Medicine (Baltimore) 1999; 78(1):26–37.
21. Keogh KA, Specks U. Churg-Strauss syndrome: clinical presentation, antineutrophil cytoplasmic antibodies, and leukotriene receptor antagonists. Am J Med 2003;115(4):284–90.
22. Comarmond C, Pagnoux C, Khellaf M, et al. Eosinophilic granulomatosis with polyangiitis (Churg-Strauss): clinical characteristics and long-term followup of the 383 patients enrolled in the French Vasculitis Study Group Cohort. Arthritis Rheum 2013;65(1):270–81.
23. Neumann T, Manger B, Schmid M, et al. Cardiac involvement in Churg-Strauss syndrome: impact of endomyocarditis. Medicine (Baltimore) 2009;88(4):236–43.
24. Sinico RA, Di Toma L, Maggiore U, et al. Renal involvement in Churg-Strauss syndrome. Am J Kidney Dis 2006;47(5):770–9.
25. Sable-Fourtassou R, Cohen P, Mahr A, et al. Antineutrophil cytoplasmic antibodies and the Churg-Strauss syndrome. Ann Intern Med 2005;143(9):632–8.
26. Valent P, Klion AD, Horny HP, et al. Contemporary consensus proposal on criteria and classification of eosinophilic disorders and related syndromes. J Allergy Clin Immunol 2012;130(3):607–12.e9.
27. Ogbogu PU, Bochner BS, Butterfield JH, et al. Hypereosinophilic syndrome: a multicenter, retrospective analysis of clinical characteristics and response to therapy. J Allergy Clin Immunol 2009;124(6):1319–25.e3.
28. Ribi C, Cohen P, Pagnoux C, et al. Treatment of Churg-Strauss syndrome without poor-prognosis factors: a multicenter, prospective, randomized, open-label study of seventy-two patients. Arthritis Rheum 2008;58(2):586–94.
29. Guillevin L, Pagnoux C, Seror R, et al. The five-factor score revisited: assessment of prognoses of systemic necrotizing vasculitides based on the French Vasculitis Study Group (FVSG) cohort. Medicine (Baltimore) 2011;90(1):19–27.
30. Guillevin L, Lhote F, Gayraud M, et al. Prognostic factors in polyarteritis nodosa and Churg-Strauss syndrome. A prospective study in 342 patients. Medicine (Baltimore) 1996;75(1):17–28.
31. Gayraud M, Guillevin L, le Toumelin P, et al. Long-term followup of polyarteritis nodosa, microscopic polyangiitis, and Churg-Strauss syndrome: analysis of four prospective trials including 278 patients. Arthritis Rheum 2001;44(3): 666–75.
32. Gayraud M, Guillevin L, Cohen P, et al. Treatment of good-prognosis polyarteritis nodosa and Churg-Strauss syndrome: comparison of steroids and oral or pulse

cyclophosphamide in 25 patients. French Cooperative Study Group for vasculitides. Br J Rheumatol 1997;36(12):1290–7.

33. Samson M, Puechal X, Devilliers H, et al. Long-term outcomes of 118 patients with eosinophilic granulomatosis with polyangiitis (Churg-Strauss syndrome) enrolled in two prospective trials. J Autoimmun 2013;43:60–9.

34. Mohammad AJ, Hot A, Arndt F, et al. Rituximab for the treatment of eosinophilic granulomatosis with polyangiitis (Churg-Strauss). Ann Rheum Dis 2014. [Epub ahead of print].

35. Kim S, Marigowda G, Oren E, et al. Mepolizumab as a steroid-sparing treatment option in patients with Churg-Strauss syndrome. J Allergy Clin Immunol 2010; 125(6):1336–43.

36. Moosig F, Gross WL, Herrmann K, et al. Targeting interleukin-5 in refractory and relapsing Churg-Strauss syndrome. Ann Intern Med 2011;155(5):341–3.

37. ROSE GA. The natural history of polyarteritis. Br Med J 1957;2(5054): 1148–52.

38. Kamisawa T, Egawa N, Nakajima H. Autoimmune pancreatitis is a systemic autoimmune disease. Am J Gastroenterol 2003;98(12):2811–2.

39. Brito-Zeron P, Ramos-Casals M, Bosch X, et al. The clinical spectrum of IgG4-related disease. Autoimmun Rev 2014;13(12):1203–10.

40. Deshpande V, Zen Y, Chan JK, et al. Consensus statement on the pathology of IgG4-related disease. Mod Pathol 2012;25(9):1181–92.

41. Stone JH, Khosroshahi A, Deshpande V, et al. Recommendations for the nomenclature of IgG4-related disease and its individual organ system manifestations. Arthritis Rheum 2012;64(10):3061–7.

42. Kamisawa T, Zen Y, Pillai S, et al. IgG4-related disease. Lancet 2015;385(9976): 1460–71.

43. Kanno A, Nishimori I, Masamune A, et al. Nationwide epidemiological survey of autoimmune pancreatitis in Japan. Pancreas 2012;41(6):835–9.

44. Umemura T, Ota M, Hamano H, et al. Genetic association of Fc receptor-like 3 polymorphisms with autoimmune pancreatitis in Japanese patients. Gut 2006; 55(9):1367–8.

45. Ota M, Katsuyama Y, Hamano H, et al. Two critical genes (HLA-DRB1 and ABCF1) in the HLA region are associated with the susceptibility to autoimmune pancreatitis. Immunogenetics 2007;59(1):45–52.

46. Umemura T, Ota M, Hamano H, et al. Association of autoimmune pancreatitis with cytotoxic T-lymphocyte antigen 4 gene polymorphisms in Japanese patients. Am J Gastroenterol 2008;103(3):588–94.

47. Ota M, Ito T, Umemura T, et al. Polymorphism in the KCNA3 gene is associated with susceptibility to autoimmune pancreatitis in the Japanese population. Dis Markers 2011;31(4):223–9.

48. Tanaka A, Moriyama M, Nakashima H, et al. Th2 and regulatory immune reactions contribute to IgG4 production and the initiation of Mikulicz disease. Arthritis Rheum 2012;64(1):254–63.

49. Barron L, Wynn TA. Fibrosis is regulated by Th2 and Th17 responses and by dynamic interactions between fibroblasts and macrophages. Am J Physiol Gastrointest Liver Physiol 2011;300(5):G723–8.

50. Ohta N, Makihara S, Okano M, et al. Roles of IL-17, Th1, and Tc1 cells in patients with IgG4-related sclerosing sialadenitis. Laryngoscope 2012; 122(10):2169–74.

51. Tabata T, Kamisawa T, Takuma K, et al. Serum IgG4 concentrations and IgG4-related sclerosing disease. Clin Chim Acta 2009;408(1–2):25–8.

52. Ghazale A, Chari ST, Smyrk TC, et al. Value of serum IgG4 in the diagnosis of autoimmune pancreatitis and in distinguishing it from pancreatic cancer. Am J Gastroenterol 2007;102(8):1646–53.

53. Carruthers MN, Khosroshahi A, Augustin T, et al. The diagnostic utility of serum IgG4 concentrations in IgG4-related disease. Ann Rheum Dis 2015;74(1):14–8.

54. Shimosegawa T, Chari ST, Frulloni L, et al. International consensus diagnostic criteria for autoimmune pancreatitis: guidelines of the International Association of Pancreatology. Pancreas 2011;40(3):352–8.

55. Haroche J, Arnaud L, Cohen-Aubart F, et al. Erdheim-Chester disease. Rheum Dis Clin North Am 2013;39(2):299–311.

56. Hart PA, Topazian MD, Witzig TE, et al. Treatment of relapsing autoimmune pancreatitis with immunomodulators and rituximab: the Mayo Clinic experience. Gut 2013;62(11):1607–15.

57. Hart PA, Kamisawa T, Brugge WR, et al. Long-term outcomes of autoimmune pancreatitis: a multicentre, international analysis. Gut 2013;62(12):1771–6.

58. Khosroshahi A, Bloch DB, Deshpande V, et al. Rituximab therapy leads to rapid decline of serum IgG4 levels and prompt clinical improvement in IgG4-related systemic disease. Arthritis Rheum 2010;62(6):1755–62.

59. Khosroshahi A, Carruthers MN, Deshpande V, et al. Rituximab for the treatment of IgG4-related disease: lessons from 10 consecutive patients. Medicine (Baltimore) 2012;91(1):57–66.

60. Takahashi N, Ghazale AH, Smyrk TC, et al. Possible association between IgG4-associated systemic disease with or without autoimmune pancreatitis and non-Hodgkin lymphoma. Pancreas 2009;38(5):523–6.

61. Shiokawa M, Kodama Y, Yoshimura K, et al. Risk of cancer in patients with autoimmune pancreatitis. Am J Gastroenterol 2013;108(4):610–7.

62. Shulman LE. Diffuse fasciitis with eosinophilia: a new syndrome? Trans Assoc Am Physicians 1975;88:70–86.

63. Lakhanpal S, Ginsburg WW, Michet CJ, et al. Eosinophilic fasciitis: clinical spectrum and therapeutic response in 52 cases. Semin Arthritis Rheum 1988;17(4):221–31.

64. Bujold J, Boivin C, Amin M, et al. Eosinophilic fasciitis occurring under treatment with natalizumab for multiple sclerosis. J Cutan Med Surg 2014;18(1):69–71.

65. Sheu J, Kattapuram SV, Stankiewicz JM, et al. Eosinophilic fasciitis-like disorder developing in the setting of multiple sclerosis therapy. J Drugs Dermatol 2014; 13(9):1144–7.

66. Choquet-Kastylevsky G, Kanitakis J, Dumas V, et al. Eosinophilic fasciitis and simvastatin. Arch Intern Med 2001;161(11):1456–7.

67. DeGiovanni C, Chard M, Woollons A. Eosinophilic fasciitis secondary to treatment with atorvastatin. Clin Exp Dermatol 2006;31(1):131–2.

68. Cantini F, Salvarani C, Olivieri I, et al. Possible association between eosinophilic fasciitis and subcutaneous heparin use. J Rheumatol 1998;25(2):383–5.

69. Biasi D, Caramaschi P, Carletto A, et al. Scleroderma and eosinophilic fasciitis in patients taking fosinopril. J Rheumatol 1997;24(6):1242.

70. Buchanan RR, Gordon DA, Muckle TJ, et al. The eosinophilic fasciitis syndrome after phenytoin (dilantin) therapy. J Rheumatol 1980;7(5):733–6.

71. Hayashi N, Igarashi A, Matsuyama T, et al. Eosinophilic fasciitis following exposure to trichloroethylene: successful treatment with cyclosporin. Br J Dermatol 2000;142(4):830–2.

72. Sillo P, Pinter D, Ostorhazi E, et al. Eosinophilic fasciitis associated with mycoplasma arginini infection. J Clin Microbiol 2012;50(3):1113–7.

73. Granter SR, Barnhill RL, Duray PH. Borrelial fasciitis: diffuse fasciitis and peripheral eosinophilia associated with Borrelia infection. Am J Dermatopathol 1996; 18(5):465–73.

74. Hashimoto Y, Takahashi H, Matsuo S, et al. Polymerase chain reaction of Borrelia burgdorferi flagellin gene in Shulman syndrome. Dermatology 1996;192(2): 136–9.

75. Bischoff L, Derk CT. Eosinophilic fasciitis: demographics, disease pattern and response to treatment: report of 12 cases and review of the literature. Int J Dermatol 2008;47(1):29–35.

76. Tallman MS, McGuffin RW, Higano CS, et al. Bone marrow transplantation in a patient with myelodysplasia associated with diffuse eosinophilic fasciitis. Am J Hematol 1987;24(1):93–9.

77. Fleming CJ, Clarke P, Kemmett D. Eosinophilic fasciitis with myelodysplasia responsive to treatment with cyclosporin. Br J Dermatol 1997;136(2):297–8.

78. Brito-Babapulle F. Patients with eosinophilic fasciitis should have a bone marrow examination to identify myelodysplasia. Br J Dermatol 1997;137(2):316–7.

79. Farrell AM, Ross JS, Bunker CB. Eosinophilic fasciitis associated with autoimmune thyroid disease and myelodysplasia treated with pulsed methylprednisolone and antihistamines. Br J Dermatol 1999;140(6):1185–7.

80. Kim H, Kim MO, Ahn MJ, et al. Eosinophilic fasciitis preceding relapse of peripheral T-cell lymphoma. J Korean Med Sci 2000;15(3):346–50.

81. Eklund KK, Anttila P, Leirisalo-Repo M. Eosinophilic fasciitis, myositis and arthritis as early manifestations of peripheral T-cell lymphoma. Scand J Rheumatol 2003;32(6):376–7.

82. Chan LS, Hanson CA, Cooper KD. Concurrent eosinophilic fasciitis and cutaneous T-cell lymphoma. Eosinophilic fasciitis as a paraneoplastic syndrome of T-cell malignant neoplasms? Arch Dermatol 1991;127(6):862–5.

83. Castellanos-Gonzalez M, Velasco Rodriguez D, Blanco Echevarria A, et al. Eosinophilic fasciitis as a manifestation of a cutaneous T-cell lymphoma not otherwise specified. Am J Dermatopathol 2013;35(6):666–70.

84. Antic M, Lautenschlager S, Itin PH. Eosinophilic fasciitis 30 years after—what do we really know? Report of 11 patients and review of the literature. Dermatology 2006;213(2):93–101.

85. Khanna D, Verity A, Grossman JM. Eosinophilic fasciitis with multiple myeloma: a new haematological association. Ann Rheum Dis 2002;61(12):1111–2.

86. Michaels RM. Eosinophilic fasciitis complicated by Hodgkin's disease. J Rheumatol 1982;9(3):473–6.

87. de Boysson H, Cheze S, Chapon F, et al. Eosinophilic fasciitis with paroxysmal nocturnal hemoglobinuria. Joint Bone Spine 2013;80(2):208–10.

88. Barnes L, Rodnan GP, Medsger TA, et al. Eosinophilic fasciitis. A pathologic study of twenty cases. Am J Pathol 1979;96(2):493–518.

89. Toquet C, Hamidou MA, Renaudin K, et al. In situ immunophenotype of the inflammatory infiltrate in eosinophilic fasciitis. J Rheumatol 2003;30(8): 1811–5.

90. Viallard JF, Taupin JL, Ranchin V, et al. Analysis of leukemia inhibitory factor, type 1 and type 2 cytokine production in patients with eosinophilic fasciitis. J Rheumatol 2001;28(1):75–80.

91. Jinnin M, Ihn H, Yamane K, et al. Serum levels of tissue inhibitor of metalloproteinase-1 and 2 in patients with eosinophilic fasciitis. Br J Dermatol 2004;151(2):407–12.

92. Lebeaux D, Sene D. Eosinophilic fasciitis (Shulman disease). Best Pract Res Clin Rheumatol 2012;26(4):449–58.
93. Pinal-Fernandez I, Selva-O'Callaghan A, Grau JM. Diagnosis and classification of eosinophilic fasciitis. Autoimmun Rev 2014;13(4–5):379–82.
94. Herson S, Brechignac S, Piette JC, et al. Capillary microscopy during eosinophilic fasciitis in 15 patients: distinction from systemic scleroderma. Am J Med 1990;88(6):598–600.
95. Nashel J, Steen V. Scleroderma mimics. Curr Rheumatol Rep 2012;14(1):39–46.
96. Belongia EA, Mayeno AN, Osterholm MT. The eosinophilia-myalgia syndrome and tryptophan. Annu Rev Nutr 1992;12:235–56.
97. Kaufman LD, Krupp LB. Eosinophilia-myalgia syndrome, toxic-oil syndrome, and diffuse fasciitis with eosinophilia. Curr Opin Rheumatol 1995;7(6):560–7.
98. Alonso-Ruiz A, Zea-Mendoza AC, Salazar-Vallinas JM, et al. Toxic oil syndrome: a syndrome with features overlapping those of various forms of scleroderma. Semin Arthritis Rheum 1986;15(3):200–12.
99. Lebeaux D, Frances C, Barete S, et al. Eosinophilic fasciitis (Shulman disease): new insights into the therapeutic management from a series of 34 patients. Rheumatology (Oxford) 2012;51(3):557–61.
100. Tzaribachev N, Holzer U, Schedel J, et al. Infliximab effective in steroid-dependent juvenile eosinophilic fasciitis. Rheumatology (Oxford) 2008;47(6):930–2.
101. Khanna D, Agrawal H, Clements PJ. Infliximab may be effective in the treatment of steroid-resistant eosinophilic fasciitis: report of three cases. Rheumatology (Oxford) 2010;49(6):1184–8.
102. Poliak N, Orange JS, Pawel BR, et al. Eosinophilic fasciitis mimicking angioedema and treatment response to infliximab in a pediatric patient. Ann Allergy Asthma Immunol 2011;106(5):444–5.
103. Heidary N, Cheung W, Wang N, et al. Eosinophilic fasciitis/generalized morphea overlap. Dermatol Online J 2009;15(8):2.
104. Scheinberg M, Hamerschlak N, Kutner JM, et al. Rituximab in refractory autoimmune diseases: Brazilian experience with 29 patients (2002–2004). Clin Exp Rheumatol 2006;24(1):65–9.
105. Hertzman PA, Blevins WL, Mayer J, et al. Association of the eosinophilia-myalgia syndrome with the ingestion of tryptophan. N Engl J Med 1990;322(13):869–73.
106. Centers for Disease Control (CDC). Eosinophilia-myalgia syndrome and L-tryptophan-containing products–New Mexico, Minnesota, Oregon, and New York, 1989. MMWR Morb Mortal Wkly Rep 1989;38(46):785–8.
107. Eidson M, Philen RM, Sewell CM, et al. L-tryptophan and eosinophilia-myalgia syndrome in New Mexico. Lancet 1990;335(8690):645–8.
108. Swygert LA, Back EE, Auerbach SB, et al. Eosinophilia-myalgia syndrome: mortality data from the US national surveillance system. J Rheumatol 1993;20(10):1711–7.
109. Allen JA, Peterson A, Sufit R, et al. Post-epidemic eosinophilia-myalgia syndrome associated with L-tryptophan. Arthritis Rheum 2011;63(11):3633–9.
110. Belongia EA, Hedberg CW, Gleich GJ, et al. An investigation of the cause of the eosinophilia-myalgia syndrome associated with tryptophan use. N Engl J Med 1990;323(6):357–65.
111. Slutsker L, Hoesly FC, Miller L, et al. Eosinophilia-myalgia syndrome associated with exposure to tryptophan from a single manufacturer. JAMA 1990;264(2):213–7.
112. Hill RH Jr, Caudill SP, Philen RM, et al. Contaminants in L-tryptophan associated with eosinophilia myalgia syndrome. Arch Environ Contam Toxicol 1993;25(1):134–42.

113. Love LA, Rader JI, Crofford LJ, et al. Pathological and immunological effects of ingesting L-tryptophan and 1,1'-ethylidenebis (L-tryptophan) in Lewis rats. J Clin Invest 1993;91(3):804–11.
114. Mayeno AN, Belongia EA, Lin F, et al. 3-(Phenylamino)alanine, a novel aniline-derived amino acid associated with the eosinophilia-myalgia syndrome: a link to the toxic oil syndrome? Mayo Clin Proc 1992;67(12):1134–9.
115. Silver RM. Pathophysiology of the eosinophilia-myalgia syndrome. J Rheumatol Suppl 1996;46:26–36.
116. Kaufman LD, Seidman RJ, Gruber BL. L-tryptophan-associated eosinophilic perimyositis, neuritis, and fasciitis. A clinicopathologic and laboratory study of 25 patients. Medicine (Baltimore) 1990;69(4):187–99.
117. Blauvelt A, Falanga V. Idiopathic and L-tryptophan-associated eosinophilic fasciitis before and after L-tryptophan contamination. Arch Dermatol 1991;127(8): 1159–66.
118. Martin RW, Duffy J, Lie JT. Eosinophilic fasciitis associated with use of L-tryptophan: a case-control study and comparison of clinical and histopathologic features. Mayo Clin Proc 1991;66(9):892–8.
119. Umbert I, Winkelmann RK, Wegener L. Comparison of the pathology of fascia in eosinophilic myalgia syndrome patients and idiopathic eosinophilic fasciitis. Dermatology 1993;186(1):18–22.
120. Hertzman PA, Clauw DJ, Kaufman LD, et al. The eosinophilia-myalgia syndrome: status of 205 patients and results of treatment 2 years after onset. Ann Intern Med 1995;122(11):851–5.
121. Kaufman LD, Kephart GM, Seidman RJ, et al. The spectrum of eosinophilic myositis. Clinical and immunopathogenic studies of three patients, and review of the literature. Arthritis Rheum 1993;36(7):1014–24.
122. Kamm MA, Dennett X, Byrne E. Relapsing eosinophilic myositis–a cause of pseudothrombophlebitis in an alcoholic. J Rheumatol 1987;14(4):831–4.
123. Sladek GD, Vasey FB, Sieger B, et al. Relapsing eosinophilic myositis. J Rheumatol 1983;10(3):467–70.
124. Hall FC, Krausz T, Walport MJ. Idiopathic eosinophilic myositis. QJM 1995;88(8): 581–6.
125. Cantarini L, Volpi N, Carbotti P, et al. Eosinophilia-associated muscle disorders: an immunohistological study with tissue localisation of major basic protein in distinct clinicopathological forms. J Clin Pathol 2009;62(5):442–7.
126. Murata K, Sugie K, Takamure M, et al. Eosinophilic major basic protein and interleukin-5 in eosinophilic myositis. Eur J Neurol 2003;10(1):35–8.
127. Selva-O'Callaghan A, Trallero-Araguas E, Grau JM. Eosinophilic myositis: an updated review. Autoimmun Rev 2014;13(4–5):375–8.
128. Pickering MC, Walport MJ. Eosinophilic myopathic syndromes. Curr Opin Rheumatol 1998;10(6):504–10.
129. Kobayashi Y, Fujimoto T, Shiiki H, et al. Focal eosinophilic myositis. Clin Rheumatol 2001;20(5):369–71.
130. Serratrice G, Pellissier JF, Roux H, et al. Fasciitis, perimyositis, myositis, polymyositis, and eosinophilia. Muscle Nerve 1990;13(5):385–95.
131. Van den Enden E, Praet M, Joos R, et al. Eosinophilic myositis resulting from sarcocystosis. J Trop Med Hyg 1995;98(4):273–6.
132. Arness MK, Brown JD, Dubey JP, et al. An outbreak of acute eosinophilic myositis attributed to human sarcocystis parasitism. Am J Trop Med Hyg 1999;61(4):548–53.

133. Gherardi R, Baudrimont M, Lionnet F, et al. Skeletal muscle toxoplasmosis in patients with acquired immunodeficiency syndrome: a clinical and pathological study. Ann Neurol 1992;32(4):535–42.
134. Esposito DH, Stich A, Epelboin L, et al. Acute muscular sarcocystosis: an international investigation among ill travelers returning from Tioman Island, Malaysia, 2011-2012. Clin Infect Dis 2014;59(10):1401–10.
135. Italiano CM, Wong KT, AbuBakar S, et al. Sarcocystis nesbitti causes acute, relapsing febrile myositis with a high attack rate: description of a large outbreak of muscular sarcocystosis in Pangkor Island, Malaysia, 2012. PLoS Negl Trop Dis 2014;8(5):e2876.
136. Suresh E, Dhillon VB, Smith C, et al. Churg-Strauss vasculitis diagnosed on muscle biopsy. J Clin Pathol 2004;57(3):334.
137. Weinstock A, Green C, Cohen BH, et al. Becker muscular dystrophy presenting as eosinophilic inflammatory myopathy in an infant. J Child Neurol 1997;12(2):146–7.
138. Krahn M, Lopez de Munain A, Streichenberger N, et al. CAPN3 mutations in patients with idiopathic eosinophilic myositis. Ann Neurol 2006;59(6):905–11.
139. Brown RH Jr, Amato A. Calpainopathy and eosinophilic myositis. Ann Neurol 2006;59(6):875–7.
140. Amato AA. Adults with eosinophilic myositis and calpain-3 mutations. Neurology 2008;70(9):730–1.
141. Baumeister SK, Todorovic S, Milic-Rasic V, et al. Eosinophilic myositis as presenting symptom in gamma-sarcoglycanopathy. Neuromuscul Disord 2009; 19(2):167–71.
142. Meyer A, Lannes B, Carapito R, et al. Eosinophilic myositis as first manifestation in a patient with type 2 myotonic dystrophy CCTG expansion mutation and rheumatoid arthritis. Neuromuscul Disord 2015;25(2):149–52.
143. Oflazer PS, Gundesli H, Zorludemir S, et al. Eosinophilic myositis in calpainopathy: could immunosuppression of the eosinophilic myositis alter the early natural course of the dystrophic disease? Neuromuscul Disord 2009;19(4):261–3.
144. Schroder T, Fuchss J, Schneider I, et al. Eosinophils in hereditary and inflammatory myopathies. Acta Myol 2013;32(3):148–53.

Eosinophilia in Pulmonary Disorders

Kerry Woolnough, MBChB, MRCP(resp)[a,b], Andrew J. Wardlaw, MD, PhD[a,b],*

KEYWORDS

- Asthma • AFAD • Eosinophilic pneumonia
- Eosinophilic granulomatosis with polyangiitis (EGPA) • Hypereosinophilic syndrome

KEY POINTS

- The presence of lung disease can aid in the diagnosis, investigation, and management of eosinophilic disorders.
- Sputum eosinophilia has been shown to be associated with persistent airway inflammation, uncontrolled asthma, lung function decline, future risk of exacerbations, and asthma severity.
- Eosinophilic pneumonia (EP) may represent a relapse of chronic EP and is rarely simple or acute unless caused by a defined and avoidable trigger (usually a drug reaction).
- A better classification of EP in the authors' opinion would be by cause: parasitic migration, allergic (including drug allergy) or idiopathic (the most common form).
- The boundaries between nonatopic eosinophil-predominant asthma, EP, eosinophilic granulomatosis with polyangiitis (EGPA), and hypereosinophilic syndrome (HES) with respiratory involvement are blurred, and they may all be part of the same condition, possibly driven by Type 2 innate lymphoid cells (ILC2) cells in response to an unknown antigen.

GENERAL CONSIDERATIONS
Introduction

Lung disease associated with marked peripheral blood or tissue eosinophilia is an unusual event and almost always points toward a diagnosis. For example, florid allergic fungal airway disease (AFAD) with pulmonary masses, upper lobe shadowing, or large airway collapse is commonly misdiagnosed as lung cancer or tuberculosis but invariably is associated with a peripheral blood eosinophilia that is unusual in these other conditions. The peripheral blood eosinophil count is a balance between eosinophil

The authors were supported by the National Institute for Health Research Leicester Respiratory Biomedical Research Unit. The views expressed are those of the authors and not necessarily those of the NHS, the NIHR, or the Department of Health.

a Department of Infection Immunity and Inflammation, Institute for Lung Health, University of Leicester, Groby Road, Leicester LE3 9QP, UK; b Department of Respiratory Medicine and Allergy, University Hospitals of Leicester NHS Trust, Groby Road, Leicester LE3 9QP, UK
* Corresponding author. Institute for Lung Health, Glenfield Hospital, Groby Road, Leicester LE3 9QP, UK.
E-mail address: aw24@le.ac.uk

production and the rate of entry of eosinophils into the tissue. If there is a strong inflammatory stimulus in the lung recruiting eosinophils into the tissue, then the tissue eosinophilia may be marked to a modest or even normal peripheral blood eosinophil count. In other situations such as drug allergy in which there is a systemic stimulus for eosinophilopoiesis, the latter may be the case with a modest tissue eosinophilia in the context of a marked peripheral blood eosinophilia. This review is written from the perspective of expertise gained in a tertiary level specialist clinic for people with an unexplained peripheral blood eosinophilia (>1.5 × 10^9/L), set within a respiratory and allergy department with an ethnically mixed catchment of about 1,000,000 and a regional catchment of about 5,000,000. The most common causes of an eosinophilia affecting the respiratory system seen in this clinic are severe asthma, AFAD, HES, EGPA, and chronic idiopathic EP. The patient's medical history including a detailed drug history and geographic background is therefore important in guiding investigations when trying to elicit a cause.

Eosinophilia has been associated with several diseases that affect the small and large airways. It can be detected as an increased percentage of the differential cell count on peripheral blood, induced sputum and bronchoalveolar lavage (BAL) samples, or as eosinophilic infiltration seen on lung biopsy specimens. Its presence or absence is used to endotype patients and guide treatment intensity during exacerbations and stable state in asthma[1] and chronic obstructive pulmonary disease (COPD)[2,3] and is likely to form part of the criteria for treatment with new drugs, such as mepolizumab, an anti-interleukin (IL)-5 antibody developed for treatment of asthma.[4] The common causes of an eosinophilia associated with respiratory disease seen in the authors' clinic are listed in **Table 1**. The degree of eosinophilia seen in each condition varies and is not helpful for diagnosis, although an eosinophil count of greater than 5 × 10^9/L is not often seen in severe asthma without another complication such as fungal allergy. This list does not include conditions such as eosinophilic bronchitis or idiopathic pulmonary fibrosis in which there is a sputum or BAL eosinophilia without a peripheral blood eosinophilia.

Mechanisms of Eosinophil Migration into the Lung

Eosinophils are one of the key effector cells of allergic inflammation. Their maturation, recruitment, and survival are closely associated with cytokines and chemokines generated in the context of the immune pathway involving T$_H$2 lymphocytes in the adaptive system and ILC2 cells in the innate system, with IL-5 and IL-13 being central to the process. Epithelial-derived Thymic stromal lymphopoietin (TSLP), IL-33, and IL-25 seem to orchestrate this pathway to a significant extent.[5,6] Differentiation of eosinophils also occurs in the lung with increased numbers of CD34$^+$ Interleukin 5 receptor, alpha (IL5Rα) cells seen in sputum in response to allergen challenge, although the physiologic importance of this is uncertain.[7,8]

Although IL-3 and Granulocyte macrophage colony-stimulating factor (GM-CSF) are involved in the eosinophil maturational pathway, IL-5 is essential for the late differentiation of eosinophils. Eosinophilia is reactive in most cases (as opposed to being due to a malignant transformation of the eosinophil) and has been shown to be responsive to antibody therapy directed against IL-5, which causes a marked decrease (although not a complete ablation) in the peripheral blood eosinophil count.[9,10] Antieosinophil therapies are much more effective at reducing the eosinophilia in the blood than in the tissue. Thus, mepolizumab, an antieosinophilic antibody that binds IL-5, preventing it from binding to the IL-5 receptor, reduced the blood eosinophil count by 90% but the eosinophil count in the bronchial mucosa by only 50%.[11] A marked reduction in the blood eosinophil count by mepolizumab is associated with a prevention of asthma

Table 1

Causes of an eosinophilia linked to respiratory disease seen in a specialist hypereosinophilia clinic during a 10-year period

General Diagnosis	Specific Diagnosis	Number of Cases	Comment	Gender (M:F)	Highest Eosinophil Count ×10⁹/L	Mean Eosinophil Count ×10⁹/L
Hypereosinophilic syndromes	Myeloproliferative	8	Not all have respiratory symptoms	5:3	49.6	23.8
	EGPA	19	—	13:6	33.4	10.1
	HES general	25	Not all have respiratory symptoms	17:7	28	11.5
Chronic infection with helminthic parasites	Strongyloides, schistosomiasis, filariasis	37	Cough occasionally associated with strongyloides but mostly asymptomatic		25.8	4.3
Primary respiratory disease	Severe asthma	35	—	11:24	5.31	3.4
	Allergic fungal airway disease	32	—	19:13	42.34	5.5
	Chronic eosinophilic pneumonia	16	—	4:12	30	6.5
	COPD	3	—	3:0	2.9	2.2
Drug allergy	—	15	Some have respiratory symptoms	7:8	20.9	13.7
Malignant disease	Lung cancer and lymphoma	7	—	5:2	7.0	20.1
Miscellaneous*		6	—	1:4	2.5	2.3

* A heterogenous group that do not fit into any particular diagnostic group.

exacerbations and a reduction in the bronchial lumen eosinophilic infiltration, without much effect on the sputum eosinophilia.[4]

Migration of eosinophils into the lung is a multistep process, with the exact mechanism depending on the location of the tissue eosinophilia (**Fig. 1**).[12] Trafficking associated with an eosinophilia affecting the alveolar compartment as seen in EP is likely to occur through the low-pressure pulmonary circulation via the pulmonary capillaries into the alveolar compartment and mediated primarily by a chemoattractant-driven process. Migration into the bronchial tree through the high-pressure bronchial artery system follows the multistep paradigm involving capture in the postcapillary endothelium followed by activation-mediated arrest and transendothelial migration.[13] Interactions with the extracellular matrix are involved in eosinophil persistence and survival in tissue before migration through the bronchial epithelium into the bronchial lumen results in apoptosis and removal by macrophage phagocytosis.[14] IL-5 prevents apoptosis and extends eosinophil survival by acting upstream of Bax translocation to the mitochondria to inhibit cytochrome C release and caspases 9, 3, and 7 activation.[15] IL-5 and interferon (IFN) γ have also been shown to increase eosinophil survival by inhibiting Fas-mediated apoptosis and caspases 3 and 8 activation.[16]

A marked tissue eosinophilia often occurs without a neutrophilia, emphasizing the dichotomy between T_H1-T_H17 (neutrophilic) and T_H2 immune processes. An important

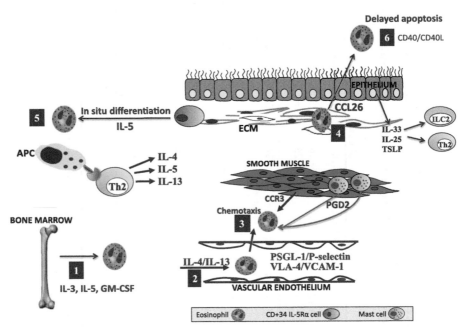

Fig. 1. Selective accumulation of eosinophils is a multistep process. (1) Eosinophil differentiation and maturation from pluripotent CD34$^+$ stem cells. (2) Primed eosinophils bind IL-5 to the IL-5R and upregulate P-selectin. (3) Eosinophil chemotaxis occurs by release of CCR3 from smooth muscle and PGD2 from mast cells. (4) Eosinophil trafficking from ECM into the airspace. (5) CD34$^+$ IL-5Rα cells differentiate into eosinophils in the lung. (6) IL-5 prolongs survival by preventing eosinophil caspase release and Fas-mediated apoptosis. APC, antigen presenting cell; CCR, chemokine receptors; ECM, extra-cellular matrix; GM-CSF, granulocyte macrophage colony-stimulating factor; ILC, innate lymphoid cell; PGD, prostaglandin; PSGL, P-selectin glycoprotein ligand; TSLP, thymic stromal lymphopoietin; VCAM, vascular cell adhesion molecule; VLA, very late antigen.

selection point for eosinophil, as compared with neutrophil, migration occurs in the postcapillary endothelium where IL-13 (a hub cytokine in asthma) increases expression of P-selectin and vascular cell adhesion molecule 1 on endothelial cells, directing eosinophil migration via PSGL-1 and VLA-4, respectively (see **Fig. 1**).[17–19] Consistent with this model, anti-IL-13 monoclonal antibodies caused an increase in the peripheral blood eosinophil count.[20] The mediators involved in the activation step of eosinophil adhesion to endothelium are uncertain, although β2 integrins, particularly CD11b-CD18, are the adhesion receptors involved.[21] The CCR3-associated chemokines, chemokine ligand (CCL)11 (eotaxin 1), CCL24 (eotaxin 2), and CCL26 (eotaxin 3), have been regarded as being central to this process, but the lack of efficacy of potent CCR3 antagonists calls this into question.[22] There are several other chemoattractants that could be involved, including PGD_2 released by mast cells, which is a ligand for CRTH2, a chemoattractant receptor expressed on eosinophils, basophils, ILC2 cells, and a subset of T_H2 lymphocytes.[23] This topic is of current interest, because several potent CRTH2 antagonists are in clinical development.

Role of Eosinophils in Lung Disease

Theories about the role of eosinophils in host defense and lung injury have oscillated over the decades between the concept that they are tissue damaging, primarily because of the effects of granule proteins on bronchial epithelial integrity, and the idea that they are simply markers of allergic inflammation without any active role in disease and more recently a resurgence in the view that they are important in maintaining immune homeostasis.[24,25] Studies of mepolizumab demonstrate a causal link between eosinophilia and severe exacerbations in asthma.[26] The mechanism by which eosinophils are implicated in severe exacerbations is unclear, although it is thought that they promote hypersecretion of viscid mucus, which blocks the airway and is a prominent feature of deaths due to asthma. The benefit of mepolizumab in patients with idiopathic HES also supports the idea that they are directly involved in disease pathogenesis.[27]

CLINICAL FEATURES
Asthma

Asthma is diagnosed by the presence of bronchial hyperresponsiveness and variable airflow obstruction, which may become fixed in long-standing disease.[28] Although not all asthma is eosinophilic, an airway eosinophilia remains a hallmark of the condition with a sputum eosinophilia (>2%) 80% sensitive and 95% specific as a diagnostic test.[29] A sputum eosinophilia is a risk factor for the development of severe exacerbations of asthma, and suppression of the eosinophilia either by glucocorticoids or by anti-IL-5 agents prevents severe exacerbations.[30] Eosinophilic airway inflammation has been linked to airway remodeling, increased basement membrane thickness, and smooth muscle hypertrophy but is not closely associated with variable airflow obstruction.[31–33] Patients with atopic asthma, and in particular those who are sensitized to fungi, are known to have more severe disease with a reduced postbronchodilator forced expiration volume in the first second of respiration; sensitization to fungi is also known to be a risk factor for life-threatening asthma.[34–36]

In mild to moderate disease, the peripheral blood eosinophil count is often normal or only slightly increased. However, a more striking peripheral blood eosinophilia is seen in association with severe exacerbations and an endotype of hypereosinophilic asthma characterized by adult onset, lack of atopy (defined as a positive specific IgE to common aeroallergens), and nasal polyposis. These patients often present with cough and congestion and recurrent severe exacerbations rather than complaints of wheeze and chest tightness. The methacholine Pc20 may be normal.

Severe asthma is characterized by persistent airway inflammation despite maximal medical treatment and affects approximately 5% of asthmatics.[37] Sputum eosinophilia has been shown to be associated with persistent airway inflammation, uncontrolled asthma, lung function decline, future risk of exacerbations, and asthma severity.[38–40] Those with an eosinophilic endotype respond better to corticosteroids than those who have a noneosinophilic, neutrophilic endotype.[41] A subgroup of patients with eosinophilic bronchitis presents with cough and has an airway eosinophilia but no airway hyperresponsiveness or blood eosinophilia.[42]

Allergic Fungal Airway Disease

IgE sensitization to thermotolerant filamentous fungi (particularly *Aspergillus* [mainly *Aspergillus fumigatus*] and *Penicillium* genera) and yeasts (particularly *Candida albicans*) is one of the most common causes of lung disease in association with an eosinophilia. Although this usually occurs in the context of asthma, it is also a common complication of cystic fibrosis and smoking-related obstructive airway disease (COPD). In severe asthma, it is frequently associated with childhood-onset atopic asthma, but it presents heterogeneously sometimes complicating adult-onset disease whereby a characteristic presentation is late-onset fixed airflow obstruction. Lobar collapse due to viscid mucus, a fungal pneumonitis associated with heavy fungal exposure, and a fungal bronchitis characterized by a purulent cough with heavy fungal growth, not necessarily in the context of either IgE sensitization or asthma, are characteristic presentations.[43] Fleeting shadows on the chest x-ray are also characteristic but less often seen with the advent of high-dose inhaled corticosteroids, which suppress the inflammatory response in the large airways, although they may predispose to fungal colonization in the lower airways. Aspergilloma, although classically linked to increased *A fumigatus* IgG levels, is also often accompanied by IgE sensitization to *A fumigatus*. The immunologically and clinically florid end of the allergic fungal lung disease spectrum is termed allergic bronchopulmonary aspergillosis (ABPA), the criteria for which may exclude people in whom the fungal sensitization is relevant to their disease process.[44] The authors therefore prefer the more inclusive term allergic fungal airway disease (defined as airway disease in the context of IgE sensitization to a thermotolerant fungus), qualified in terms of the amount of lung damage and the underlying lung disease (if present) such as asthma, cystic fibrosis, or COPD.[45,46] **Fig. 2** shows a computed tomographic (CT) scan of a patient with AFAD.

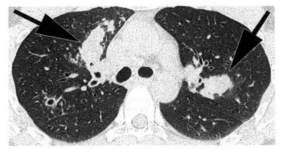

Fig. 2. Computed tomographic scan showing inflammatory masses and bronchiectasis associated with AFAD. The arrows show airways filled by mucoid secretions resulting in mucoid impaction often seen as inflammatory masses on CT.

Eosinophilic Pneumonia

The terminology around EP (pneumonic shadowing associated with, and presumably caused by, a marked tissue eosinophilia) is confusing. Loeffler syndrome was initially described in the context of lung migrating parasitic larvae and is probably best restricted to this condition, which is rare in industrialized countries, even in communities where chronic parasitic infection with worms is not uncommon. Some researchers divide EP into simple, acute, and chronic. In the authors' practice EP is rarely simple, and acute EP, unless caused by a defined and avoidable trigger (usually drug reactions), may represent a relapse of chronic EP. A wide variety of drugs have been implicated in causing EP mainly involving antibiotics, including antimalarials, sulfonamides, tetracyclines, nitrofurantoin, antituberculous drugs, and daptomycin.[47] Chronic idiopathic EP is not uncommon, mostly occurs in women (aged 20–50 years), and is associated with asthma and nasal polyposis, with pneumonic shadowing differentiating it from adult-onset eosinophilic asthma.

A better classification of EP would be by cause: parasitic migration, allergic (including drug allergy), or idiopathic (the most common form). Patients with acute EP are unwell, with type 1 respiratory failure (defined as an arterial partial pressure of oxygen [Pao_2] of <8 kPa [60 mm Hg], equivalent to oxygen saturations of less than 90%, with a normal or low arterial partial pressure of carbon dioxide [$Paco_2$][48]) and florid lung shadowing, which classically shows a peripheral distribution (**Fig. 3**). A nonproductive cough, low-grade fever, weight loss, and general malaise are common symptoms. The hallmark is a blood eosinophilia (bacterial and viral pneumonias are almost invariably associated with an eosinopenia), although the blood eosinophil count can be transiently normal on presentation, presumably due to the rapid migration of eosinophils into the lung.[49] Both the blood and lung eosinophilia start to resolve within 48 hours with high-dose systemic corticosteroids. EP can unusually be associated with endomyocardial fibrosis, and cardiac MRI should be performed. The differential diagnosis includes EGPA, and it is sometimes difficult to distinguish between these 2 conditions.

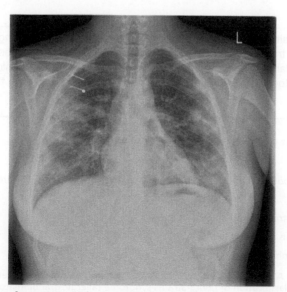

Fig. 3. Chest x-ray of a patient with acute EP, showing florid lung shadowing, which classically shows a peripheral distribution.

Eosinophilic Granulomatosis with Polyangiitis (Formerly Churg-Strauss Syndrome)

Churg-Strauss syndrome affects small to medium-sized vessels. It has been renamed EGPA.[50] The American College of Rheumatology criteria have been shown to be 85% sensitive and 99.7% specific for its diagnosis when any 4 of the 6 criteria are present (**Box 1**).[51]

EGPA is mostly seen in refractory late-onset eosinophilic asthma with fixed airflow obstruction and in association with chronic rhinosinusitis/nasal polyposis.[52] Nodules, purpura, or urticaria is seen in 70% of individuals and mononeuritis multiplex in 66%.[53] Individuals who are p-Anti-neutrophil cytoplasmic antibody (ANCA) positive (40%) have a higher rate of alveolar hemorrhage, glomerulonephritis, and mononeuritis multiplex.[54]

Idiopathic Hypereosinophilic Syndrome

Idiopathic HES is defined by a persistent blood eosinophilia of 1.5×10^9/L or more, with no secondary cause identified and evidence of eosinophil-related end organ damage.[55] It is heterogeneous in its presentation, but respiratory involvement (usually involving airway symptoms and airflow obstruction, although parenchymal abnormalities are common on CT scanning) is common both at the time of diagnosis and during the course of the illness.[55] The most common form of HES is reactive with the eosinophilia secondary to overproduction of IL-5. In some cases, this is due to an aberrant/clonal T-cell population. Myeloproliferative variants account for 10% of HES, of which the most common is a form of chronic eosinophilic leukemia (due to a constitutively active tyrosine kinase FIP1-like-1platelet-derived growth factor receptor-α [FIP1L1-PDGFRα]). This condition has a striking 9:1 male predominance and until the advent of imatinib mesylate, which is effective at inducing and maintaining remission, had a poor prognosis.[55] The subtype of reactive HES does not seem to influence the pattern of respiratory disease, which can usually be controlled with corticosteroids. Cardiac involvement accounts for most of the morbidity and mortality, especially endomyocardial fibrosis.[56]

Infections

Helminthic parasites and fungal infections can cause eosinophilic lung disease. Parasites can cause transient pulmonary infiltrates, a significant blood eosinophilia, and a rash during the larval migration. Serology, guided by travel to endemic areas, is more sensitive than stool examination, as symptoms often appear before the adult worms

---

Box 1
American College of Rheumatology criteria for Churg-Strauss syndrome

1. Asthma

2. Peripheral blood eosinophilia greater than 10% of white blood cell differential count

3. Neuropathy

4. Migratory or transient pulmonary opacities

5. Paranasal sinus abnormalities

6. Tissue eosinophilia

Data from Masi AT, Hunder GG, Lie JT, et al. The American College of Rheumatology 1990 criteria for the classification of Churg-Strauss syndrome (allergic granulomatosis and angiitis). Arthritis Rheum 1990;33(8):1094–100.

develop. Fungal infections include primary coccidioidomycosis, which presents with pulmonary infiltrates[57]; *Pneumocystis jiroveci*, which presents with profound hypoxia (correlating to the degree of BAL eosinophilia)[58]; and colonization with *A fumigatus*, which may lead to a fungal bronchitis. Viral and bacterial infections almost invariably are associated with eosinopenia, although *Mycobacterium tuberculosis* is known to cause an eosinophilic picture in those presenting with a pleural effusion from tuberculous pleuritis.[59]

Malignancy

Lymphoma affecting the lung is well described as being associated with both a blood and tissue eosinophilia unresponsive to steroids. Primary and secondary solid tumors affecting the lung can also be associated with a marked peripheral blood eosinophilia, but this is usually in the context of advanced disease.

DIAGNOSTIC TESTS

Eosinophils reside mainly in the tissues and are present in the blood only for 8 to 12 hours.[60] Thus, a more accurate appreciation of tissue infiltration can be gained from more direct measurements using sputum, BAL samples, or lung biopsy specimens. Sputum cell differential counting on induced sputum is a noninvasive method of measuring airway inflammation and can be used in routine clinical practice in a range of chronic lung diseases to detect the degree of eosinophilia present.[61] Sputum eosinophilia correlates with the degree of clinical improvement to inhaled corticosteroids and predicts response, and relapse, to corticosteroid reduction.[62] Lung biopsies demonstrate eosinophilic infiltration but are rarely diagnostic of the underlying condition unless vasculitic changes or fungal elements are seen. Tests of lung physiology may be less valuable than in asthma, but the development of fixed airflow obstruction is not uncommon so regular spirometry is required. All patients with a lung eosinophilia should be screened for allergy to thermotolerant fungi, including *A fumigatus*, *Penicillium chrysogenum*, *C albicans*, and *Malassezia* species. Other investigations including ANCA, serum tryptase, EMG studies, cardiac MRI, and lymphocyte phenotype testing should be undertaken as per the investigation of HES.[63] **Fig. 4** illustrates a suggested diagnostic pathway to aid in the workup of someone with an unexplained eosinophilia, and **Table 2** describes some characteristic radiologic appearances of eosinophilic disease.

MANAGEMENT

The use of sputum cell counts to control eosinophilic airway inflammation by titration of corticosteroid is recognized as part of the standard of care for asthma in the American Thoracic Society/European Respiratory Society guidelines[64] and has been proved in a meta-analysis to reduce exacerbations.[65]

Anti-IL-5 agents (mepolizumab and reslizumab) have been shown to reduce tissue eosinophilia and exacerbation frequency and have allowed reduction in oral corticosteroid dose in refractory eosinophilic asthma.[26,66] Improvement in lung function has been seen with both CRTH2 antagonists and lebrikizumab (anti-IL-13) in patients with severe asthma with high pretreatment periostin levels.[20,23] Mepolizumab is going through licensing procedures, but the other agents are in earlier phases of clinical development.

Steroids are the mainstay of treatment in eosinophilic pulmonary disorders. In unresponsive cases, intravenous methylprednisolone can be used in acute EP until resolution of hypoxemia and lung shadowing and then medication switched to a tapering course of oral prednisolone.[67] Chronic idiopathic eosinophilic pneumonia requires

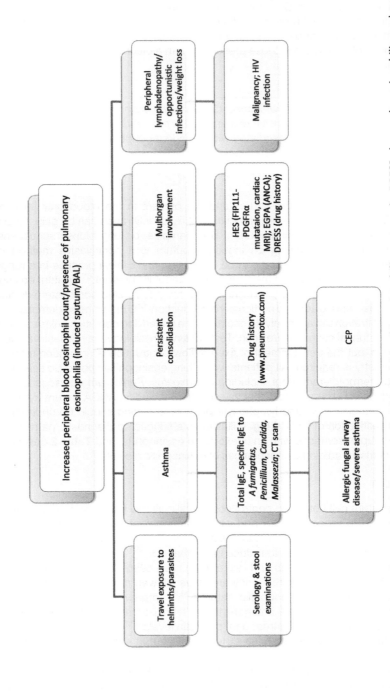

Fig. 4. Diagnostic pathway for eosinophilic lung disease. CEP, chronic idiopathic eosinophilic pneumonia; DRESS, drug rash, eosinophilia, and systemic symptoms; HIV, human immunodeficiency virus.

Table 2
Radiologic appearances of eosinophilic pulmonary disorders

Disorder	Characteristics	Location
AEP	Diffuse ground glass opacities Reticular densities Interlobular septal thickening Pleural effusions	Bilateral and peripheral
CEP	Small areas of nonsegmental airspace consolidation or ground glass shadowing seen on CT scan Nodules are common	May have upper lobe predominance
Eosinophilic granulomatosis with polyangiitis	No specific features	
Allergic fungal airway disease	Central bronchiectasis Transient pulmonary opacities Tubular bronchial gloved-finger opacities Centrilobular nodules Tree-in-bud opacities Mucoid impaction and high attenuation mucus Isolated lobar or segmental atelectasis	Central and upper zones
Idiopathic HES	Focal or diffuse interstitial or alveolar nonlobular opacities Focal/diffuse ground glass associated with nodules Pleural effusions (~50%)	Peripheral

Eosinophilia associated with allergic fungal airway disease does produce some characteristic appearances; however, the radiographic presentation of other lung diseases associated with an eosinophilia is varied and often nonspecific.

Abbreviations: AEP, acute eosinophilic pneumonia; CEP, chronic idiopathic eosinophilic pneumonia.

Data from Jeong YJ, Kim KI, Seo IJ, et al. Eosinophilic lung diseases: a clinical, radiologic, and pathologic overview. Radiographics 2007;27(3):617–37. [discussion: 637–9].

long-term oral corticosteroids (generally low dose, 5–10 mg).[68] There are no double-blind prospective clinical trials of treatment of EGPA in the acute phase, and the use of cyclophosphamide is based on other vasculitic conditions such as granulomatosis with polyangiitis (formerly Wegener granulomatosis). Patients with primarily lung and cardiac disease respond to high-dose oral corticosteroids, but those with renal involvement and a positive ANCA (40%) who have a more vasculitic component often are given cyclophosphamide to induce remission. Prednisolone is used as a single agent to control chronic disease.[54] Patients with AFAD may require long-term oral corticosteroids. Antifungals can be used to control disease activity in addition to oral steroids if there is active fungal bronchitis.[69] However, in the absence of heavy fungal colonization of the airways, the role of antifungals in AFAD remains uncertain.[70,71] About 85% of HES cases show a good response when corticosteroids are used as monotherapy.[55,72] Hydroxyurea and IFN-α have been used as second-line agents to control disease activity in HES.

CURRENT CONTROVERSIES

Classification of eosinophilic lung disease is problematic in the absence of a clear understanding of its pathogenesis. Eosinophilic predominant asthma may have a limited degree of variable airflow obstruction and little objective reversibility, with severe exacerbations being the most prominent feature. A nonproductive cough and secretion of viscid mucus is often more of a problem than wheeze or episodic shortness of breath. These patients may not fit the criteria for asthma used for inclusion into clinical trials. AFAD is a common cause of eosinophilic lung disease, but understanding of the role of fungi in airway disease has been complicated by the criteria used to define ABPA, which needs to be revisited. The current classification of EP into simple, acute, and chronic does not aid diagnosis or management and should be changed to a system based on etiology. The boundaries between nonatopic eosinophil predominant asthma, EP, EGPA, and HES with respiratory involvement are blurred, and they may all be part of the same condition, possibly driven by ILC2 cells in response to an unknown antigen. It is hoped that anti-IL-5 biological therapies can be prescribed within the asthma envelope for use in these rare overlap conditions so that the drugs can be used as tools to enhance understanding of the etiology and pathogenesis of eosinophilic lung disease as well as help the patients.

FUTURE CONSIDERATIONS/SUMMARY

Lung disease associated with a marked peripheral blood eosinophilia is unusual and nearly always clinically significant, providing important pointers to the diagnosis. Based on the authors' experience in a specialist hypereosinophilia clinic set within a large secondary and tertiary care respiratory and allergy service, the most common lung conditions causing a blood eosinophilia of greater than 1.5×10^9/L are severe eosinophilic asthma especially during exacerbations, AFAD, idiopathic EP, EGPA, and HES. Once recognized, these conditions are generally easy to manage, albeit with long-term systemic corticosteroids, which can lead to troublesome side effects. A failure to respond to oral steroids in the context of good compliance suggests a malignant cause for the eosinophilia. An important development is the introduction of antieosinophil therapies, particularly those directed against the IL-5 pathway, which is hoped to provide benefit in the full spectrum of eosinophilic lung disease as well as asthma, reducing the burden of side effects and resultant comorbidities in this group of patients.

REFERENCES

1. Haldar P, Pavord ID, Shaw DE, et al. Cluster analysis and clinical asthma phenotypes. Am J Respir Crit Care Med 2008;178(3):218–24.
2. Brightling CE, Monteiro W, Ward R, et al. Sputum eosinophilia and short-term response to prednisolone in chronic obstructive pulmonary disease: a randomised controlled trial. Lancet 2000;356(9240):1480–5.
3. Bafadhel M, McKenna S, Terry S, et al. Acute exacerbations of chronic obstructive pulmonary disease: identification of biologic clusters and their biomarkers. Am J Respir Crit Care Med 2011;184(6):662–71.
4. Pavord ID, Korn S, Howarth P, et al. Mepolizumab for severe eosinophilic asthma (DREAM): a multicentre, double-blind, placebo-controlled trial. Lancet 2012; 380(9842):651–9.
5. Mjosberg J, Eidsmo L. Update on innate lymphoid cells in atopic and non-atopic inflammation in the airways and skin. Clin Exp Allergy 2014;44(8):1033–43.
6. Scanlon ST, McKenzie AN. The messenger between worlds: the regulation of innate and adaptive type-2 immunity by innate lymphoid cells. Clin Exp Allergy 2015;45(1):9–20.

7. Dorman SC, Efthimiadis A, Babirad I, et al. Sputum CD34+IL-5Ralpha+ cells increase after allergen: evidence for in situ eosinophilopoiesis. Am J Respir Crit Care Med 2004;169(5):573–7.

8. Radinger M, Lotvall J. Eosinophil progenitors in allergy and asthma - do they matter? Pharmacol Ther 2009;121(2):174–84.

9. Rosenberg HF, Phipps S, Foster PS. Eosinophil trafficking in allergy and asthma. J Allergy Clin Immunol 2007;119(6):1303–10 [quiz: 1311–2].

10. Fabian I, Lass M, Kletter Y, et al. Differentiation and functional activity of human eosinophilic cells from an eosinophil HL-60 subline: response to recombinant hematopoietic growth factors. Blood 1992;80(3):788–94.

11. Flood-Page PT, Menzies-Gow AN, Kay AB, et al. Eosinophil's role remains uncertain as anti-interleukin-5 only partially depletes numbers in asthmatic airway. Am J Respir Crit Care Med 2003;167(2):199–204.

12. Wardlaw AJ. Molecular basis for selective eosinophil trafficking in asthma: a multistep paradigm. J Allergy Clin Immunol 1999;104(5):917–26.

13. Kariyawasam HH, Robinson DS. The eosinophil: the cell and its weapons, the cytokines, its locations. Semin Respir Crit Care Med 2006;27(2): 117–27.

14. Muessel MJ, Scott KS, Friedl P, et al. CCL11 and GM-CSF differentially use the Rho GTPase pathway to regulate motility of human eosinophils in a three-dimensional microenvironment. J Immunol 2008;180(12):8354–60.

15. Dewson G, Cohen GM, Wardlaw AJ. Interleukin-5 inhibits translocation of Bax to the mitochondria, cytochrome c release, and activation of caspases in human eosinophils. Blood 2001;98(7):2239–47.

16. Letuve S, Druilhe A, Grandsaigne M, et al. Involvement of caspases and of mitochondria in Fas ligation-induced eosinophil apoptosis: modulation by interleukin-5 and interferon-gamma. J Leukoc Biol 2001;70(5):767–75.

17. Woltmann G, McNulty CA, Dewson G, et al. Interleukin-13 induces PSGL-1/P-selectin-dependent adhesion of eosinophils, but not neutrophils, to human umbilical vein endothelial cells under flow. Blood 2000;95(10):3146–52.

18. Symon FA, Walsh GM, Watson SR, et al. Eosinophil adhesion to nasal polyp endothelium is P-selectin-dependent. J Exp Med 1994;180(1):371–6.

19. Fukuda T, Fukushima Y, Numao T, et al. Role of interleukin-4 and vascular cell adhesion molecule-1 in selective eosinophil migration into the airways in allergic asthma. Am J Respir Cell Mol Biol 1996;14(1):84–94.

20. Corren J, Lemanske RF, Hanania NA, et al. Lebrikizumab treatment in adults with asthma. N Engl J Med 2011;365(12):1088–98.

21. Johansson MW. Activation states of blood eosinophils in asthma. Clin Exp Allergy 2014;44(4):482–98.

22. Neighbour H, Boulet LP, Lemiere C, et al. Safety and efficacy of an oral CCR3 antagonist in patients with asthma and eosinophilic bronchitis: a randomized, placebo-controlled clinical trial. Clin Exp Allergy 2014;44(4):508–16.

23. Barnes N, Pavord I, Chuchalin A, et al. A randomized, double-blind, placebo-controlled study of the CRTH2 antagonist OC000459 in moderate persistent asthma. Clin Exp Allergy 2012;42(1):38–48.

24. Jacobsen EA, Lee NA, Lee JJ. Re-defining the unique roles for eosinophils in allergic respiratory inflammation. Clin Exp Allergy 2014;44(9):1119–36.

25. Wardlaw AJ, Kay AB. The role of the eosinophil in the pathogenesis of asthma. Allergy 1987;42(5):321–35.

26. Haldar P, Brightling CE, Hargadon B, et al. Mepolizumab and exacerbations of refractory eosinophilic asthma. N Engl J Med 2009;360(10):973–84.

27. Rothenberg ME, Klion AD, Roufosse FE, et al. Treatment of patients with the hyper-eosinophilic syndrome with mepolizumab. N Engl J Med 2008;358(12):1215–28.
28. Hargreave FE, Nair P. The definition and diagnosis of asthma. Clin Exp Allergy 2009;39(11):1652–8.
29. Hunter CJ, Brightling CE, Woltmann G, et al. A comparison of the validity of different diagnostic tests in adults with asthma. Chest 2002;121(4):1051–7.
30. Green RH, Brightling CE, McKenna S, et al. Asthma exacerbations and sputum eosinophil counts: a randomised controlled trial. Lancet 2002;360(9347): 1715–21.
31. Elliot JG, Jones RL, Abramson MJ, et al. Distribution of airway smooth muscle re-modelling in asthma: relation to airway inflammation. Respirology 2015;20(1): 66–72.
32. Ward C, Pais M, Bish R, et al. Airway inflammation, basement membrane thick-ening and bronchial hyperresponsiveness in asthma. Thorax 2002;57(4): 309–16.
33. Gonem S, Raj V, Wardlaw AJ, et al. Phenotyping airways disease: an A to E approach. Clin Exp Allergy 2012;42(12):1664–83.
34. Agbetile J, Fairs A, Desai D, et al. Isolation of filamentous fungi from sputum in asthma is associated with reduced post-bronchodilator FEV1. Clin Exp Allergy 2012;42(5):782–91.
35. Fairs A, Agbetile J, Hargadon B, et al. IgE sensitization to *Aspergillus fumigatus* is associated with reduced lung function in asthma. Am J Respir Crit Care Med 2010;182(11):1362–8.
36. Black PN, Udy AA, Brodie SM. Sensitivity to fungal allergens is a risk factor for life-threatening asthma. Allergy 2000;55(5):501–4.
37. Bousquet J, Mantzouranis E, Cruz AA, et al. Uniform definition of asthma severity, control, and exacerbations: document presented for the World Health Organiza-tion Consultation on Severe Asthma. J Allergy Clin Immunol 2010;126:926–38.
38. Louis R, Lau LC, Bron AO, et al. The relationship between airways inflammation and asthma severity. Am J Respir Crit Care Med 2000;161(1):9–16.
39. Newby C, Agbetile J, Hargadon B, et al. Lung function decline and variable airway inflammatory pattern: longitudinal analysis of severe asthma. J Allergy Clin Immunol 2014;134(2):287–94.
40. Lemiere C, Ernst P, Olivenstein R, et al. Airway inflammation assessed by invasive and noninvasive means in severe asthma: eosinophilic and noneosinophilic phe-notypes. J Allergy Clin Immunol 2006;118(5):1033–9.
41. Bacci E, Cianchetti S, Bartoli M, et al. Low sputum eosinophils predict the lack of response to beclomethasone in symptomatic asthmatic patients. Chest 2006; 129(3):565–72.
42. Chung KF, Pavord ID. Prevalence, pathogenesis, and causes of chronic cough. Lancet 2008;371(9621):1364–74.
43. Woolnough K, Fairs A, Pashley CH, et al. Allergic fungal airway disease: patho-physiologic and diagnostic considerations. Curr Opin Pulm Med 2015;21(1): 39–47.
44. Agarwal R, Chakrabarti A, Shah A, et al. Allergic bronchopulmonary aspergillosis: review of literature and proposal of new diagnostic and classification criteria. Clin Exp Allergy 2013;43(8):850–73.
45. Hinson KF, Moon AJ, Plummer NS. Broncho-pulmonary aspergillosis; a review and a report of eight new cases. Thorax 1952;7(4):317–33.
46. Patterson R, Greenberger PA, Radin RC, et al. Allergic bronchopulmonary asper-gillosis: staging as an aid to management. Ann Intern Med 1982;96(3):286–91.

47. Phillips J, Cardile AP, Patterson TF, et al. Daptomycin-induced acute eosinophilic pneumonia: analysis of the current data and illustrative case reports. Scand J Infect Dis 2013;45(10):804–8.
48. O'Driscoll BR, Howard LS, Davison AG, et al, British Thoracic Society. BTS guidelines for emergency oxygen use in adult patients. Thorax 2008;63(Suppl VI):vi1–68.
49. Buelow BJ, Kelly BT, Zafra HT, et al. Absence of peripheral eosinophilia on initial clinical presentation does not rule out the diagnosis of acute eosinophilic pneumonia. J Allergy Clin Immunol Pract 2015;15:S2213–98.
50. Jennette JC, Falk RJ, Bacon PA, et al. 2012 Revised International Chapel Hill Consensus Conference Nomenclature of Vasculitides. Arthritis Rheum 2013; 65(1):1–11.
51. Masi AT, Hunder GG, Lie JT, et al. The American College of Rheumatology 1990 criteria for the classification of Churg-Strauss syndrome (allergic granulomatosis and angiitis). Arthritis Rheum 1990;33(8):1094–100.
52. Khoury P, Grayson PC, Klion AD. Eosinophils in vasculitis: characteristics and roles in pathogenesis. Nat Rev Rheumatol 2014;10(8):474–83.
53. Mouthon L, Le Toumelin P, Andre MH, et al. Polyarteritis nodosa and Churg-Strauss angiitis: characteristics and outcome in 38 patients over 65 years. Medicine (Baltimore) 2002;81(1):27–40.
54. Guillevin L, Cohen P, Gayraud M, et al. Churg-Strauss syndrome. Clinical study and long-term follow-up of 96 patients. Medicine (Baltimore) 1999;78(1):26–37.
55. Ogbogu PU, Bochner BS, Butterfield JH, et al. Hypereosinophilic syndrome: a multicenter, retrospective analysis of clinical characteristics and response to therapy. J Allergy Clin Immunol 2009;124(6):1319–25.e3.
56. Spry CJ, Davies J, Tai PC, et al. Clinical features of fifteen patients with the hypereosinophilic syndrome. Q J Med 1983;52(205):1–22.
57. Lombard CM, Tazelaar HD, Krasne DL. Pulmonary eosinophilia in coccidioidal infections. Chest 1987;91(5):734–6.
58. Fleury-Feith J, Van Nhieu JT, Picard C, et al. Bronchoalveolar lavage eosinophilia associated with *Pneumocystis carinii* pneumonitis in AIDS patients. Comparative study with non-AIDS patients. Chest 1989;95(6):1198–201.
59. Martinez-Garcia MA, Cases-Viedma E, Cordero-Rodriguez P, et al. Diagnostic utility of eosinophils in the pleural fluid. Eur Respir J 2000;15:166–9.
60. Wenzel SE, Schwartz LB, Langmack EL, et al. Evidence that severe asthma can be divided pathologically into two inflammatory subtypes with distinct physiologic and clinical characteristics. Am J Respir Crit Care Med 1999;160(3):1001–8.
61. Ward R, Woltmann G, Wardlaw AJ, et al. Between-observer repeatability of sputum differential cell counts. Influence of cell viability and squamous cell contamination. Clin Exp Allergy 1999;29(2):248–52.
62. Leuppi JD, Salome CM, Jenkins CR, et al. Predictive markers of asthma exacerbation during stepwise dose reduction of inhaled corticosteroids. Am J Respir Crit Care Med 2001;163(2):406–12.
63. Roufosse F, Weller PF. Practical approach to the patient with hypereosinophilia. J Allergy Clin Immunol 2010;126(1):39–44.
64. Chung KF, Wenzel SE, Brozek JL, et al. International ERS/ATS guidelines on definition, evaluation and treatment of severe asthma. Eur Respir J 2014;43:343–73.
65. Petsky HL, Cates CJ, Lasserson TJ, et al. A systematic review and meta-analysis: tailoring asthma treatment on eosinophilic markers (exhaled nitric oxide or sputum eosinophils). Thorax 2012;67:199–208.
66. Nair P, Pizzichini MM, Kjarsgaard M, et al. Mepolizumab for prednisone-dependent asthma with sputum eosinophilia. N Engl J Med 2009;360:985–93.

67. Pope-Harman AL, Davis WB, Allen ED, et al. Acute eosinophilic pneumonia. A summary of 15 cases and review of the literature. Medicine (Baltimore) 1996; 75(6):334–42.
68. Marchand E, Reynaud-Gaubert M, Lauque D, et al. Idiopathic chronic eosinophilic pneumonia. A clinical and follow-up study of 62 cases. The Groupe d'Etudes et de Recherche sur les Maladies "Orphelines" Pulmonaires (GERM"O"P). Medicine (Baltimore) 1998;77(5):299–312.
69. Wark PA, Gibson PG, Wilson AJ. Azoles for allergic bronchopulmonary aspergillosis associated with asthma. Cochrane Database Syst Rev 2004;(3):CD001108.
70. Denning DW, O'Driscoll BR, Powell G, et al. Randomized controlled trial of oral antifungal treatment for severe asthma with fungal sensitization: The Fungal Asthma Sensitization Trial (FAST) study. Am J Respir Crit Care Med 2009;179: 11–8.
71. Agbetile J, Bourne M, Fairs A, et al. Effectiveness of voriconazole in the treatment of *Aspergillus fumigatus*-associated asthma (EVITA3 study). J Allergy Clin Immunol 2014;134:33–9.
72. Katzenstein AL, Liebow AA, Friedman PJ. Bronchocentric granulomatosis, mucoid impaction, and hypersensitivity reactions to fungi. Am Rev Respir Dis 1975;111(4):497–537.

Eosinophilia in Infectious Diseases

Elise M. O'Connell, MD*, Thomas B. Nutman, MD

KEYWORDS

- Eosinophilia • Infection • Fever • Travel • Immigrant • Refugee

KEY POINTS

- Eosinophilia greater than 1000/μL in the setting of acute illness essentially excludes bacteria or viruses as an etiology for the acute illness.
- Strongyloidiasis is found worldwide, including in areas of the United States. Anyone with eosinophilia who comes from an endemic area should have a serologic test performed if available.
- Acute schistosomiasis should be suspected in any traveler returning from Africa with eosinophilia and fever.
- Immigrants or refugees can have very subtle or no symptoms from parasitic infections and often have very mild eosinophilia.
- Some helminth infections can persist for many years after acquisition.

INTRODUCTION

Eosinophilia can be caused by both infectious and noninfectious processes, many of which may be clinically indistinguishable. Narrowing the differential diagnosis can be achieved by considering the type of patient, accompanying symptoms, duration of eosinophilia, and, to a certain extent, the degree of eosinophilia. In general, refugees/immigrants originally from resource-limited countries, along with travelers/expatriates to these same areas, have a high likelihood of eosinophilia being caused by parasitic helminth infections. Patients from high-income countries without a significant travel history are much more likely to have allergic, autoimmune, malignancy-related, or other underlying causes for their eosinophilia.

The authors have nothing to disclose.

This work was supported by the Division of Intramural Research, National Institute of Allergy and Infectious Diseases.

Helminth Immunology Section, Laboratory of Parasitic Diseases, National Institute of Allergy and Infectious Diseases, National Institutes of Health, 4 Center Drive, Building 4, Room B105, Bethesda, MD 20892, USA

* Corresponding author.

E-mail address: oconnellem@mail.nih.gov

Immunol Allergy Clin N Am 35 (2015) 493–522

http://dx.doi.org/10.1016/j.iac.2015.05.003

0889-8561/15/$ – see front matter Published by Elsevier Inc.

immunology.theclinics.com

Thus, in this review, we discuss the infectious causes of eosinophilia in travelers, nontravelers, and immigrants separately, and examine the causes in the context of symptom location and/or organ system involvement. Because most *infectious* causes of peripheral blood eosinophilia are parasitic, this review has an emphasis on eosinophilia in the traveler and immigrant/refugee, who are most likely to acquire these infections. For simplicity, we define eosinophilia as an absolute eosinophil count of greater than 500/μL and classify less than 1000/μL as being mild and those greater than 1500/μL as being marked.

INITIAL APPROACH

Eosinophilia is often identified as part of a complete blood count done either routinely or as part of an evaluation for a particular symptom complex. It is helpful to know whether the eosinophilia has developed acutely or is chronic (**Table 1**), although this is not always possible. In the setting of an acute febrile illness with eosinophilia, however, historical eosinophil counts become less important. If eosinophilia (particularly >1000/μL) is found in the context of fever, the same process driving the eosinophilia is most likely causing the acute illness. Studies have demonstrated suppression of peripheral eosinophil counts in patients during acute bacterial and viral infections.[2,3] Therefore, eosinophilia in the context of an acute illness points toward a noninfectious (eg, autoimmune), parasitic (eg, acute schistosomiasis), or fungal (eg, coccidiomycosis) etiology as the cause of the illness.[2]

In helminth infections, eosinophilia is usually most pronounced early in infection, coinciding with the larval migration through tissues, which then slowly decreases over time. Protozoa, in general, do not cause eosinophilia, with the exception of *Cystisospora belli* and *Sarcocystis* spp. Although human immunodeficiency virus (HIV) alone is unlikely to be a significant cause of eosinophilia, HIV status should be assessed in all patients presenting with eosinophilia, as it increases suspicion for eosinophilia-associated diseases not seen in immunocompetent patients (eg, eosinophilic folliculitis, *C belli*).[4–6]

A thorough review of symptoms and physical examination should be performed on every patient with eosinophilia of unknown etiology. A detailed travel history, including residence abroad should be assessed to classify the type of patient and guide the evaluation, as some helminth infections can persist for decades after leaving endemic areas (eg, the filariae, schistosomes, Echinococcus, *Strongyloides stercoralis*). Medications (including over the counter and dietary supplements) must be reviewed, as they are a common cause of otherwise asymptomatic eosinophilia. Notably, a stool ova and parasite examination can be helpful in diagnosing some hepatobiliary/intestinal parasites (**Table 2**), but is a relatively insensitive test. Symptoms often do not correspond with when eggs will be found in the stool, and many parasites that cause eosinophilia are not found in the stool.

EOSINOPHILIA IN THE SHORT-TERM TRAVELER

The locations of (see **Table 1**) and exposures during (including consumption of raw/undercooked meat or seafood and water contact) travel and symptoms should guide the clinical evaluation with respect to infectious diseases. Although many of the following infections can be subclinical in some patients, we discuss them with their most typical presenting characteristics. Notably, however, ascariasis most commonly presents without any symptoms. Rarely, Loeffler syndrome (cough, low-grade fevers, transient lung infiltrates, and mild to marked eosinophilia) occurs 3 to 9 days after infection with *Ascaris*.[15,16]

Table 1
Infectious causes of eosinophilia and likelihood of seeing listed etiologies in practice in North America or Europe as well as geographic locations of acquisition, duration of eosinophilia, and main anatomic site affected

Eosinophilia Cause (Infectious Etiology)	Main Geographic Location(s)	Duration of Eosinophilia[a]		Main Anatomic Site(s) of Infection
		Acute	Chronic	
Common causes of acute eosinophilia seen in clinical practice in North America and Europe[a,b]				
Coccidioides spp[c]	Southwest United States	X	—	Lungs, skin, CNS, liver
Echinococcus granulosus (days following rupture)	Europe, South America, Australia	X	—	Liver, lung
Fasciola spp	South America, Europe, Asia, Egypt	X	—	Liver
Schistosoma haematobium	Throughout Africa, specifically the Nile, large rivers and lakes as well as smaller bodies of freshwater	X	X	Genitourinary tract
Schistosoma mansoni	Africa, South America, Caribbean	X	X	Liver, GI
Trichinella spp	Worldwide	X	X	Muscle, GI
Causes of acute eosinophilia rarely seen in clinical practice in North America and Europe				
Anisakis spp[d]	Japan, Europe	X	—	GI
Ascaris lumbricoides	Latin America, Sub-Saharan Africa, Asia, Western Pacific	X	—	GI
Angiostrongylus cantonensis	Southeast Asia, Pacific Basin, Africa, Caribbean, Central America	X	—	CNS
Cystoisospora belli (formerly Isospora belli)	Tropical regions	X	X	—
Dirofilaria immitis	Worldwide	X	—	Lung
Gnathostoma spp	Southeast Asia, Latin America	X	X	Subcutaneous tissue, CNS
Hookworm (Ancylostoma duodenale and Necator americanus)	Latin America, Sub-Saharan Africa, Asia, Western Pacific	X	X	GI
Paragonimus kellicotti	Mississippi River drainage basin, United States,[1] most from Missouri	X	X	Lungs, subcutaneous tissue, CNS

(continued on next page)

Table 1
(continued)

Eosinophilia Cause (Infectious Etiology)	Main Geographic Location(s)	Duration of Eosinophilia[a]		Main Anatomic Site(s) of Infection
		Acute	Chronic	
Sarcocystis spp	Southeast Asia, especially Malaysia	X	—	Muscle, GI; Subcutaneous, skin
Causes of acute eosinophilia extremely rarely seen in clinical practice in North America and Europe				
Schistosoma intercalatum	Central and West Africa	X	X	Liver, GI
Schistosoma japonicum	Indonesia, China, Southeast Asia	X	X	Liver, GI
Schistosoma mekongi	Cambodia, Laos	X	X	Liver, GI
Toxocara spp (visceral larval migrans)	Worldwide	X	X	Liver, eye, lung
Basidiobolus ranarum	Worldwide, especially South US	X	—	GI
Baylisascaris procyonis	North America	X	—	CNS, eye, liver, lung
Capillaria hepatica	Worldwide	X	—	Liver
Dicrocoeliasis (*Dicrocoelium dendriticum*)	Europe, Middle East, northern Asia, North America, northern Africa	X	—	Hepatobiliary, GI
Echinostoma spp	Asia	X	—	GI
Myiasis (especially *Hypoderma* spp)	Northern Hemisphere	X	—	Subcutaneous, skin, rarely deeper tissues
Sparganosis (*Spirometra* spp, *Sparganum proliferum*)	Asia, rare sporadic reports worldwide	X	—	Subcutaneous, skin, eye, CNS
Tropical pulmonary eosinophilia	South Asia	X	X	Lungs
Trichostrongyloides spp	Worldwide	X	X	GI
Causes of chronic eosinophilia commonly seen in clinical practice in North America and Europe				
Strongyloides stercoralis[e]	Worldwide	X	X	GI, skin
Clonorchis spp	East Asia	X	X	Hepatobiliary
Opisthorchis spp	Southeast Asia, former Soviet Union	X	X	Hepatobiliary
Paragonimus spp (non-kellicotti)	Southeast Asia, Central/West Africa, Latin America	X	X	Hepatobiliary

Causes of chronic eosinophilia rarely seen in clinical practice in North America and Europe

Loa loa	Central/West Africa	X	X	Subcutaneous tissue, eye
Lymphatic filariasis (Wuchereria bancrofti, Brugia malayi)	Sub-Saharan Africa, Southeast Asia (Including India), Western Pacific	X	X	Lymphatics, blood
Mansonella ozzardi	Latin America, the Caribbean	X	X	Blood
Mansonella perstans	Sub-Saharan Africa, South America	X	X	Blood
Mansonella streptocerca	Africa	X	X	Skin
Onchocerca volvulus	Sub-Saharan Africa	X	X	Skin, subcutaneous tissue

Abbreviations: CNS, central nervous system; GI, gastrointestinal; X, applicable.

a Although many diseases listed here can present as either chronic or acute eosinophilia (as indicated by this column), disease etiologies have been grouped by their most common presentations.

b Some listed processes are more likely to cause eosinophilia than others. This table is organized by what the clinician in North America or Europe is most likely to see in terms of causes of eosinophilia in their clinical practice (which takes into account generally how often the organism causes eosinophilia and how common people are infected and seek medical attention).

c Most often seen in Western United States, very rare in Europe.

d When seen in Europe, it is mostly in the Netherlands, Spain, and Italy, extremely rare in the United States.

e Strongyloidiasis is by far the most common infectious cause of chronic eosinophilia.

Table 2
Parasitic causes of eosinophilia and diagnostic tests of choice

Parasite	Diagnostic Test
Angiostrongylus	Larvae in CSF, PCR of CSF (CDC)
Anisakis spp	<12 h from raw fish/squid ingestion: EGD for visualization of larvae >12 h from ingestion: anti-Anisakis IgG and IgA[7]
Ascaris lumbricoides	Eggs in stool, serology
Baylisascaris procyonis	Larva or larval tracks seen on ocular examination Serology (EIA, reference laboratory)
Basidiobolus ranarum	Fungal elements on histopathologic examination, fungal culture of surgical specimen
Brachylaima spp	Eggs in stool
Capillaria hepatica	Eggs/worms on liver biopsy Serology—high titer (low titer indicates spurious infection from ingesting infected liver)
Coccidioides spp	Fungal elements on histopathologic examination, fungal culture of surgical specimen, serology (complement fixation)
Clonorchis spp	Eggs in stool, serology (not available in United States)
Cystoisospora belli (formerly Isospora belli)	Oocysts in stool
Dicrocoelium dendriticum	Ova in stool (after abstaining from ingestion of liver)
Dirofilaria immitis	Worm in surgical specimen, appearance on radiograph
Echinococcus granulosus	Combination of imaging (appearance on ultrasound or CT) and serology (50%–75% sensitive)[8]
Fasciola spp	Serology Eggs in stool (late in disease)
Gnathostoma spp	Larvae in biopsy, serology (reference laboratory tests)
Hookworm (Ancylostoma duodenale and Necator americanus)	Eggs in stool
Loa loa	MF in midday blood (concentrate with filtration) Serology (nonspecific filarial antibody, reference laboratory tests) Presence of eyeworm

Lymphatic filariasis (*Wuchereria bancrofti, Brugia malayi*)	MF in nighttime blood (concentrate with filtration) Serology (nonspecific filarial antibody, reference laboratory tests) Circulating filarial antigen card test (not available in United States)
Mansonella perstans, Mansonella ozzardi	MF in blood (concentrate with filtration)
Mansonella streptocerca	Skin snips
Onchocerca volvulus	Skin snips, serology (nonspecific filarial antibody, reference laboratory tests)
Opisthorchis spp	Eggs in stool
Paragonimus spp	Serology (ELISA or immunoblot)[9,10] Eggs in sputum (sensitivity 60%, 2 samples)[11] Eggs in stool (insensitive)[12]
Sarcocystis spp	Muscle biopsy
Schistosoma haematobium	Eggs in urine, serology
Schistosoma intercalatum	Eggs in stool, serology
Schistosoma japonicum	Eggs in stool, serology
Schistosoma mansoni	Eggs in stool/rectal biopsy, serology
Schistosoma mekongi	Eggs in stool
Strongyloides stercoralis	Serology (SSIR and NIE IgG LIPS sensitivity 100%, spec 100%),[13] larvae in stool (insensitive except in hyperinfection)
Sparganosis (*Spirometra* spp, *Sparganum proliferum*)	Sparganum in infected tissue For CNS disease, positive CSF ELISA, typical CT findings, and history of eating frogs or snakes from endemic area strongly supports diagnosis[14]
Toxocara canis (visceral larva migrans)	Serology, larvae in liver biopsy (rarely seen)
Trichinella spp	Serology, muscle biopsy
Trichostrongyloides spp	Eggs in stool

Abbreviations: CDC, Centers for Disease Control and Prevention; CNS, central nervous system; CSF, cerebrospinal fluid; CT, computed tomography; EGD, esophagogastroduodenoscopy; EIA, enzyme immunoassay; ELISA, enzyme-linked immunosorbent assay; Ig, immunoglobulin; LIPS, Luciferase Immunoprecipitation Systems; MF, Microfilariae; PCR, polymerase chain reaction.

Infectious Causes of Eosinophilia and Fevers in the Traveler

Fevers associated with peripheral eosinophilia in a traveler are most commonly associated with acute schistosomiasis, infections with other flukes, or with a drug reaction. We discuss, in turn, those infections in which fever and eosinophilia are associated with particular symptom complexes.

Eosinophilia with fevers and abdominal and/or pulmonary symptoms in the traveler

Acute schistosomiasis ("Katayama fever") Acute schistosomiasis ("Katayama fever") is one of the most common causes of travel-acquired eosinophilia.[17] Although symptom onset varies slightly depending on the schistosome species, symptoms often begin 3 to 4 weeks (range 2–9) after infection[18] that occurs through contact with cercarial-containing fresh water. The most common presenting complaints are a combination of malaise, myalgia, diarrhea, cough, abdominal pain, fevers, and/or headache.[17–22] A minority of patients develop urticaria with the onset of symptoms. Despite its eponym, up to 30% of patients never have fever.[17] Hepatomegaly and mild liver enzyme elevations may be seen. Eosinophilia is present in nearly all patients, commonly ranging between 3000 to 7000/μL.[17,19] Symptoms improve over several weeks to months,[20] even in the absence of treatment. Eggs are only detectable in the urine/stool at approximately 6 weeks after exposure, whereas schistosome-specific immunoglobulin (Ig) M is detectable at 4 to 5 weeks and IgG at 5 to 8 weeks after exposure.[18] With treatment, eosinophil counts often normalize within 4 to 12 months.[17,19]

Fascioliasis Fascioliasis is acquired by ingesting contaminated freshwater vegetables or water (see **Table 1**). Patients typically present with fevers, leukocytosis, high-grade eosinophilia, and right upper quadrant pain.[23–25] Elevated serum transaminases with normal bilirubin levels are commonly seen. Computed tomography (CT) during this time shows non–contrast-enhancing, low-attenuated liver lesions,[26] and liver biopsy often shows eosinophilic granulomas.[23] Over 2 to 4 months without treatment, symptoms and eosinophilia may slowly improve as the larvae migrate to the biliary tree, at which time intermittent elevations in bilirubin and liver transaminases may be seen as a reflection of biliary obstruction.[27] At this stage, eggs may be seen on stool examination.

Opisthorchiasis Opisthorchiasis is endemic to Southeast Asia and the states of the former Soviet Union, although in recent years outbreaks in visitors to Italy have been reported.[28,29] Two to 3 weeks after ingestion of raw fish, symptoms of fever, abdominal pain, headache, diarrhea, nausea, and vomiting can be seen, occasionally accompanied by jaundice. Laboratory abnormalities may lag slightly behind the clinical course and consist of cholestatic liver enzyme abnormalities with peripheral eosinophilia. The severity of cholestasis correlates with degree of eosinophilia, which is typically very marked and commonly exceeds 10,000/μL. CT can reveal hypodense lesions in the liver. Eggs are not detected in the stool until at least 5 weeks following infection. Symptoms respond quickly to treatment and eosinophilia normalizes within 3 months.[28–31]

Clonorchiasis Clonorchiasis is endemic to East and Southeast Asia. Unlike opisthorchiasis, acute infections with *Clonorchis* spp are typically clinically asymptomatic or with subtle, nonspecific complaints.[32] However, particularly in travelers, an acute syndrome with right upper quadrant pain, nausea, and occasional fever or cough may develop.[32,33] Eosinophilia is typically greater than 1500/μL, and eggs appear in the stool 3 to 4 weeks after infection.[33]

Gnathostomiasis Gnathostomiasis is endemic in most Asian countries and is increasing in prevalence in Latin America. Larvae are ingested from raw fish, shellfish, eel, frog, or chicken. Within 24 to 48 hours following ingestion of contaminated food, patients may develop severe abdominal pain with nausea, vomiting, and diarrhea along with generalized malaise, urticaria, headache, and fever. Often there is a marked eosinophilia during this time.[34–37] After this acute stage, migratory swellings typically develop (see later in this article). Occasionally, visceral involvement may occur in the setting of migration of larvae through the lungs (effusions, cough, hemoptysis), the abdomen (mass, abdominal pain, hematuria), the eyes (anterior uveitis), and even the central nervous system (CNS) (**Table 3**).[34]

Paragonimiasis Paragonimiasis is most commonly caused by *Paragonimus westermani* in Southeast Asia (other species are found elsewhere). Infection is usually acquired through ingestion of uncooked crab or crayfish. Fever is a frequent (but not universal) finding, along with dyspnea, chest pain, cough, and hemoptysis that begin several months after exposure.[64–66] Eosinophilia is typically marked,[9] and peaks 1 to 2 months following the onset of illness (correlates with pleural involvement). The eosinophilia slowly decreases as the parenchymal disease evolves.[67]

Capillariasis Capillariasis due to *Capillaria hepatica* is an extremely unusual illness (<100 reported cases) that can be acquired through ingestion of contaminated soil.[68,69] Patients present with fevers (83%), hepatomegaly (87%), and eosinophilia (87%).[70] Liver transaminases are commonly elevated, and very rarely, elevations of bilirubin and jaundice are seen.[70] The severity of infection appears proportional to the number of mature eggs ingested.[71,72] Imaging reveals space-occupying lesions,[68,72,73] and liver biopsies can show adult worms, eggs, and/or inflammatory cells with eosinophils and granulomata.[70]

Eosinophilia with fevers and myositis in the traveler
Trichinellosis Trichinellosis is caused by consumption of undercooked domestic pork, wild boar, bear, deer, and walrus.[74–77] The average incubation period is 1 to 4 weeks depending on larval load and the *Trichinella* species.[74,75,78,79] Approximately 90% of patients present with an absolute eosinophil count greater than 1000/μL. Nearly all patients have fever and myalgia as presenting complaints (occasionally preceded by diarrhea), and edema (including periorbital or facial) is seen in most patients. Creatine phosphokinase (CPK) is elevated in 60% to 85%, and liver transaminases may be elevated 5 to 10 times above normal levels. The acute illness typically improves in 2 to 5 weeks, but myalgia can take months to resolve. Eosinophilia can take 6 months or longer to normalize.[74,75,78–81]

Muscular sarcocystosis Muscular sarcocystosis has occurred in travelers in several recent outbreaks after visiting rural peninsular Malaysia,[82] Pangkor Island,[83] and Tioman Island.[84] In these outbreaks, 2 to 8 weeks following exposure patients developed fever and myalgia, sometimes preceded by a short diarrheal illness. Other prominent symptoms were fatigue and headache. Less commonly seen was weakness, rash, or muscle swelling (including facial swelling). Commonly the muscles of mastication, back muscles, and calf muscles were involved. Eosinophilia and CPK elevations are very frequently seen (although not universally), and may not develop until after initial clinical presentation. Symptoms usually last for approximately 2 months (although relapse is possible). Cardiac involvement has been reported.[85,86]

Eosinophilia with fevers and central nervous system symptoms in the traveler
See section titled "Eosinophilic meningitis."

Table 3
Infectious causes and symptoms of eosinophilic meningitis

| | | | MRI Abnormalities | | | Eosinophilia | |
| | | | White Matter Increased Signal on T2/FLAIR | Hydrocephalus | Mass Lesion(s) | Frequency of Peripheral Eosinophilia | CSF Degree of Eosinophilia |
Organism	Risk	Symptoms					
Angiostrongylus cantonensis[38-40]	Consumption of raw snails, frogs, shellfish, fish, or contaminated vegetables or water	HA, NV	X	—	—	77%–90%	+++
Baylisascaris procyonis[41-43]	Ingestion of eggs in raccoon feces (toddlers/young children)	Fever, ataxia, developmental regression, SZ	X	X	—	5%–45%	+++
Coccidioides spp[44-48]	Residing in endemic area; males of Hispanic, African, and Asian ethnicity; immunocompromised (HIV, steroid use)	HA, AMS, fever	—	X	X	19%–75%	+/−
Gnathostoma spp[34,49]	Ingestion of uncooked fish, amphibians, reptiles, poultry, pork from endemic area (see **Table 1**)	Sudden pain followed by limb paralysis, urinary retention, AMS	X	—	—	~50%	++
Paragonimus spp[50]	Consuming uncooked freshwater crabs or crayfish	HA, NV, paralysis, SZ	—	—	X	~88%	+/−
Schistosoma spp[51-55]	Freshwater contact in an endemic area (see **Table 1**)	HA, AMS, SZ, limb weakness	—	—	X	>50%	+/−
Spirometra spp, *Sparganum proliferum*[14,56]	Ingestion of snakes, frogs, or untreated freshwater	SZ, hemiparesis, HA	X	X	X	~25%	ND
Taenia solium (Neurocysticercosis)[57-61]	Ingestion of stool from a human infected with pig tapeworm	SZ, HA, NV, AMS	—	X	X	—	+
Toxocara canis or *Toxocara cati*[62,63]	Ingestion of eggs in dog/cat feces	AMS, SZ, paralysis	—	—	X	>50%	++

Abbreviations: +, fewer than 50 eosinophils/μL; ++, 50–500 eosinophils/μL; +++, more than 500 eosinophils/μL; +/−, eosinophils may or may not be seen; AMS, altered mental status; HA, Headache; ND, no data; NV, nausea/vomiting; SZ, seizure; X, applicable.

Infectious Causes of Eosinophilia and Gastrointestinal Symptoms (Without Fever) in the Traveler

Travel-associated diarrhea is overwhelmingly associated with bacterial causes.[87] However, in travelers returning from low-income and middle-income countries, helminth infections are the most common etiology of abdominal complaints when accompanied by eosinophilia.[88,89]

Hookworm infections

Hookworm infections are endemic worldwide and typically cause abdominal pain, increased flatus, nausea, vomiting, and diarrhea approximately 30 to 45 days following infection, coinciding with a significant rise in peripheral blood eosinophils.[90] Loeffler syndrome (transient pulmonary infiltrates due to larval migration through the lungs) with low-grade fevers may occur before the development of abdominal symptoms (approximately 8 to 21 days after infection) in some cases, but most people are asymptomatic in the prepatent period.[90] Marked eosinophilia frequently develops (1500 to 4000/μL) and often diminishes to a small degree at the time of patency. Eggs appear in the stool 1 to 2 months after exposure. Following treatment, eosinophil counts typically normalize within 2 to 3 months.[90]

Strongyloidiasis

Strongyloidiasis is rarely acquired in the short-term traveler,[91] likely due to the need for bare skin to have prolonged contact with soil for transmission to occur, as well as the reduced relative frequency of travel to Africa and Asia, where it is most frequently acquired. It causes mild eosinophilia (in 88% of infected patients)[92] that can be associated with diarrhea, abdominal discomfort, or no symptoms at all.[93]

Cystoisospora belli (formerly Isospora belli)

Cystoisospora belli (formerly Isospora belli) is a protozoan found worldwide, especially in tropical and subtropical areas. In the otherwise healthy host, it causes a self-limited diarrheal illness with transient fever and weight loss that can last 2 to 6 weeks, but can take longer to resolve in rare cases.[94–97] In the setting of immunosuppression, diarrhea with malabsorption, dehydration, and weight loss are common. Symptoms may persist for months, and may be the presenting manifestation of underlying malignancy, HIV, or primary immunodeficiency.[98–101] In approximately 50% of patients, a mild eosinophilia is seen over the course of illness.[102,103]

Echinostomiasis

Echinostomiasis (Echinostoma spp) is caused by intestinal flukes endemic in East Asia and is acquired through ingesting uncooked freshwater or brackish water fish, shellfish, and amphibians.[104] Within a few weeks, a diarrheal illness with abdominal pain can be seen with accompanying eosinophilia that peaks 4 weeks after infection.[105]

Infectious Causes of Eosinophilia and Allergic or Dermatologic/Soft Tissue Symptoms in the Traveler

Anisakiasis

Anisakiasis is most common in Japan and Europe (mostly Spain). It causes a spectrum of illness that ranges from severe acute abdominal pain secondary to edema of the stomach or small intestine to a purely allergic reaction (ie, urticaria, angioedema, or anaphylaxis) without abdominal symptoms. Some patients present with an overlapping symptom complex that includes abdominal pain and urticaria or angioedema (rarely anaphylaxis).[106] The key to the diagnosis is eliciting the history of recent raw fish ingestion. In the case of acute upper gastrointestinal (GI) symptoms, raw fish was often ingested within hours of symptom development, whereas those with more lower GI tract symptoms may present several days after raw fish consumption. Typical CT imaging in the cases with abdominal symptoms reveals thickened, edematous walls of the stomach or proximal small intestine.[7] Eosinophilia typically does not develop until several days after the onset of clinical symptoms.[107]

Ascariasis

Ascariasis is endemic worldwide and is acquired through fecal-oral contamination. With heavy inoculum, *Ascaris lumbricoides* infection can cause generalized urticaria shortly after infection,[16] although typically the infection is subclinical.

Cutaneous larva migrans

Cutaneous larva migrans is a common travel-related infection acquired on beaches in tropical areas. Days to weeks following skin contact with contaminated sand, linear, serpiginous, highly pruritic cutaneous lesions develop due to dog/cat hookworm (*Ancylostoma canium*, *Ancylostoma braziliense*) larvae penetrating intact skin. Pruritus and lesions last several weeks to months if not treated. Mild peripheral blood eosinophilia is seen in fewer than 10% of patients.[108–110]

Onchocerciasis

Onchocerciasis is transmitted by the bite of the black fly in much of Africa. In travelers, symptoms often start within months following exposure, but there may be a significant time interval between exposure and symptom development.[111–113] The most common manifestations are pruritus, rash (commonly a papular dermatitis), and fixed extremity swelling.[112–115] In 80% of travelers, marked eosinophilia is seen (1000 to 2000/μL),[89,113,114] but microfilariae are difficult to find in skin snips from travelers because of the relatively low burden of infection that results from a short exposure.[113,116]

Lymphatic filariasis

Lymphatic filariasis is rarely found in returned travelers, although it has been reported.[111,117] Symptoms usually develop 1 to 2 months following infection.[118] Extremity edema (proximal > distal) or scrotal swelling, which may be associated with a painful lymph node and mild to marked eosinophilia, are the most notable findings.[117]

Loiasis

Loiasis, caused by *Loa loa* in travelers to Central/West Africa, is frequently very symptomatic in those acquiring the infection through travel.[119] However, microfilariae are not often detected in the blood in these patients.[120,121] The minimum latency period appears to be 4 to 6 months,[121] but it may take years[122] after infection for symptoms to develop. In the visitor and expatriate, Calabar swellings (migratory angioedema) on the limbs and/or face are the most common symptoms. The swellings are nonpainful and nonpruritic, but can occasionally appear erythematous, and typically resolve in 1 to 3 days.[123] Other symptoms commonly seen are pruritus and urticaria.[121] Eosinophilia is essentially universal in nonendemic patients, typically marked (average is 3000 to 4000/μL)[119,120,122] and may mediate some of the pathologic findings in this infection.

Gnathostomiasis

Gnathostomiasis, acquired most commonly from uncooked fish in Southeast Asia or Latin America, causes subcutaneous nodules or swellings, which migrate to various areas of the body and can last for years. It may begin shortly after an acute febrile gastrointestinal illness, but this stage may be subclinical or occur weeks to months before onset of cutaneous symptoms.[34] The swellings frequently last 1 to 2 weeks at a time and are associated with pruritus, erythema, pain,[34,124] or without other symptoms.[120] In one series of patients with chronic migratory swellings, only 50% had eosinophilia (900 to 2000/μL), which normalized following treatment.[125]

Paragonimiasis
Paragonimiasis can cause nontender, migratory subcutaneous nodules that rarely appear at the time of pulmonary involvement,[9,66] but more commonly precede lung symptoms, or can occur without other symptoms altogether.[9,126] Lesions are typically on the abdominal wall,[127] and have rarely been reported in travelers.[126]

Eosinophilia in the traveler conclusions
Despite extensive evaluation, up to 60% of travelers with eosinophilia never have an underlying cause defined for their eosinophilia identified.[89,92] In the cases in which patients remain asymptomatic and testing is negative, it is reasonable to simply monitor the eosinophil count periodically, as most eosinophilia in these cases will self-resolve. Another approach is to treat empirically for soil-transmitted helminths and flukes with a 1-day treatment of albendazole, ivermectin, and praziquantel, and monitor for eosinophil resolution.

EOSINOPHILIA IN INDIGENOUS POPULATIONS (IMMIGRANT/REFUGEES) AND LONG-TERM RESIDENTS

All of the short-term travel-associated infections can be seen in these patients, particularly in immigrants who return abroad to visit friends and relatives, as they are more likely to acquire new helminth infections on short trips compared with tourists.[128] Patients with chronic, long-standing exposure to parasitic infections typically have more subtle or different symptoms, and eosinophilia, when present, is less impressive. Therefore, for some infections already mentioned, we again discuss them here, highlighting the differences in symptom complexes in the immigrant/refugee.[19,119,120,129,130]

Infectious Causes of Eosinophilia and Gastrointestinal Symptoms in the Immigrant

Echinococcosis
Echinococcosis due to *Echinococcus granulosus* (hydatid cysts), while not commonly associated with eosinophilia,[131,132] can cause intermittent eosinophilia[8,133–136] likely due to spontaneous cyst leakage or occult intrabiliary rupture.[137] However, immediately following a clinically significant cyst rupture (often iatrogenic), eosinophil counts are transiently suppressed (<500) and neutrophils significantly increase.[138–140] Eosinophils then progressively rise to moderately high levels over the next several days to weeks.[140–142] Abdominal pain with an elevated bilirubin is seen if the cyst ruptures into the biliary tree. Cysts also can grow large and cause symptoms related to mass effect. Less commonly, cysts develop in the lungs causing respiratory symptoms or pain.[131] *Echinococcus multilocularis* is associated with eosinophilia less frequently that with *E. granulosis,* but rarely, mild eosinophil elevations may be seen.[143–146]

Ascariasis
Ascariasis, particularly in children, can cause abdominal complaints in patients from endemic areas due to heavy worm burdens, which can cause intestinal obstruction,[147] appendicitis,[148] or cholangitis.[149] In chronic infection, eosinophilia is not common and when present is mild.[150–152]

Trichuriasis
Trichuriasis can, in situations in which there are extremely large worm burdens, cause a dysentery syndrome that is associated with a mild to marked eosinophilia, severe

iron deficiency anemia, and rectal prolapse (the latter 2 more commonly seen in children).[153–155]

Strongyloidiasis

Strongyloidiasis can persist for many decades after infection because of its autoinfective cycle. Although chronic strongyloidiasis is typically asymptomatic, clinical findings, including chronic abdominal discomfort, excessive flatus, and/or diarrhea, are present in up to 16% of patients.[156,157] Refugees with proven S stercoralis infection have eosinophilia approximately 25% of the time.[129]

Opisthorchis and Clonorchis

Opisthorchis and Clonorchis are biliary flukes that, although distributed differently geographically, in chronic form are largely indistinguishable clinically. Chronic infections are typically asymptomatic or accompanied by nonspecific abdominal symptoms (pain, flatulence, dyspepsia). Alterations in liver enzymes or bilirubin are not seen unless complications develop (ie, cholangitis, cholelithiasis, cholangiocarcinoma). Most patients have a mild eosinophilia (<1000/µL). Ultrasound findings of increased periductal echogenicity (indicating periductal fibrosis) are specific for these flukes. It is important to make the diagnosis given the significantly elevated well-established risk of cholangiocarcinoma caused by chronic infection.[158–162]

Hymenolepis nana

Hymenolepis nana is a common intestinal tapeworm found in tropical and subtropical countries.[163–166] It can be transmitted person to person and has an autoinfective cycle.[166] Although typically asymptomatic, it can cause diarrhea and abdominal pain, and has highest rates in children.[165] Eosinophilia may be absent[167,168] or be marked (up to 2000/µL).[169]

Schistosoma mansoni infection

Chronic S mansoni infection may result in what has been termed "hepatosplenic schistosomiasis," which is caused by schistosome eggs occluding the portal venules, causing periportal fibrosis and presinusoidal portal hypertension. With lifelong exposure, hepatomegaly and/or splenomegaly peaks in the second to third decade of life along with symptoms of bloody stools and colicky abdominal pain.[170,171] Varices can develop but cirrhosis is not seen.[172] Mild eosinophilia (<1000/µL) is seen in approximately 50% of patients.[171]

Infectious Causes of Eosinophilia and Pulmonary Symptoms in the Immigrant

Paragonimiasis

Paragonimiasis is acquired in East Asia, the Americas, and Central/West Africa through ingesting uncooked crabs, crayfish, or wild boar flesh. Patients from endemic areas frequently present with a subacute to chronic cough, often mildly productive with blood-streaked sputum.[12,173–175] Up to 17% of patients with lung infections have no symptoms.[67] The most common imaging findings are effusions (20% to 60%) or pleural thickening seen adjacent to a pulmonary nodule. Consolidation or cavitary lesions also can be seen[173,176,177] and may be mistaken for tuberculosis. Moderate to marked eosinophilia helps distinguish paragonimiasis from tuberculosis, although up to 25% of patients can have a normal peripheral eosinophil count.[9,67,178,179]

Echinococcal cyst

Echinococcal cyst of the lung causes a rise in eosinophils several days after rupture. Patients are symptomatic with chest pain and/or cough. Radiographs frequently misdiagnose ruptured lung cysts as pneumonia[140] or pneumothorax.[180]

Tropical pulmonary eosinophilia

Tropical pulmonary eosinophilia is an immunologically mediated hypersensitivity to *Wuchereria bancrofti* or *Brugia malayi* seen rarely in patients from regions in which lymphatic filariasis is endemic. Patients present with an asthmalike illness, with nocturnal cough, wheezing, and dyspnea, but have a much higher eosinophilia (nearly always >3000/µL, often 10,000 to 20,000/µL). Radiographs often demonstrate an interstitial infiltrate. Symptoms and eosinophilia have a dramatic improvement with treatment for lymphatic filariasis.[181,182]

Chronic schistosomiasis

Chronic schistosomiasis can result in eggs traveling anywhere in the body, where they are encased in an eosinophil-rich granuloma. Therefore, rarely in chronic schistosomiasis pulmonary angiopathy and cor pulmonale have been described due to migration of eggs to the lungs.[183]

Infectious Causes of Eosinophilia and Genitourinary Symptoms in the Immigrant

Chronic schistosomiasis

Chronic schistosomiasis caused by *Schistosoma haematobium* is a common infection in Africa and should be suspected in a patient from there with symptoms of hematuria, chronic suprapubic pain, or obstructive uropathy.[20,183] Hematuria and dysuria can develop within months of infection (due to bladder ulcerations), occur intermittently, and hydronephrosis may develop within the first 3 years of infection.[20,172] In women, eggs also can deposit around the cervix, vagina, and ovaries,[183] and has been associated with infertility and increased susceptibility to HIV.[184,185] Although eosinophils may be elevated early in chronic infection, it typically decreases over subsequent years.

Infectious Causes of Allergic and/or Dermatologic Symptoms in the Immigrant

Echinococcal cyst

Echinococcal cyst can cause anaphylaxis after rupture into the peritoneal or pleural cavity.[132]

Strongyloidiasis

Strongyloidiasis can cause chronic urticaria or "larva currens," presumably as a reaction to migrating filariform larvae. These cause extremely pruritic serpiginous lesions found typically on the buttocks, thighs, or lower torso.[157] *Larva currens* is extremely uncommon in an acute infection, and is more often seen years after the infection was initiated.[156,186] If the patient becomes immunosuppressed with steroid use or HTLV-1, dissemination can occur, and dissemination to the skin causes purpuric lesions.[157] Eosinophilia is rarely seen (approximately 16% of cases)[187] in the setting of dissemination.

Sparganosis

Sparganosis is most often acquired in East Asia from ingesting uncooked amphibian or reptile meat or drinking unpurified stream water.[188] In its most common form, sparganosis causes a firm subcutaneous mass; however, this is not associated with eosinophilia.[188-192] Leukocytosis and marked eosinophilia is seen, however, with the proliferative form (*Sparganum proliferum*) that is accompanied by systemic illness and disseminated serpiginous cutaneous lesions that are extremely pruritic.[193-195] This form also has been reported to manifest years after the typical subcutaneous nodules have resolved.[194] Eosinophilia can also be seen with CNS manifestations (see **Table 3**).

Onchocerciasis

Onchocerciasis usually presents with chronic pruritic papular dermatitis (mimicking atopic dermatitis). Depigmentation, scaling, lichenification, and diffuse papules may be seen on the lower extremities in chronic infection,[196–198] and there may be enlarged inguinal lymph nodes as well.[199] Approximately 80% will have mild eosinophilia.[197] However, there is an immunologically hyperreactive form termed localized onchocercal dermatitis (or "sowda") that is associated with hyperpigmentation, reactive edema, and few (if any) microfilariae in the skin. Eosinophilia is typically marked in these patients,[200–202] but the diagnosis is difficult to make definitively and often relies on serology or a typical posttreatment response.

Loiasis

Loiasis in immigrants from endemic areas is often clinically asymptomatic, although it can present as an eyeworm or with Calabar swellings. Only approximately 50% have mild eosinophilia (<1000/μL) although usually microfilaremia can be detected on midday blood examination.[119,120,203]

Lymphatic filariasis

Lymphatic filariasis is a chronic filarial infection that may present acutely with retrograde adenolymphangitis or subacutely with lymphedema of the extremities or scrotum.[204–206] Approximately 20% of patients chronically infected will have eosinophilia.[207]

Eosinophilia in the immigrant/refugee conclusion

The immigrant/refugee coming from parasitic-endemic areas with unexplained eosinophilia, even without symptoms, should have an infectious workup targeting previous exposures.

INFECTIOUS CAUSES OF EOSINOPHILIA IN THE PATIENT IRRESPECTIVE OF TRAVEL/ EXPOSURE HISTORY

Important considerations in approaching eosinophilia in these patients are preexisting diagnoses and medications (even if started years ago). Mild eosinophilia commonly can be caused by atopic dermatitis and asthma. However, in patients with eosinophilia higher than 1500/μL, an alternative diagnosis should be sought. Asymptomatic eosinophilia in a patient without a history of travel outside of the United States and Europe is unlikely to have an infectious cause, with one exception being strongyloidiasis in areas of the United States and Europe where it is still endemic (see later in this article).

Infectious Causes of Eosinophilia and Pulmonary Symptoms

Allergic bronchopulmonary aspergillosis

Allergic bronchopulmonary aspergillosis (ABPA) results in increased airway hyperresponsiveness secondary to allergic hypersensitivity to *Aspergillus* spp colonizing the airways. Patients with chronic lung disease and bronchiectasis, particularly patients with cystic fibrosis, are more likely to develop ABPA. Blood eosinophilia (>500/μL) is a criterion to make the diagnosis, but the eosinophils in the peripheral blood are commonly greater than 3000/μL, particularly during exacerbations.[208]

Coccidioidomycosis

Coccidioidomycosis has been increasing in the Southwest United States in recent years.[209] In localized pulmonary infection, mild eosinophilia may be seen in 30% to 50% of cases.[44,210] In disseminated (particularly liver and skin) disease, marked eosinophilia can be seen.[44,45,211]

Tuberculosis

Tuberculosis (TB) in North America and Europe today is typically seen in the context of HIV or immigration, and so patients may have multiple reasons for developing eosinophilia. In a series before 1943, approximately 10% of patients with TB had a very mild eosinophilia (6% to 10%), but it was never seen in the setting of high fevers[212] (ie, TB is not in the differential diagnosis of fever and eosinophilia).

Paragonimiasis

Paragonimiasis acquired in the United States is caused by infection with *Paragonimus kellicotti*. In recent years, nearly all cases have been acquired in Missouri[213] as a result of eating raw infected crayfish. The average incubation period was approximately 4 weeks (range 2 to 12 weeks). All patients had cough, pleural effusion, and eosinophilia (mean 1600, range 800 to 3600/µL), and most had fever and weight loss.[213] Imaging revealed a nodule ("worm nodule") connected to the pleura by a linear track in 50% of patients, and rarely patients had pneumothoraces.[214] Unlike *P westermani* acquired outside of the United States, paragonimiasis acquired in the United States was not found to have cavitary lesions or bronchiectasis.[214]

Dirofilaria immitis

Dirofilaria immitis, the dog heartworm, is a zoonosis that can be transmitted from dogs to humans through mosquitos. It causes an asymptomatic pulmonary nodule in 50% of people. Those with symptoms experience cough, chest pains, and fevers. Only approximately 10% of patients have eosinophilia.[215]

Myiasis

Myiasis is the term given to the development of fly larvae in human tissues. Most commonly this occurs in subcutaneous sites due to *Dermatobia* spp (botfly in South/Central America) and *Cordylobia anthropophaga* (tumbu fly in Africa); however, these do not cause eosinophilia. Invasive fly larvae that have the ability to penetrate beyond subcutaneous tissues, however, can cause marked eosinophilia so dramatic it can mimic hypereosinophilic syndrome. Although *Hypoderma bovis* and *Hypoderma lineatum* are the most common cause of invasive myiasis, it is altogether an extremely rare entity. *Hypoderma* spp are found in the Northern Hemisphere (including the United States and Canada), primarily where cattle are raised. After eggs are inadvertently laid on human skin, hatched larvae burrow and migrate through subcutaneous tissues for weeks, occasionally to deeper tissues (pleura, pericardium, brain).[216–221]

Infectious Causes of Eosinophilia and Abdominal Symptoms

Basidiobolomycosis

Basidiobolomycosis is an emerging fungal infection that causes mass or inflammatory lesions in the GI tract, most commonly the colon. Sporadic cases have occurred worldwide, but 40% have been in the southwestern part of the United States. Patients present with abdominal pain and GI symptoms concordant with the location of their lesion(s). Eosinophilia has been seen in all published cases, typically between 1000 and 2000/µL.[222,223]

Visceral larva migrans

Visceral larva migrans is caused by ingesting dirt contaminated with dog/cat feces containing *Toxocara canis* or *Toxocara cati*. This is primarily seen in children with pica (average age 1 to 4 years). Symptoms are proportional to ingested inoculum, and fevers, abdominal pain with hepatomegaly (due to eosinophilic abscesses), and asthmalike difficulty breathing is frequently seen. Eosinophilia is very pronounced, with counts as high as 15,000 to 100,000/μL, and the eosinophilia can take years to fully resolve. In older children (7 to 10 years old) and rarely adults, ocular involvement with eosinophilia can be seen without other systemic symptoms. Ingesting a very low inoculum can cause an asymptomatic eosinophilia that can persist for more than a year.[224–227] Extremely rarely, cardiac[228,229] or neurologic complications (see **Table 3**) may result.

Strongyloidiasis

Strongyloidiasis is endemic worldwide and remains one of the few helminth parasites capable of being acquired in the United States. It is found in areas of low socioeconomic status in the Appalachian regions of Kentucky,[230] Tennessee, North Carolina, and Virginia,[231] and possibly other areas in the southern United States that have not been surveyed recently. Patients can have nonspecific abdominal bloating, but frequently have no symptoms whatsoever. Eosinophilia (typically mild) is seen in fewer than half of patients.[231]

Infectious Causes of Eosinophilia and Dermatologic Symptoms

Eosinophilic folliculitis

Eosinophilic folliculitis is seen in the setting of HIV/AIDS, but has been reported after bone marrow transplantation and hematologic malignancy. Pruritus typically develops on the trunk. In the setting of HIV, eosinophilic folliculitis causes mild eosinophilia.[232]

Crusted scabies

Crusted scabies results from a significant infestation of the mite and the failure of the host to mount an adequate immune response. Thus, it is seen in patients with HIV/AIDS or other underlying diseases associated with immunosuppression. In approximately 50% of patients, marked eosinophilia can develop along with overt skin abnormalities.[233]

Eosinophilia in the nontraveler conclusion

The asymptomatic nontraveler with an eosinophil count less than 1500/μL can be safely monitored periodically to ensure eosinophils are not rising over time. However, patients with symptoms or with marked eosinophilia should undergo further evaluation to determine an etiology, which commonly will be allergic (eg, eosinophilic enteritis), autoimmune (eg, sarcoidosis), myeloproliferative (eg, mastocytosis), or malignant (eg, Hodgkin lymphoma) in nature.

EOSINOPHILIC MENINGITIS

Eosinophilic meningitis, which may or may not be associated with peripheral eosinophilia, has a limited number of possible infectious etiologies. The most common infectious causes, presenting features, and cerebral spinal fluid (CSF) features are presented in **Table 3**. It is important to note that occasionally CSF will not be eosinophil-rich very early in the course. Therefore, if there is suspicion of one of the causes from **Table 3** as the etiology for meningitis, repeat lumbar puncture several days into illness may be necessary to identify CNS eosinophilia.

FINAL REMARKS

In summary, the type of patient, the patient's exposure history, and symptom complex (or lack thereof) should guide the evaluation of unexplained eosinophilia. Rarely, in the case of immune dysfunction/immunodeficiency, eosinophilia may be present in the context of an infection that by itself does not normally cause eosinophilia. Therefore, in complicated cases, it is often necessary for the infectious disease specialist to work alongside colleagues with differing expertise in determining the etiologies for both infectious and noninfectious eosinophilia.

REFERENCES

1. Diaz JH. Paragonimiasis acquired in the United States: native and nonnative species. Clin Microbiol Rev 2013;26:493–504.
2. Pitman MC, Anstey NM, Davis JS. Eosinophils in severe sepsis in northern Australia: do the usual rules apply in the tropics? Crit Care Med 2013;41: e286–8.
3. Farmakiotis D, Varughese J, Sue P, et al. Typhoid fever in an inner city hospital: a 5-year retrospective review. J Travel Med 2013;20:17–21.
4. Cohen AJ, Steigbigel RT. Eosinophilia in patients infected with human immunodeficiency virus. J Infect Dis 1996;174:615–8.
5. Abate E, Belayneh M, Gelaw A, et al. The impact of asymptomatic helminth coinfection in patients with newly diagnosed tuberculosis in north-west Ethiopia. PLoS One 2012;7:e42901.
6. Assefa S, Erko B, Medhin G, et al. Intestinal parasitic infections in relation to HIV/AIDS status, diarrhea and CD4 T-cell count. BMC Infect Dis 2009;9:155.
7. Takabayashi T, Mochizuki T, Otani N, et al. Anisakiasis presenting to the ED: clinical manifestations, time course, hematologic tests, computed tomographic findings, and treatment. Am J Emerg Med 2014;32:1485–9.
8. Fahim F, Al Salamah SM. Cystic echinococcosis in central Saudi Arabia: a 5-year experience. Turk J Gastroenterol 2007;18:22–7.
9. Obara A, Nakamura-Uchiyama F, Hiromatsu K, et al. Paragonimiasis cases recently found among immigrants in Japan. Intern Med 2004;43:388–92.
10. Fischer PU, Curtis KC, Folk SM, et al. Serological diagnosis of North American Paragonimiasis by Western blot using Paragonimus kellicotti adult worm antigen. Am J Trop Med Hyg 2013;88:1035–40.
11. Belizario V Jr, Totanes FI, Asuncion CA, et al. Integrated surveillance of pulmonary tuberculosis and paragonimiasis in Zamboanga del Norte, the Philippines. Pathog Glob Health 2014;108:95–102.
12. Yokogawa M. Paragonimus and paragonimiasis. Adv Parasitol 1965;3:99–158.
13. Ramanathan R, Burbelo P, Groot S, et al. A luciferase immunoprecipitation systems assay enhances the sensitivity and specificity of diagnosis of Strongyloides stercoralis infection. The Journal of infectious diseases 2008;198: 444–51.
14. Chang KH, Chi JG, Cho SY, et al. Cerebral sparganosis: analysis of 34 cases with emphasis on CT features. Neuroradiology 1992;34:1–8.
15. Nemir RL, Heyman A, Gorvoy JD, et al. Pulmonary infiltration and blood eosinophilia in children (Loeffler's syndrome); a review with report of 8 cases. J Pediatr 1950;37:819–43.
16. Barlow JB, Pocock WA, Tabatznik BA. An epidemic of 'acute eosinophilic pneumonia' following 'beer drinking' and probably due to infestation with *Ascaris lumbricoides*. S Afr Med J 1961;35:390–4.
17. Leshem E, Maor Y, Meltzer E, et al. Acute schistosomiasis outbreak: clinical features and economic impact. Clin Infect Dis 2008;47:1499–506.
18. Visser LG, Polderman AM, Stuiver PC. Outbreak of schistosomiasis among travelers returning from Mali, West Africa. Clin Infect Dis 1995;20:280–5.

19. de Jesus AR, Silva A, Santana LB, et al. Clinical and immunologic evaluation of 31 patients with acute *Schistosomiasis mansoni*. J Infect Dis 2002;185:98–105.
20. Fairley NH. Egyptian bilharziasis: its recent pathology, symptomatology and treatment. Proc R Soc Med 1920;13:1–18.
21. Schwartz E, Rozenman J, Perelman M. Pulmonary manifestations of early schistosome infection among nonimmune travelers. Am J Med 2000;109:718–22.
22. Bottieau E, Clerinx J, de Vega MR, et al. Imported Katayama fever: clinical and biological features at presentation and during treatment. J Infect 2006;52: 339–45.
23. el-Shabrawi M, el-Karaksy H, Okasha S, et al. Human fascioliasis: clinical features and diagnostic difficulties in Egyptian children. J Trop Pediatr 1997;43: 162–6.
24. Price TA, Tuazon CU, Simon GL. Fascioliasis: case reports and review. Clin Infect Dis 1993;17:426–30.
25. Fica A, Dabanch J, Farias C, et al. Acute fascioliasis–clinical and epidemiological features of four patients in Chile. Clin Microbiol Infect 2012;18:91–6.
26. Aksoy DY, Kerimoglu U, Oto A, et al. *Fasciola hepatica* infection: clinical and computerized tomographic findings of ten patients. Turk J Gastroenterol 2006; 17:40–5.
27. Gulsen MT, Savas MC, Koruk M, et al. Fascioliasis: a report of five cases presenting with common bile duct obstruction. Neth J Med 2006;64:17–9.
28. Armignacco O, Caterini L, Marucci G, et al. Human illnesses caused by *Opisthorchis felineus* flukes, Italy. Emerg Infect Dis 2008;14:1902–5.
29. Traverso A, Repetto E, Magnani S, et al. A large outbreak of *Opisthorchis felineus* in Italy suggests that opisthorchiasis develops as a febrile eosinophilic syndrome with cholestasis rather than a hepatitis-like syndrome. Eur J Clin Microbiol Infect Dis 2012;31:1089–93.
30. Wunderink HF, Rozemeijer W, Wever PC, et al. Foodborne trematodiasis and *Opisthorchis felineus* acquired in Italy. Emerg Infect Dis 2014;20:154–5.
31. Tselepatiotis E, Mantadakis E, Papoulis S, et al. A case of *Opisthorchis felineus* infestation in a pilot from Greece. Infection 2003;31:430–2.
32. Wang KX, Zhang RB, Cui YB, et al. Clinical and epidemiological features of patients with clonorchiasis. World J Gastroenterol 2004;10:446–8.
33. Koenigstein RP. Observations on the epidemiology of infections with *Clonorchis sinensis*. Trans R Soc Trop Med Hyg 1949;42:503–6.
34. Rusnak JM, Lucey DR. Clinical gnathostomiasis: case report and review of the English-language literature. Clin Infect Dis 1993;16:33–50.
35. Li DM, Chen XR, Zhou JS, et al. Short report: case of gnathostomiasis in Beijing, China. Am J Trop Med Hyg 2009;80:185–7.
36. Migasena S, Pitisuttithum P, Desakorn V. *Gnathostoma* larva migrans among guests of a New Year party. Southeast Asian J Trop Med Public Health 1991; 22(Suppl):225–7.
37. Diaz Camacho SP, Willms K, de la Cruz Otero Mdel C, et al. Acute outbreak of gnathostomiasis in a fishing community in Sinaloa, Mexico. Parasitol Int 2003;52: 133–40.
38. Punyagupta S, Juttijudata P, Bunnag T. Eosinophilic meningitis in Thailand. Clinical studies of 484 typical cases probably caused by *Angiostrongylus cantonensis*. Am J Trop Med Hyg 1975;24:921–31.
39. Tseng YT, Tsai HC, Sy CL, et al. Clinical manifestations of eosinophilic meningitis caused by *Angiostrongylus cantonensis*: 18 years' experience in a medical center in southern Taiwan. J Microbiol Immunol Infect 2011;44:382–9.

40. Graeff-Teixeira C, da Silva AC, Yoshimura K. Update on eosinophilic meningo-encephalitis and its clinical relevance. Clin Microbiol Rev 2009;22:322–48.
41. Rowley HA, Uht RM, Kazacos KR, et al. Radiologic-pathologic findings in raccoon roundworm (Baylisascaris procyonis) encephalitis. AJNR Am J Neuro-radiol 2000;21:415–20.
42. Gavin PJ, Kazacos KR, Shulman ST. Baylisascariasis. Clin Microbiol Rev 2005; 18:703–18.
43. Sorvillo F, Ash LR, Berlin OG, et al. Baylisascaris procyonis: an emerging hel-minthic zoonosis. Emerg Infect Dis 2002;8:355–9.
44. Echols RM, Palmer DL, Long GW. Tissue eosinophilia in human coccidioidomy-cosis. Rev Infect Dis 1982;4:656–64.
45. Harley WB, Blaser MJ. Disseminated coccidioidomycosis associated with extreme eosinophilia. Clin Infect Dis 1994;18:627–9.
46. Drake KW, Adam RD. Coccidioidal meningitis and brain abscesses: analysis of 71 cases at a referral center. Neurology 2009;73:1780–6.
47. Thompson GR 3rd, Bays D, Taylor SL, et al. Association between serum 25-hy-droxyvitamin D level and type of coccidioidal infection. Med Mycol 2013;51: 319–23.
48. Ragland AS, Arsura E, Ismail Y, et al. Eosinophilic pleocytosis in coccidioidal meningitis: frequency and significance. Am J Med 1993;95:254–7.
49. Punyagupta S, Bunnag T, Juttijudata P. Eosinophilic meningitis in Thailand. Clin-ical and epidemiological characteristics of 162 patients with myeloencephalitis probably caused by Gnathostoma spinigerum. J Neurol Sci 1990;96:241–56.
50. Xia Y, Ju Y, Chen J, et al. Cerebral paragonimiasis: a retrospective analysis of 27 cases. J Neurosurg Pediatr 2015;15:101–6.
51. Ferrari TC, Faria LC, Vilaca TS, et al. Identification and characterization of im-mune complexes in the cerebrospinal fluid of patients with spinal cord schisto-somiasis. J Neuroimmunol 2011;230:188–90.
52. Scrimgeour EM, Gajdusek DC. Involvement of the central nervous system in Schistosoma mansoni and S. haematobium infection. A review. Brain 1985; 108(Pt 4):1023–38.
53. Houdon L, Flodrops H, Rocaboy M, et al. Two patients with imported acute neu-roschistosomiasis due to Schistosoma mansoni. J Travel Med 2010;17:274–7.
54. Ferrari TC, Moreira PR, Cunha AS. Clinical characterization of neuroschistoso-miasis due to Schistosoma mansoni and its treatment. Acta Trop 2008;108: 89–97.
55. Pittella JE, Gusmao SN, Carvalho GT, et al. Tumoral form of cerebral Schistoso-miasis mansoni. A report of four cases and a review of the literature. Clin Neurol Neurosurg 1996;98:15–20.
56. Hong D, Xie H, Zhu M, et al. Cerebral sparganosis in mainland Chinese patients. J Clin Neurosci 2013;20:1514–9.
57. Sotelo J, Guerrero V, Rubio F. Neurocysticercosis: a new classification based on active and inactive forms. A study of 753 cases. Arch Intern Med 1985;145: 442–5.
58. Earnest MP, Reller LB, Filley CM, et al. Neurocysticercosis in the United States: 35 cases and a review. Rev Infect Dis 1987;9:961–79.
59. Shandera WX, White AC Jr, Chen JC, et al. Neurocysticercosis in Houston, Texas. A report of 112 cases. Medicine (Baltimore) 1994;73:37–52.
60. Castillo-Iglesias H, Mouly S, Ducros A, et al. Late-onset eosinophilic chronic meningitis occurring 30 years after Taenia solium infestation in a white Cauca-sian woman. J Infect 2006;53:e35–8.

61. Monteiro L, Almeida-Pinto J, Stocker A, et al. Active neurocysticercosis, parenchymal and extraparenchymal: a study of 38 patients. J Neurol 1993;241:15–21.
62. Xinou E, Lefkopoulos A, Gelagoti M, et al. CT and MR imaging findings in cerebral toxocaral disease. AJNR Am J Neuroradiol 2003;24:714–8.
63. Moreira-Silva SF, Rodrigues MG, Pimenta JL, et al. Toxocariasis of the central nervous system: with report of two cases. Rev Soc Bras Med Trop 2004;37:169–74.
64. Johnson JR, Falk A, Iber C, et al. Paragonimiasis in the United States. A report of nine cases in Hmong immigrants. Chest 1982;82:168–71.
65. Kan H, Ogata T, Taniyama A, et al. Extraordinarily high eosinophilia and elevated serum interleukin-5 level observed in a patient infected with *Paragonimus westermani*. Pediatrics 1995;96:351–4.
66. Ashitani J, Kumamoto K, Matsukura S. *Paragonimiasis westermani* with multifocal lesions in lungs and skin. Intern Med 2000;39:433–6.
67. Nakamura-Uchiyama F, Onah DN, Nawa Y. Clinical features of paragonimiasis cases recently found in Japan: parasite-specific immunoglobulin M and G antibody classes. Clin Infect Dis 2001;32:e151–3.
68. Klenzak J, Mattia A, Valenti A, et al. Hepatic capillariasis in Maine presenting as a hepatic mass. Am J Trop Med Hyg 2005;72:651–3.
69. Camargo LM, de Souza Almeida Aranha Camargo J, Vera LJ, et al. Capillariaisis (trichurida, trichinellidae, *Capillaria hepatica*) in the Brazilian Amazon: low pathogenicity, low infectivity and a novel mode of transmission. Parasit Vectors 2010; 3:11.
70. Fuehrer HP, Igel P, Auer H. *Capillaria hepatica* in man–an overview of hepatic capillariasis and spurious infections. Parasitol Res 2011;109:969–79.
71. Choe G, Lee HS, Seo JK, et al. Hepatic capillariasis: first case report in the Republic of Korea. Am J Trop Med Hyg 1993;48:610–25.
72. Kohatsu H, Zaha O, Shimada K, et al. A space-occupying lesion in the liver due to *Capillaria* infection. Am J Trop Med Hyg 1995;52:414–8.
73. Tesana S, Puapairoj A, Saeseow O. Granulomatous, hepatolithiasis and hepatomegaly caused by *Capillaria hepatica* infection: first case report of Thailand. Southeast Asian J Trop Med Public Health 2007;38:636–40.
74. Fichi G, Stefanelli S, Pagani A, et al. Trichinellosis outbreak caused by meat from a wild boar hunted in an Italian region considered to be at negligible risk for trichinella. Zoonoses Public Health 2015;62:285–91.
75. Hall RL, Lindsay A, Hammond C, et al. Outbreak of human trichinellosis in Northern California caused by *Trichinella murrelli*. Am J Trop Med Hyg 2012;87: 297–302.
76. Wilson NO, Hall RL, Montgomery SP, et al. Trichinellosis surveillance—United States, 2008-2012. MMWR Surveill Summ 2015;64(Suppl 1):1–8.
77. McAuley JB, Michelson MK, Schantz PM. Trichinella infection in travelers. J Infect Dis 1991;164:1013–6.
78. Turk M, Kaptan F, Turker N, et al. Clinical and laboratory aspects of a trichinellosis outbreak in Izmir, Turkey. Parasite 2006;13:65–70.
79. Sharma RK, Raghavendra N, Mohanty S, et al. Clinical & biochemical profile of trichinellosis outbreak in north India. Indian J Med Res 2014;140:414–9.
80. Pozio E, Varese P, Morales MA, et al. Comparison of human trichinellosis caused by *Trichinella spiralis* and by *Trichinella britovi*. Am J Trop Med Hyg 1993;48: 568–75.
81. Calcagno MA, Bourlot I, Taus R, et al. Description of an outbreak of human trichinellosis in an area of Argentina historically regarded as trichinella-free: the importance of surveillance studies. Vet Parasitol 2014;200:251–6.

82. Arness MK, Brown JD, Dubey JP, et al. An outbreak of acute eosinophilic myositis attributed to human Sarcocystis parasitism. Am J Trop Med Hyg 1999;61:548–53.

83. Abubakar S, Teoh BT, Sam SS, et al. Outbreak of human infection with *Sarcocystis nesbitti*, Malaysia, 2012. Emerg Infect Dis 2013;19:1989–91.

84. Esposito DH, Stich A, Epelboin L, et al. Acute muscular sarcocystosis: an international investigation among ill travelers returning from Tioman Island, Malaysia, 2011-2012. Clin Infect Dis 2014;59:1401–10.

85. Jeffrey HC. Sarcosporidiosis in man. Trans R Soc Trop Med Hyg 1974;68:17–29.

86. Beaver PC, Gadgil K, Morera P. Sarcocystis in man: a review and report of five cases. Am J Trop Med Hyg 1979;28:819–44.

87. Kendall ME, Crim S, Fullerton K, et al. Travel-associated enteric infections diagnosed after return to the United States, foodborne diseases active surveillance network (FoodNet), 2004–2009. Clin Infect Dis 2012;54:S480–7.

88. O'Brien DP, Leder K, Matchett E, et al. Illness in returned travelers and immigrants/refugees: the 6-year experience of two Australian infectious diseases units. J Travel Med 2006;13:145–52.

89. Harries AD, Myers B, Bhattacharrya D. Eosinophilia in Caucasians returning from the tropics. Trans R Soc Trop Med Hyg 1986;80:327–8.

90. Maxwell C, Hussain R, Nutman TB, et al. The clinical and immunologic responses of normal human volunteers to low dose hookworm (*Necator americanus*) infection. Am J Trop Med Hyg 1987;37:126–34.

91. Soonawala D, van Lieshout L, den Boer MA, et al. Post-travel screening of asymptomatic long-term travelers to the tropics for intestinal parasites using molecular diagnostics. Am J Trop Med Hyg 2014;90:835–9.

92. Schulte C, Krebs B, Jelinek T, et al. Diagnostic significance of blood eosinophilia in returning travelers. Clin Infect Dis 2002;34:407–11.

93. Baaten GG, Sonder GJ, van Gool T, et al. Travel-related schistosomiasis, strongyloidiasis, filariasis, and toxocariasis: the risk of infection and the diagnostic relevance of blood eosinophilia. BMC Infect Dis 2011;11:84.

94. Perez-Ayala A, Monge-Maillo B, Diaz-Menendez M, et al. Self-limited travelers' diarrhea by *Isospora belli* in a patient with dengue infection. J Travel Med 2011;18:212–3.

95. Agnamey P, Djeddi D, Oukachbi Z, et al. *Cryptosporidium hominis* and *Isospora belli* diarrhea in travelers returning from West Africa. J Travel Med 2010;17:141–2.

96. Butler T, Middleton FG, Earnest DL, et al. Chronic and recurrent diarrhea in American servicemen in Vietnam. An evaluation of etiology and small bowel structure and function. Arch Intern Med 1973;132:373–7.

97. Brandborg LL, Goldberg SB, Breidenbach WC. Human coccidiosis–a possible cause of malabsorption. N Engl J Med 1970;283:1306–13.

98. Silva GB, Fernandes KP, Segundo GR. Common variable immunodeficiency and isosporiasis: first report case. Rev Soc Bras Med Trop 2012;45:768–9.

99. DeHovitz JA, Pape JW, Boncy M, et al. Clinical manifestations and therapy of *Isospora belli* infection in patients with the acquired immunodeficiency syndrome. N Engl J Med 1986;315:87–90.

100. Resiere D, Vantelon JM, Bouree P, et al. *Isospora belli* infection in a patient with non-Hodgkin's lymphoma. Clin Microbiol Infect 2003;9:1065–7.

101. Ud Din N, Torka P, Hutchison RE, et al. Severe *Isospora* (*Cystoisospora*) *belli* diarrhea preceding the diagnosis of human T-cell-leukemia-virus-1-associated T-cell lymphoma. Case Rep Infect Dis 2012;2012:640104.

102. Apt WB. Eosinophilia in Isospora infections. Parasitol Today 1986;2:22.
103. Junod C. *Isospora belli* coccidiosis in immunocompetent subjects (a study of 40 cases seen in Paris). Bull Soc Pathol Exot Filiales 1988;81:317–25 [in French].
104. Graczyk TK, Fried B. Echinostomiasis: a common but forgotten food-borne disease. Am J Trop Med Hyg 1998;58:501–4.
105. Miyamoto K, Nakao M, Ohnishi K, et al. Studies on the zoonoses in Hokkaido, Japan. 6. Experimental human echinostomiasis. Hokkaido Igaku Zasshi 1984; 59:696–700 [in Japanese].
106. Mattiucci S, Fazii P, De Rosa A, et al. Anisakiasis and gastroallergic reactions associated with *Anisakis pegreffii* infection, Italy. Emerg Infect Dis 2013;19:496–9.
107. Pampiglione S, Rivasi F, Criscuolo M, et al. Human anisakiasis in Italy: a report of eleven new cases. Pathol Res Pract 2002;198:429–34.
108. Jelinek T, Maiwald H, Nothdurft HD, et al. Cutaneous larva migrans in travelers: synopsis of histories, symptoms, and treatment of 98 patients. Clin Infect Dis 1994;19:1062–6.
109. Blackwell V, Vega-Lopez F. Cutaneous larva migrans: clinical features and management of 44 cases presenting in the returning traveller. Br J Dermatol 2001; 145:434–7.
110. Davies HD, Sakuls P, Keystone JS. Creeping eruption. A review of clinical presentation and management of 60 cases presenting to a tropical disease unit. Arch Dermatol 1993;129:588–91.
111. Lipner EM, Law MA, Barnett E, et al. Filariasis in travelers presenting to the GeoSentinel surveillance network. PLoS Negl Trop Dis 2007;1:e88.
112. Ezzedine K, Malvy D, Dhaussy I, et al. Onchocerciasis-associated limb swelling in a traveler returning from Cameroon. J Travel Med 2006;13:50–3.
113. McCarthy JS, Ottesen EA, Nutman TB. Onchocerciasis in endemic and nonendemic populations: differences in clinical presentation and immunologic findings. J Infect Dis 1994;170:736–41.
114. Pryce D, Behrens R, Davidson R, et al. Onchocerciasis in members of an expedition to Cameroon: role of advice before travel and long term follow up. BMJ 1992;304:1285–6.
115. Wolfe MS, Petersen JL, Neafie RC, et al. Onchocerciasis presenting with swelling of limb. Am J Trop Med Hyg 1974;23:361–8.
116. Connor DH, George GH, Gibson DW. Pathologic changes of human onchocerciasis: implications for future research. Rev Infect Dis 1985;7:809–19.
117. Bean B, Ellman MH, Kagan IG. Acute lymphatic filariasis in an American traveler. Diagn Microbiol Infect Dis 1992;15:345–7.
118. Kumaraswami V. The clinical manifestations of lymphatic filariasis. In: Nutman TB, editor. Lymphatic filariasis. London: Imperial College Press; 1991. p. 103–18.
119. Herrick JA, Metenou S, Makiya MA, et al. Eosinophil-associated processes underlie differences in clinical presentation of loiasis between temporary residents and those indigenous to Loa-endemic areas. Clin Infect Dis 2015;60:55–63.
120. Klion AD, Massougbodji A, Sadeler BC, et al. Loiasis in endemic and nonendemic populations: immunologically mediated differences in clinical presentation. J Infect Dis 1991;163:1318–25.
121. Nutman TB, Miller KD, Mulligan M, et al. *Loa loa* infection in temporary residents of endemic regions: recognition of a hyperresponsive syndrome with characteristic clinical manifestations. J Infect Dis 1986;154:10–8.
122. Antinori S, Schifanella L, Million M, et al. Imported *Loa loa* filariasis: three cases and a review of cases reported in non-endemic countries in the past 25 years. Int J Infect Dis 2012;16:e649–62.

123. Rakita RM, White AC Jr, Kielhofner MA. *Loa loa* infection as a cause of migratory angioedema: report of three cases from the Texas medical center. Clin Infect Dis 1993;17:691–4.
124. Vanegas ES, Cendejas RF, Mondragon A. A 41-year-old woman with migratory panniculitis. Am J Trop Med Hyg 2014;90:786–7.
125. Moore DA, McCroddan J, Dekumyoy P, et al. Gnathostomiasis: an emerging imported disease. Emerg Infect Dis 2003;9:647–50.
126. Malvy D, Ezzedine KH, Receveur MC, et al. Extra-pulmonary paragonimiasis with unusual arthritis and cutaneous features among a tourist returning from Gabon. Travel Med Infect Dis 2006;4:340–2.
127. Shim SS, Kim Y, Lee JK, et al. Pleuropulmonary and abdominal paragonimiasis: CT and ultrasound findings. Br J Radiol 2012;85:403–10.
128. Boggild AK, Yohanna S, Keystone JS, et al. Prospective analysis of parasitic infections in Canadian travelers and immigrants. J Travel Med 2006;13: 138–44.
129. Naidu P, Yanow SK, Kowalewska-Grochowska KT. Eosinophilia: a poor predictor of *Strongyloides* infection in refugees. Can J Infect Dis Med Microbiol 2013;24: 93–6.
130. Carranza-Rodriguez C, Pardo-Lledias J, Muro-Alvarez A, et al. Cryptic parasite infection in recent West African immigrants with relative eosinophilia. Clin Infect Dis 2008;46:e48–50.
131. Taguri S, Dar FK. Serological and clinical investigations of human hydatid case in Libya. Trans R Soc Trop Med Hyg 1978;72:338–41.
132. Aytac A, Yurdakul Y, Ikizler C, et al. Pulmonary hydatid disease: report of 100 patients. Ann Thorac Surg 1977;23:145–51.
133. Baykal K, Onol Y, Iseri C, et al. Diagnosis and treatment of renal hydatid disease: presentation of four cases. Int J Urol 1996;3:497–500.
134. Calma CL, Neghina AM, Moldovan R, et al. Cystic echinococcosis in Arad county, Romania. Vector Borne Zoonotic Dis 2012;12:333–5.
135. Cappello E, Cacopardo B, Caltabiano E, et al. Epidemiology and clinical features of cystic hydatidosis in Western Sicily: a ten-year review. World J Gastroenterol 2013;19:9351–8.
136. Kaya K, Gokce G, Kaya S, et al. Isolated renal and retroperitoneal hydatid cysts: a report of 23 cases. Trop Doct 2006;36:243–6.
137. Prousalidis J, Kosmidis C, Kapoutzis K, et al. Intrabiliary rupture of hydatid cysts of the liver. Am J Surg 2009;197:193–8.
138. Li Y, Zheng H, Cao X, et al. Demographic and clinical characteristics of patients with anaphylactic shock after surgery for cystic echinococcosis. Am J Trop Med Hyg 2011;85:452–5.
139. Constantin V, Popa F, Socea B, et al. Spontaneous rupture of a splenic hydatid cyst with anaphylaxis in a patient with multi-organ hydatid disease. Chirurgia (Bucur) 2014;109:393–5.
140. Sekiguchi H, Suzuki J, Pritt BS, et al. Coughing up a diagnosis: a cavitary lung lesion with worsening eosinophilia. Am J Med 2013;126:297–300.
141. Lv H, Jiang Y, Liu G, et al. Surgical treatment of multiple hydatid cysts in the liver of a pediatric patient. Am J Trop Med Hyg 2015;92:595–8.
142. Raptou G, Pliakos I, Hytiroglou P, et al. Severe eosinophilic cholangitis with parenchymal destruction of the left hepatic lobe due to hydatid disease. Pathol Int 2009;59:395–8.
143. Dulger AC, Esen R, Begenik H, et al. Alveolar echinococcosis of the liver: a single center experience. Pol Arch Med Wewn 2012;122:133–8.

144. Sturm D, Menzel J, Gottstein B, et al. Interleukin-5 is the predominant cytokine produced by peripheral blood mononuclear cells in alveolar echinococcosis. Infect Immun 1995;63:1688–97.

145. Vuitton DA, Bresson-Hadni S, Lenys D, et al. IgE-dependent humoral immune response in *Echinococcus multilocularis* infection: circulating and basophil-bound specific IgE against *Echinococcus* antigens in patients with alveolar echinococcosis. Clin Exp Immunol 1988;71:247–52.

146. Vuitton DA, Lassegue A, Miguet JP, et al. Humoral and cellular immunity in patients with hepatic alveolar echinococcosis. A 2 year follow-up with and without flubendazole treatment. Parasite Immunol 1984;6:329–40.

147. Lopez L, Caceres R, Servin J, et al. Surgical diagnosis and management of intestinal obstruction due to *Ascaris lumbricoides*. Surg Infect (Larchmt) 2010;11: 183–5.

148. Wani I, Maqbool M, Amin A, et al. Appendiceal ascariasis in children. Ann Saudi Med 2010;30:63–6.

149. Hamaloglu E. Biliary ascariasis in fifteen patients. Int Surg 1992;77:77–9.

150. Aderele WI. Bronchial asthma in Nigerian children. Arch Dis Child 1979;54: 448–53.

151. Katz Y, Varsano D, Siegal B, et al. Intestinal obstruction due to *Ascaris lumbricoides* mimicking intussusception. Dis Colon Rectum 1985;28:267–9.

152. Guzman GE, Teves PM, Monge E. Ascariasis as a cause of recurrent abdominal pain. Dig Endosc 2010;22:156–7.

153. Khuroo MS, Khuroo MS, Khuroo NS. Trichuris dysentery syndrome: a common cause of chronic iron deficiency anemia in adults in an endemic area (with videos). Gastrointest Endosc 2010;71:200–4.

154. Azira NM, Zeehaida M. Severe chronic iron deficiency anaemia secondary to trichuris dysentery syndrome—a case report. Trop Biomed 2012;29: 626–31.

155. Krishnamurthy S, Samanta D, Yadav S. Trichuris dysentery syndrome with eosinophilic leukemoid reaction mimicking inflammatory bowel disease. J Postgrad Med 2009;55:76–7.

156. Gill GV, Welch E, Bailey JW, et al. Chronic *Strongyloides stercoralis* infection in former British Far East prisoners of war. QJM 2004;97:789–95.

157. Smith JD, Goette DK, Odom RB. Larva currens. Cutaneous strongyloidiasis. Arch Dermatol 1976;112:1161–3.

158. Upatham ES, Viyanant V, Kurathong S, et al. Relationship between prevalence and intensity of Opisthorchis viverrini infection, and clinical symptoms and signs in a rural community in north-east Thailand. Bull World Health Organ 1984;62: 451–61.

159. Stauffer WM, Sellman JS, Walker PF. Biliary liver flukes (Opisthorchiasis and Clonorchiasis) in immigrants in the United States: often subtle and diagnosed years after arrival. J Travel Med 2004;11:157–9.

160. Mairiang E, Laha T, Bethony JM, et al. Ultrasonography assessment of hepatobiliary abnormalities in 3359 subjects with *Opisthorchis viverrini* infection in endemic areas of Thailand. Parasitol Int 2012;61:208–11.

161. Choi MH, Ryu JS, Lee M, et al. Specific and common antigens of *Clonorchis sinensis* and *Opisthorchis viverrini* (Opisthorchiidae, trematoda). Korean J Parasitol 2003;41:155–63.

162. Choi MH, Ge T, Yuan S, et al. Correlation of egg counts of *Clonorchis sinensis* by three methods of fecal examination. Korean J Parasitol 2005;43: 115–7.

163. Ragunathan L, Kalivaradhan SK, Ramadass S, et al. Helminthic infections in school children in Puducherry, South India. J Microbiol Immunol Infect 2010; 43:228–32.

164. Kheirandish F, Tarahi MJ, Ezatpour B. Prevalence of intestinal parasites among food handlers in Western Iran. Rev Inst Med Trop Sao Paulo 2014;56:111–4.

165. Chero JC, Saito M, Bustos JA, et al. Hymenolepis nana infection: symptoms and response to nitazoxanide in field conditions. Trans R Soc Trop Med Hyg 2007; 101:203–5.

166. Mirdha BR, Samantray JC. Hymenolepis nana: a common cause of paediatric diarrhoea in urban slum dwellers in India. J Trop Pediatr 2002;48:331–4.

167. Marseglia GL, Marseglia A, Licari A, et al. Chronic urticaria caused by Hymenolepis nana in an adopted girl. Allergy 2007;62:821–2.

168. Maggi P, Brandonisio O, Carito V, et al. Hymenolepis nana parasites in adopted children. Clin Infect Dis 2005;41:571–2.

169. Cooper BT, Hodgson HJ, Chadwick VS. Hymenolepiasis: an unusual cause of diarrhoea in Western Europe. Digestion 1981;21:115–6.

170. Nooman ZM, Hasan AH, Waheeb Y, et al. The epidemiology of schistosomiasis in Egypt: Ismailia governorate. Am J Trop Med Hyg 2000;62:35–41.

171. Salih SY, Marshall TF, Radalowicz A. Morbidity in relation to the clinical forms and to intensity of infection in Schistosoma mansoni infections in the Sudan. Ann Trop Med Parasitol 1979;73:439–49.

172. Nash TE, Cheever AW, Ottesen EA, et al. Schistosome infections in humans: perspectives and recent findings. NIH conference. Ann Intern Med 1982;97: 740–54.

173. Kanpittaya J, Sawanyawisuth K, Vannavong A, et al. Different chest radiographic findings of pulmonary paragonimiasis in two endemic countries. Am J Trop Med Hyg 2010;83:924–6.

174. Xu HZ, Tang LF, Zheng XP, et al. Paragonimiasis in Chinese children: 58 cases analysis. Iran J Pediatr 2012;22:505–11.

175. Lemos AC, Coelho JC, Matos ED, et al. Paragonimiasis: first case reported in Brazil. Braz J Infect Dis 2007;11:153–6.

176. Im JG, Whang HY, Kim WS, et al. Pleuropulmonary paragonimiasis: radiologic findings in 71 patients. AJR Am J Roentgenol 1992;159:39–43.

177. Kim TS, Han J, Shim SS, et al. Pleuropulmonary paragonimiasis: CT findings in 31 patients. AJR Am J Roentgenol 2005;185:616–21.

178. Mukae O, Taniguchi H, Ashitani J, et al. Case report: Paragonimiasis westermani with seroconversion from immunoglobulin (Ig) m to IgG antibody with the clinical course. Am J Trop Med Hyg 2001;65:837–9.

179. Kim EA, Juhng SK, Kim HW, et al. Imaging findings of hepatic paragonimiasis: a case report. J Korean Med Sci 2004;19:759–62.

180. Shameem M, Akhtar J, Bhargava R, et al. Ruptured pulmonary hydatid cyst with anaphylactic shock and pneumothorax. Respir Care 2011;56:863–5.

181. Boggild AK, Keystone JS, Kain KC. Tropical pulmonary eosinophilia: a case series in a setting of nonendemicity. Clin Infect Dis 2004;39:1123–8.

182. Ottesen EA, Nutman TB. Tropical pulmonary eosinophilia. Annu Rev Med 1992; 43:417–24.

183. Smith JH, Christie JD. The pathobiology of Schistosoma haematobium infection in humans. Hum Pathol 1986;17:333–45.

184. Downs JA, Mguta C, Kaatano GM, et al. Urogenital schistosomiasis in women of reproductive age in Tanzania's Lake Victoria region. Am J Trop Med Hyg 2011; 84:364–9.

185. Kjetland EF, Kurewa EN, Mduluza T, et al. The first community-based report on the effect of genital *Schistosoma haematobium* infection on female fertility. Fertil Steril 2010;94:1551–3.
186. Pelletier LL Jr, Baker CB, Gam AA, et al. Diagnosis and evaluation of treatment of chronic strongyloidiasis in ex-prisoners of war. J Infect Dis 1988;157:573–6.
187. Buonfrate D, Requena-Mendez A, Angheben A, et al. Severe strongyloidiasis: a systematic review of case reports. BMC Infect Dis 2013;13:78.
188. Wiwanitkit V. A review of human sparganosis in Thailand. Int J Infect Dis 2005;9: 312–6.
189. Pampiglione S, Fioravanti ML, Rivasi F. Human sparganosis in Italy. Case report and review of the European cases. APMIS 2003;111:349–54.
190. Koo M, Kim JH, Kim JS, et al. Cases and literature review of breast sparganosis. World J Surg 2011;35:573–9.
191. Yoon HS, Jeon BJ, Park BY. Multiple sparganosis in an immunosuppressed patient. Arch Plast Surg 2013;40:479–81.
192. Chang JH, Lin OS, Yeh KT. Subcutaneous sparganosis–a case report and a review of human sparganosis in Taiwan. Kaohsiung J Med Sci 1999;15: 567–71.
193. Beaver PC, Rolon FA. Proliferating larval cestode in a man in Paraguay. A case report and review. Am J Trop Med Hyg 1981;30:625–37.
194. Moulinier R, Martinez E, Torres J, et al. Human proliferative sparganosis in Venezuela: report of a case. Am J Trop Med Hyg 1982;31:358–63.
195. Schauer F, Poppert S, Technau-Hafsi K, et al. Travel-acquired subcutaneous *Sparganum proliferum* infection diagnosed by molecular methods. Br J Dermatol 2014;170:741–3.
196. Enk CD, Anteby I, Abramson N, et al. Onchocerciasis among Ethiopian immigrants in Israel. Isr Med Assoc J 2003;5:485–8.
197. Lazarov A, Amihai B, Sion-Vardy N. Pruritus and chronic papular dermatitis in an Ethiopian man. Onchocerciasis (chronic papular onchodermatitis). Arch Dermatol 1997;133:382–3, 5–6.
198. Baum S, Greenberger S, Pavlotsky F, et al. Late-onset onchocercal skin disease among Ethiopian immigrants. Br J Dermatol 2014;171:1078–83.
199. Gibson DW, Connor DH. Onchocercal lymphadenitis: clinicopathologic study of 34 patients. Trans R Soc Trop Med Hyg 1978;72:137–54.
200. Francis H, Awadzi K, Ottesen EA. The mazzotti reaction following treatment of onchocerciasis with diethylcarbamazine: clinical severity as a function of infection intensity. Am J Trop Med Hyg 1985;34:529–36.
201. Siddiqui MA, al-Khawajah MM. The black disease of Arabia, Sowda-onchocerciasis. New findings. Int J Dermatol 1991;30:130–3.
202. Rubio de Kromer MT, Medina-De la Garza CE, Brattig NW. Differences in eosinophil and neutrophil chemotactic responses in sowda and generalized form of onchocerciasis. Acta Trop 1995;60:21–33.
203. Churchill DR, Morris C, Fakoya A, et al. Clinical and laboratory features of patients with loiasis (*Loa loa* filariasis) in the UK. J Infect 1996;33:103–9.
204. Mondal SK. Incidental detection of filaria in fine-needle aspirates: a cytologic study of 14 clinically unsuspected cases at different sites. Diagn Cytopathol 2012;40:292–6.
205. Sabageh D, Oguntola AS, Oguntola AM, et al. Incidental detection of microfilariae in a lymph node aspirate: a case report. Niger Med J 2014;55:438–40.
206. Jones RT. Non-endemic cases of lymphatic filariasis. Trop Med Int Health 2014; 19:1377–83.

207. Musso D. Relevance of the eosinophil blood count in bancroftian filariasis as a screening tool for the treatment. Pathog Glob Health 2013;107:96–102.
208. Knutsen AP, Slavin RG. Allergic bronchopulmonary aspergillosis in asthma and cystic fibrosis. Clin Dev Immunol 2011;2011:843763.
209. Centers for Disease Control and Prevention. Increase in reported coccidioido-mycosis–United States, 1998-2011. MMWR Morb Mortal Wkly Rep 2013;62: 217–21.
210. Sobonya RE, Yanes J, Klotz SA. Cavitary pulmonary coccidioidomycosis: path-ologic and clinical correlates of disease. Hum Pathol 2014;45:153–9.
211. Kuprian M, Schofield C, Bennett S. Symptomatic hepatitis secondary to dissem-inated coccidioidomycosis in an immunocompetent patient. BMJ Case Rep 2014;2014. p. 1–3.
212. Muller GL. Clinical significance of the blood in tuberculosis. New York: The Commonwealth Fund; 1943.
213. Lane MA, Marcos LA, Onen NF, et al. Paragonimus kellicotti flukes in Missouri, USA. Emerg Infect Dis 2012;18:1263–7.
214. Henry TS, Lane MA, Weil GJ, et al. Chest CT features of North American para-gonimiasis. AJR Am J Roentgenol 2012;198:1076–83.
215. Flieder DB, Moran CA. Pulmonary dirofilariasis: a clinicopathologic study of 41 lesions in 39 patients. Hum Pathol 1999;30:251–6.
216. Uttamchandani RB, Trigo LM, Poppiti RJ Jr, et al. Eosinophilic pleural effusion in cutaneous myiasis. South Med J 1989;82:1288–91.
217. Starr J, Pruett JH, Yunginger JW, et al. Myiasis due to Hypoderma lineatum infection mimicking the hypereosinophilic syndrome. Mayo Clin Proc 2000;75: 755–9.
218. Miller MJ, Lockhart JA. Hypodermal myiasis caused by larvae of the ox-warble (Hypoderma bovis). Can Med Assoc J 1950;62:592–4.
219. Puente S, Otranto D, Panadero R, et al. First diagnosis of an imported human myiasis caused by Hypoderma sinense (Diptera: Oestridae), detected in a Eu-ropean traveler returning from India. J Travel Med 2010;17:419–23.
220. Zygutiene M, Narkeviciute I, Mudeniene V, et al. A case of myiasis due to Hypo-derma bovis, Lithuania, 2004. Euro Surveill 2006;11:E1–2.
221. McGraw TA, Turiansky GW. Cutaneous myiasis. J Am Acad Dermatol 2008;58: 907–26 [quiz: 27–9].
222. Lyon GM, Smilack JD, Komatsu KK, et al. Gastrointestinal basidiobolomycosis in Arizona: clinical and epidemiological characteristics and review of the literature. Clin Infect Dis 2001;32:1448–55.
223. Vikram HR, Smilack JD, Leighton JA, et al. Emergence of gastrointestinal basi-diobolomycosis in the United States, with a review of worldwide cases. Clin Infect Dis 2012;54:1685–91.
224. Figueiredo SD, Taddei JA, Menezes JJ, et al. Clinical-epidemiological study of toxocariasis in a pediatric population. J Pediatr (Rio J) 2005;81:126–32 [in Portuguese].
225. Glickman LT, Magnaval JF, Domanski LM, et al. Visceral larva migrans in French adults: a new disease syndrome? Am J Epidemiol 1987;125:1019–34.
226. Despommier D. Toxocariasis: clinical aspects, epidemiology, medical ecology, and molecular aspects. Clin Microbiol Rev 2003;16:265–72.
227. Schantz PM, Glickman LT. Toxocaral visceral larva migrans. N Engl J Med 1978; 298:436–9.
228. Herry I, Philippe B, Hennequin C, et al. Acute life-threatening toxocaral tampo-nade. Chest 1997;112:1692–3.

229. Mok CH. Visceral larva migrans. A discussion based on review of the literature. Clin Pediatr (Phila) 1968;7:565–73.
230. Russell ES, Gray EB, Marshall RE, et al. Prevalence of *Strongyloides stercoralis* antibodies among a rural Appalachian population–Kentucky, 2013. Am J Trop Med Hyg 2014;91:1000–1.
231. Berk SL, Verghese A, Alvarez S, et al. Clinical and epidemiologic features of strongyloidiasis. A prospective study in rural Tennessee. Arch Intern Med 1987;147:1257–61.
232. Fraser SJ, Benton EC, Roddie PH, et al. Eosinophilic folliculitis: an important differential diagnosis after allogeneic bone-marrow transplant. Clin Exp Dermatol 2009;34:369–71.
233. Roberts LJ, Huffam SE, Walton SF, et al. Crusted scabies: clinical and immunological findings in seventy-eight patients and a review of the literature. J Infect 2005;50:375–81.

Eosinophilia Associated with Disorders of Immune Deficiency or Immune Dysregulation

Kelli W. Williams, MD, MPH[a], Joshua D. Milner, MD[b],
Alexandra F. Freeman, MD[c],*

KEYWORDS

- Eosinophilia • Immune • Deficiency • Dysregulation

KEY POINTS

- Eosinophilia can be seen in many disorders of immune deficiency or immune dysregulation; however, there are a few key syndromes that have eosinophilia as a consistent clinical feature.
- In these monogenic diseases of immune deficiency or immune dysregulation, peripheral and tissue eosinophil counts are variable and do not correlate with severity of disease.
- A marginal number of patients with eosinophilia have an underlying immune defect, but given the profound impact these diseases can have on morbidity and mortality, all cases of eosinophilia warrant a thorough clinical evaluation.

INTRODUCTION

Although increased peripheral eosinophilia can be found in patients with parasitic infection, significant atopic disease, drug hypersensitivity reactions, connective tissue disorders, malignancy, and rare hypereosinophilic syndromes, monogenic disorders of immune deficiency or dysregulation should be considered, particularly in the pediatric age group. Some of these syndromes include clinical manifestations of atopy,

Disclosures: the authors have nothing to disclose.
[a] Laboratory of Clinical Infectious Diseases, National Institute of Allergy and Infectious Diseases, National Institutes of Health, 33 North Drive, Building 33, Room 2W10A, Bethesda, MD 20892, USA; [b] Laboratory of Allergic Diseases, National Institute of Allergy and Infectious Diseases, National Institutes of Health, 10 Center Drive, Building 10/CRC, Room 5-3950, Bethesda, MD 20892, USA; [c] Laboratory of Clinical Infectious Diseases, National Institute of Allergy and Infectious Diseases, National Institutes of Health, 10 Center Drive, Building 10/CRC, Room 12C103, Bethesda, MD 20892, USA
* Corresponding author.
E-mail address: freemaal@mail.nih.gov

such as atopic dermatitis or food allergy, which may contribute to the eosinophilia; however, the mechanism driving the eosinophilia is not well understood. Many of these monogenic diseases are characterized by increased production of Th2 cytokines, such as interleukin 5 (IL-5), which is an essential promoter of eosinophil differentiation, maturation, and survival.[1]

In this article, several disorders of immune deficiency or dysregulation are reviewed that have documented eosinophilia as part of the syndrome (**Fig. 1**). The clinical features, common infections, laboratory findings, diagnostic methods, and genetic basis of disease of each syndrome are discussed.

SYNDROMIC CAUSES OF INCREASED IGE LEVELS AND EOSINOPHILIA
Autosomal Dominant Hyper IgE Syndrome

Job's syndrome was first described in 1966 with 2 patients who had recurrent staphylococcal abscesses, similar to the boils borne by the prophet Job in the Bible.[2] This clinical syndrome, which was first characterized as a triad of recurrent staphylococcal abscesses, pulmonary infections, and an eczematous dermatitis, was later found to be associated with increased serum IgE levels, leading to the name autosomal dominant hyper IgE syndrome (AD-HIES).[3]

Clinical features, infections, and management
AD-HIES typically presents within the first few days of life as neonatal acne or erythema toxicum neonatorum secondary to the pustular rash that often encompasses the face, scalp, and upper body.[4,5] Histologically, the skin infiltration is predominantly eosinophils.[6] The rash usually evolves to resemble an eczematous dermatitis, which is papular, pruritic, lichenified, and typically driven by *Staphylococcus aureus* colonization and superinfection.[7]

Patients with AD-HIES classically have recurrent, cold *S aureus* abscesses, which have frank pus when excised despite their lack of dolor, rubor, and calor.[2] Recurrent sinopulmonary infections generally start in the first several years of life, with *S. aureus* being the most common pathogen implicated in the pneumonias. *Streptococcus pneumoniae* and *Haemophilus influenzae* also occur frequently, and the first presentation of pneumonia in infancy may be caused by *Pneumocystis jirovecii*.[8,9] As with the cold abscesses, patients with AD-HIES with pneumonia lack systemic signs of inflammation, including fever, frequently delaying diagnosis leading to parenchymal lung damage (**Fig. 2**). Pneumatoceles and bronchiectasis increase the patients' susceptibility to difficult to treat microbes, like *Aspergillus*, *Scedosporium*, *Pseudomonas*, and nontuberculous mycobacteria, which contribute significantly to their morbidity and mortality.[9–11]

Fungal susceptibility is apparent, with more than 80% of patients having chronic mucocutaneous candidiasis (**Fig. 3**).[12] Unlike patients with dedicator of cytokinesis 8 (DOCK8) deficiency, those with AD-HIES do not commonly have severe viral infections (**Table 1**).[13,14]

Despite the increased levels of serum IgE characteristic of these patients, allergy and asthma are not typically severe or difficult to manage in AD-HIES. Siegel and colleagues[15] reported a diminished allergic phenotype in patients with AD-HIES compared with other patients with a comparably increased IgE level and atopic dermatitis, although allergies are more frequent than those with normal IgE levels.

AD-HIES is a multisystem disease with many nonimmunologic abnormalities. A characteristic facial appearance usually emerges during adolescence, with porous skin, a prominent forehead, deep-set eyes, and a bulbous and broad nose (see **Fig. 3**). Most patients fail to shed their primary teeth, requiring medical removal to

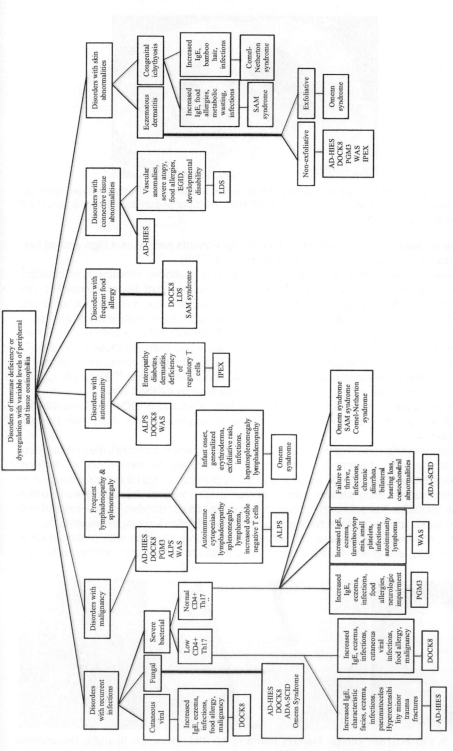

Fig. 1. Flow diagram showing disorders of immune deficiency or dysregulation with variable levels of peripheral and tissue eosinophilia. Characteristics of each disorder are listed once under the most prevalently featured category. ADA-SCID, adenosine deaminase–severe combined immunodeficiency; AD-HIES, autosomal dominant hyper IgE syndrome; ALPS, autoimmune lymphoproliferative syndrome; DOCK8, dedicator of cytokinesis 8; IPEX, immunodysregulation, polyendocrinopathy, enteropathy, X-linked syndrome; LDS, Loeys-Dietz syndrome; PGM3, phosphoglucomutase 3; SAM, severe dermatitis, multiple allergies, and metabolic wasting; WAS, Wiskott-Aldrich syndrome.

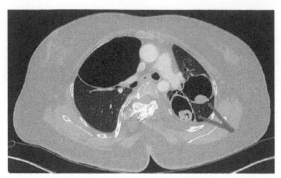

Fig. 2. Parenchymal lung findings and complications in AD-HIES. Chest computed tomography scan from a 43-year-old woman with AD-HIES, multiple pneumatoceles, and an evident aspergilloma (*arrows*).

allow the secondary teeth to emerge normally. Patients also have a high arched hard palate and palatal and lingual ridges or grooves.[8,10,16]

Extensive musculoskeletal abnormalities include scoliosis, osteopenia or osteoporosis, minimal trauma fractures, craniosynostosis, and joint hyperextensibility (see **Fig. 3**).[8,17] Joint hyperextensibility occurs in more than two-thirds of patients with AD-HIES and may contribute to the high frequency of degenerative bone disease.[12]

Recently, manifestations of gastrointestinal disease in patients with AD-HIES have been described. In a cohort of 70 individuals, nearly two-thirds of those with AD-HIES who underwent gastrointestinal endoscopy had eosinophilic esophagitis as defined by the updated consensus guidelines (Arora M, unpublished data).[18] Food allergy was not as common as in DOCK8 deficiency (Arora M, unpublished data).

As with several other primary immunodeficiency diseases (PIDDs), patients with AD-HIES are at increased risk of developing malignancy, particularly non-Hodgkin lymphoma.[13,19]

Because the clinical impact of recurrent infections can be profound, the primary focus in management is treatment of infections and prophylaxis to prevent future infections, especially with *S aureus*. Suppression of skin colonization with *S aureus* through antiseptics, such as dilute bleach baths and chlorhexidine washes, frequently leads to minimal dermatitis. Patients with chronic mucocutaneous candidiasis, or in areas endemic for *Coccidioides* or histoplasmosis, may also benefit from antifungal prophylaxis.

Parenchymal lung disease and subsequent chronic infection with molds, such as *Aspergillus*, and gram-negative bacteria, such as *Pseudomonas*, contribute to most

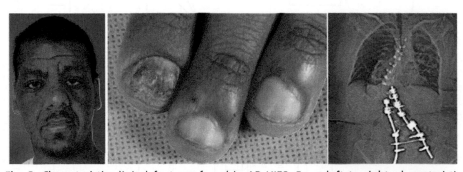

Fig. 3. Characteristic clinical features found in AD-HIES. From left to right: characteristic facies, chronic mucocutaneous candidiasis, and severe scoliosis.

Table 1
Comparison of the clinical features among the key syndromes of increased IgE levels: STAT3, DOCK8, and PGM3

	STAT3	DOCK8	PGM3
Increased serum IgE level	+++	+++	+++
Peripheral eosinophilia	+++	+++	+
Low CD4+ Th17 cells	+++	++	−
Newborn rash	+++	+	+
Eczematous dermatitis	+++	+++	+++
Recurrent skin abscesses	+++	++	++
Recurrent pneumonias	+++	++	+++
Mucocutaneous candidiasis	+++	++	−
Cutaneous viral infections	+	+++	+
Parenchymal lung changes	+++	+	++
Asthma	−	++	++
Food allergies	+	+++	++
Eosinophilic gastrointestinal disease	++	++	+
Characteristic facies	+++	−	+
Retained primary teeth	+++	−	−
Scoliosis	+++	−	++
Minimal trauma fractures	+++	−	−
Hyperextensibility	+++	−	+
Vascular abnormalities	++	−	−
Autoimmunity	+	++	++
Malignancy	++	+++	++

−, characteristic is not featured.

cases of death in AD-HIES.[11] Because of this situation, pyogenic pneumonias should be aggressively diagnosed and treated to minimize parenchymal damage.

Immunoglobulin replacement should be considered in those patients with impaired specific antibody responses, bronchiectasis, and breakthrough infections while on prophylaxis. Hematopoietic stem cell transplant (HSCT) has been performed infrequently as a possible curative treatment of AD-HIES, with varying clinical results.[20–22]

Clinical laboratory findings

In addition to the hallmark laboratory finding of increased serum IgE levels, most patients with AD-HIES have peripheral eosinophilia. IgE levels are often greater than 2000 IU/mL, although these may decrease and even normalize as adults, and absolute eosinophil counts are variable but frequently greater than 700 cells/μL. Despite this situation, the underlying cause of these increases is still unclear, and the serum eosinophil levels have not correlated with serum IgE level or clinical phenotype. In addition to the peripheral eosinophilia, increased eosinophils have been identified in sputum and abscesses.

Generally, patients with AD-HIES have normal white blood cell counts, although absolute mild neutropenia and leukopenia are common. Serum IgG and IgM levels are often normal, whereas serum IgA levels may be normal or low. Specific antibody responses to vaccines are variable in patients with AD-HIES, with some patients producing little or no response.[12,23,24]

Genetics and pathogenesis

Dominant-negative mutations in STAT3 cause AD-HIES. These mutations are primarily missense or single-codon in-frame deletions that result in single amino acid changes.[23,25]

Identifying the genetic mutation in STAT3 has offered important insight on the clinical phenotype. STAT3 is a transcription factor that plays an essential role in the signal transduction of many cytokines, including IL-6, IL-10, IL-21, IL-22, and IL-23. STAT3 is activated by Janus kinase 2 and phosphorylated to dimerize and translocate into the nucleus to initiate targeted gene transcription.[26,27] Because of its involvement with many cytokines, STAT3 plays a crucial role in immunity, inflammation, wound healing, cell survival, embryogenesis, and oncogenesis, with disruption leading to the multisystem nature of AD-HIES.

The most consistent immunologic finding in these patients is a lack of CD4+ Th17 cell differentiation.[28–31] The importance of IL-17 in the clearance of Candida, Klebsiella, and Staphylococcus aureus has been established in mice, and in humans, disruption of the IL-17 and IL-22 pathway leading to mucocutaneous Candida susceptibility is evident through several PIDDs.[32–37]

AD-HIES is also associated with diminished memory T and B lymphocytes. Decreased central memory CD4+ and CD8+ T lymphocytes are clinically evident by the reactivation of latent viral infections, resulting in an increased incidence of zoster and asymptomatic Epstein-Barr virus (EBV) viremia. Decreased memory and class switched B cells are frequently seen as well.[3,24,38]

Dedicator of Cytokinesis 8 Deficiency

Clinical features, infections, and management

DOCK8 mutations were described in 2009[39] in a subset of patients with an autosomal recessive inheritance pattern of many features of AD-HIES, although lacking most of the skeletal and connective tissue abnormalities. The many clinical characteristics of DOCK8 deficiency include atopic dermatitis, food or environmental allergies, marked IgE and eosinophil increases, recurrent sinopulmonary infections, recurrent staphylococcal skin infections or abscesses, mucocutaneous candidiasis, and, distinctly, a breadth of disseminated cutaneous viral infections. In addition, many patients with DOCK8 deficiency went on to develop malignancies, some fatal, likely resulting from the oncogenic properties of the cutaneous viruses and a dysfunction in tumor surveillance.[40,41]

Many patients with DOCK8 deficiency have an exaggerated atopic phenotype when compared with those with AD-HIES, and anaphylaxis and food allergy are more common.[15,40,42,43] Nearly all patients with DOCK8 deficiency (99%) have an eczematous dermatitis that begins in infancy, but less commonly, a newborn rash.[13,44,45] The immunologic mechanism driving their atopy and eosinophilia is unclear but is associated with a predominance of Th2 cytokine production and regulatory T-lymphocyte deficiency.[44,46]

Nearly 90% of affected patients have recurrent and even concurrent cutaneous viral infections, namely with human papillomavirus, herpes simplex virus (HSV), molluscum contagiosum virus, and varicella zoster virus (VZV) (**Fig. 4**).[40,42,43,47] Severe systemic viral infections are less frequent.[43,48]

Most patients with DOCK8 deficiency (>90%) have recurrent upper respiratory tract infections, pneumonias, sinusitis, and otitis media. Pulmonary pathogens include the more common Streptococcus pneumoniae and Haemophilus influenzae, but the spectrum broadens when bronchiectasis is present.[13,40,42,43] Fungal infections include mucocutaneous candidiasis, cryptococcal meningitis, disseminated histoplasmosis,

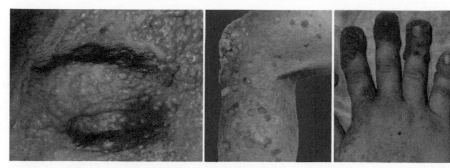

Fig. 4. Cutaneous viral infections seen in DOCK8 deficiency. From left to right: disseminated molluscum contagiosum caused by molluscum contagiosum virus and verrucous and flat warts caused by human papillomavirus.

and *Pneumocystis jirovecii*.[40,43,48] Eosinophilic pneumonias have also been seen in DOCK8 deficiency. Autoimmunity in DOCK8 deficiency has included difficult to treat autoimmune hemolytic anemia, hypothyroidism, and vasculitis.[48]

DOCK8 deficiency has a worse prognosis than AD-HIES, with most patients dying in the second and third decade of life. The only curative treatment of DOCK8 deficiency is HSCT, and this should be strongly considered for these patients. Those who have been transplanted had near or complete resolution of their cutaneous viral infections and improvement in their T-lymphocyte populations and function, eczema, and recurrent sinopulmonary within a year of transplantation.[42,49–57]

Management of DOCK8 deficiency focuses on treating and preventing infections in a manner similar to those with AD-HIES. Immunoglobulin replacement therapy is frequently indicated because of poor specific antibody production.[40,58] Acyclovir or valacyclovir should be considered for prophylaxis to prevent recurrent HSV and VZV infections. Warts and molluscum are difficult to treat in this population, and standard therapies tend to be ineffective; interferon-α has had variable benefit.[6,13,59]

Clinical laboratory findings

Peripheral eosinophilia, typically greater than 1000 cells/μL is common, as are increased serum IgE levels. The cause of the eosinophilia and increased IgE levels is not well understood. Serum levels of IgM are classically very low or even undetectable.[40,42,43,48] Serum IgG levels are often normal or slightly increased, whereas serum IgA levels are variable, with typically poor specific antibody responses.[40]

The combined immune deficiency in patients with DOCK8 is apparent with CD4+ and CD8+ T-cell lymphopenia that often worsens with age, and variability in natural killer (NK) cell and B-lymphocyte deficiency.[40,41] In addition, T-lymphocyte activation and proliferation are diminished, particularly in the CD8+ population, thus contributing their increased viral susceptibility.[40,43] Diagnosis is confirmed with DOCK8 sequencing and can be strongly suggested by absence of expression on flow cytometry.[40,60]

Genetics and pathogenesis

Mutations in DOCK8 render most patients protein negative.[40,43,48] Recently, revertant mutations have been shown, but the clinical significance remains unknown.[61] DOCK8 belongs to the DOCK180 superfamily of guanine nucleotide exchange factors.[62] These guanine nucleotide exchange factors are known to interact with the Rho family of guanosine triphosphatases, which can be found in all eukaryotic cells and have an important role in organelle and cytoskeletal development, cell migration, phagocytosis, and wound healing.[63,64] DOCK8 plays a critical immunologic role, specifically in T-lymphocyte, B-lymphocyte, and NK T-cell survival, migration, and synapse formation.[41,65,66]

Phosphoglucomutase 3 Deficiency

Clinical features, infections, and management

Mutations in phosphoglucomutase 3 (PGM3) were recently defined, leading to a multisystem disease sharing some clinical features with AD-HIES and DOCK8 deficiency. The initial clinical description of patients with this disease was the report of an autosomal recessive vasculitis-myoclonus syndrome associated with infection and severe atopy in a family with 5 affected children.[67,68] The clinical phenotype of PGM3 deficiency is still being defined, but cutaneous leukocytoclastic vasculitis, eczema-like rash, cognitive impairment and myoclonus, and delayed visual and sensory evoked potentials have all been present, as well as severe bronchiectasis.[68,69]

Poor control of viruses has presented as widespread molluscum contagiosum in 1 affected individual and poor control of EBV, with persistent EBV viremia and EBV associated Hodgkin lymphoma in 2 individuals.[68,69] Clinical variability is evident by the cohort with B and T lymphopenia similar to that seen in severe combined immunodeficiency (SCID), neutropenia, and progression to bone marrow failure.[70] Autoimmune and immune-mediated diseases have included membranoproliferative glomerulonephritis, autoimmune neutropenia, psoriasis, and vasculitis. Skeletal abnormalities have manifested as scoliosis, facial dysmorphism, and hyperextensibility. Cognitive impairment seems common, and demyelination has been observed on brain magnetic resonance imaging for several patients.[68–70]

Treatment of PGM3 deficiency is supportive. Prophylactic or suppressive antimicrobials should be considered based on clinical presentation. Immunoglobulin replacement may be considered if poor specific antibodies are present; however, anecdotal reports of improvement have been mixed. Transplant improved the bone marrow failure and immunologic phenotype in 2 patients, but the impact on the neurologic and skeletal phenotype is unclear.[70] Dietary supplementation has been used in other congenital disorders of glycosylation but has not yet been established for this defect.[71]

Clinical laboratory findings

Most individuals identified with PGM3 deficiency have had significantly increased serum IgE levels, variable eosinophilia, and immune abnormalities. Leukopenia seems common with both lymphopenia and neutropenia. The lymphopenia is predominantly from decreased CD8+ T cells and low memory B cells. IgG, IgE, and IgA levels have all been increased, and specific antibodies have been present but less robust than frequently seen in healthy controls. Consistent with the atopic clinical phenotype, the T-cell cytokine responses have a Th2 skew with increased secretion ex vivo of IL-4, IL-5, and IL-13. Compared with DOCK8 deficiency and AD-HIES, the T-lymphocyte production of IL-17 seems increased, which may explain some of the autoimmunity features and the lack of candidiasis.[62,69]

PGM3 deficiency should be suspected in an individual with an exaggerated allergic phenotype, recurrent infections, and neurologic deficits. Glycosylation defects can also be suggested by glycan profiling of urine and serum. In PGM3 deficiency, both O-linked and N-linked glycans are abnormal. Sequencing of PGM3 is key to the diagnosis.

Genetics and pathogenesis

PGM3 is an enzyme responsible for the conversion of GlcNAc-6-phosphate to GlcNAc-1-phosphate, which then converts to UDP-GlcNAc. This is a key early step in multiple glycosylation pathways, and thus essential to allow normal activity of many diverse proteins. Because most proteins require glycosylation, absence of activity is not compatible with life and is embryonic lethal in mice. The disease is autosomal recessive, and all mutations found have been hypomorphic, allowing diminished but present activity. A mouse model of PGM3 deficiency caused by hypomorphic point mutations led to lymphopenia with T lymphocytes predominantly affected, anemia, and thrombocytopenia.[72]

Wiskott-Aldrich Syndrome

Clinical features, infections, and management
Peripheral and tissue eosinophilia (eg, in lymph nodes and spleen) are characteristic of Wiskott-Aldrich syndrome (WAS).[73,74] WAS was first described in 1954 with its X-linked inheritance pattern of severe eczema, thrombocytopenia with small platelets, and recurrent infections.[75] A wide variety of infections have been reported in WAS, including *Pneumocystis jirovecii* pneumonia, severe or disseminated HSV and varicella, and invasive fungal infections.[76] Because of the significant thrombocytopenia, patients can present with bleeding, petechiae, or ecchymoses. Autoimmunity (eg, autoimmune cytopenias, inflammatory bowel disease, renal disease) and malignancy (notably, lymphoma) are seen as well.[77] Similar to those with DOCK8 deficiency, vasculitis and aortic aneurysm have also been described.[78,79]

Morbidity and mortality related to WAS are high if not properly treated. Death is usually secondary to infection, bleeding, or malignancy.[76] Because of the poor antibody responses, Immunoglobulin replacement therapy is often helpful in reducing serious infections. The immunoglobulin therapy has not shown appreciable impact on the thrombocytopenia, although splenectomy has led to normalization of platelet counts.[80,81] Those who are status post splenectomy should receive appropriate prophylaxis with vaccination and penicillin. HSCT or gene therapy should be considered.[82,83]

Clinical laboratory findings
Complete blood counts almost always show thrombocytopenia with microthrombocytes on peripheral smear. Peripheral eosinophilia and anemia are often observed, and as with other PIDD, the mechanism driving the eosinophilia is unclear. Typically, serum IgM levels are decreased, serum IgG and IgA levels are variable, and serum IgE level is increased. Poor polysaccharide vaccine responses are characteristic.[73,76,82,84]

Flow cytometry typically shows mild T-cell lymphopenia, normal circulating B lymphocytes, and normal or increased NK cells. Poor lymphocyte proliferation and NK cytotoxicity is characteristic, because WASp (WAS protein) is essential for colocalizing with actin to NK-cell activating synapses.[82,84] In addition to sequencing, flow cytometry is also used to evaluate WASp expression in suspected cases of WAS.[82]

Genetics and pathogenesis
Mutations in the gene WAS, located on the X-chromosome, have been identified as causing deficiency in WASp. WASp is a crucial regulator of platelet and lymphocyte development and is critical for cytoskeletal and immunologic synapse formation and regulatory T-cell function.[85–87] Genotype-phenotype correlations have been described, with those having X-linked thrombocytopenia and X-linked neutropenia having distinct and often milder phenotypes.[88]

SEVERE COMBINED IMMUNODEFICIENCY AND RELATED DISORDERS ASSOCIATED WITH EOSINOPHILIA
Adenosine Deaminase–Severe Combined Immunodeficiency

Clinical features, infections, and management

Although eosinophilia is not a prominent feature in all variants of SCID, peripheral eosinophilia is a commonly encountered clinical manifestation seen in adenosine deaminase (ADA)-SCID. Because of the profound T-cell, B-cell, and NK-cell lymphopenia seen in ADA-SCID, affected individuals typically present in infancy with severe opportunistic infections, such as with *Pneumocystis jirovecii* pneumonia. Recurrent or severe respiratory infections typically occur within the first few months of life, along with failure to thrive, frequent thrush, and chronic diarrhea.[84,89,90] Partial ADA deficiency has been described in a subset of patients who typically present later in life, such as in late infancy or early childhood, with a milder phenotype that may include autoimmune manifestations.[91]

Atopy is a common feature in ADA-SCID, found in about half of those with early onset disease. Of the atopic manifestations, allergic rhinitis, asthma, food allergy, mild atopic dermatitis, and urticaria were the most common identified in this population.[92]

Given the ubiquitous nature of ADA expression and the profound impacts of deoxydenosine, S-adenosylhomocysteine, and deoxyadenosine triphosphate accumulation within the tissues, patients with ADA deficiency often present with other systemic manifestations, such as hepatic degeneration and dysfunction, costochondral abnormalities, and skeletal dysplasia.[89,93] Neurologic motor and hearing impairments (ie, bilateral sensorineuronal deafness) have also been associated with ADA deficiency, and patients may have cognitive and behavioral deficits.[94,95]

Without early recognition and treatment, ADA-SCID is often fatal within the first year of life.[89,96] The treatment options for ADA deficiency include allogeneic hematopoietic stem cell therapy, enzyme replacement therapy with pegylated bovine ADA, and gene therapy.[97]

Clinical laboratory findings

Patients with ADA-SCID have a SCID with a profound deficiency of circulating T lymphocytes, B lymphocytes, and NK cells, more so than any other form of SCID.[89,96] Serum IgG levels are usually normal at presentation as a result of maternal transfer of IgG but decrease soon after. Serum IgA and IgM levels are variable, although more commonly IgM levels are low in this population.[96] Serum eosinophilia and IgE levels are also variable but frequently increased among both those with early and delayed onset, presumably because of their increased CD4+ Th2 cytokine production and their clinical features of atopy.[90,92,98]

When ADA-SCID is suspected, ADA activity should be assessed and will be low or absent. In addition, levels of S-adenosylhomocysteine and deoxyadenosine triphosphate are increased in ADA-SCID. Newborn screening for SCID through a quantitative evaluation of T-cell receptor excision circles is helpful in identifying infants with SCID who can be further screened for ADA and other causes.[99,100]

Genetics and pathogenesis

Accounting for 10% to 20% of all SCID cases, ADA-SCID results from autosomal recessive mutations in the ADA gene.[96,101] ADA is an enzyme that is crucial in the purine salvage pathway, catalyzing the deamination of deoxydenosine and adenosine to deoxyinosine and inosine. In an ADA-deficient state, there is buildup of deoxydenosine, S-adenosylhomocysteine, and deoxyadenosine triphosphate in the intracellular and extracellular compartments, leading to impaired T-lymphocyte and B-lymphocyte development. In addition to inducing thymocyte apoptosis, deoxyadenosine triphosphate interferes with terminal deoxynucleotidyl transferase activity and restricts V(D)J recombination.[96,102,103]

Omenn Syndrome

Clinical features, infections, and management
Similar to early onset ADA-SCID, Omenn syndrome presents in infancy with peripheral eosinophilia, high serum IgE levels, and rash. The rash is typically a generalized and often exfoliative erythroderma in contrast to the pustular or erythema toxicum neonatorum rash seen in AD-HIES.[104] Impairment of V(D)J recombination leads to abnormally expanded T lymphocytes. Affected infants commonly present with recurrent and severe infection, chronic diarrhea, lymphadenopathy, hepatosplenomegaly, and failure to thrive.[46]

HSCT can be curative in Omenn syndrome, and without early transplant, the disease is often fatal; however, in addition to pretransplant supportive care with immunoglobulin replacement therapy and prophylactic antimicrobials, these patients also require systemic immunosuppression for their marked lymphoproliferation and inflammation.[83,99,105–107]

Clinical laboratory findings
Patients with Omenn syndrome have increased serum Ig levels and profound eosinophilia, likely resulting from Th2 skewing, despite the low or absent circulating B lymphocytes, decreased IgG, decreased IgM, and decreased IgA levels.[104] In contrast to classic SCID, patients have normal or even markedly increased circulating activated T-lymphocyte levels; however, they are oligoclonal and associated with poor antigenic responses.[108–110]

Genetics and pathogenesis
Omenn syndrome seems to be caused by hypomorphic mutations in genes associated with SCID. These mutations have included include RAG1/2, Artemis, IL-7Rα, DNA ligase IV, RNA-processing endoribonuclease, ADA, and γc.[84,110] Patients with atypical DiGeorge syndrome (caused by a microdeletion at chromosome 22q11.2) may also present with a clinical phenotype that resembles Omenn syndrome.[111–113]

IMMUNE DYSREGULATORY SYNDROMES ASSOCIATED WITH EOSINOPHILIA
Autoimmune Lymphoproliferative Syndrome

Clinical features, infections, and management
Although eosinophilia is often not the clinical feature driving presentation of patients with autoimmune lymphoproliferative syndrome (ALPS), eosinophilia is a common manifestation. ALPS typically presents in childhood, with marked splenomegaly, generalized lymphadenopathy, and chronic cytopenias. Autoimmune hemolytic anemia, neutropenia, and thrombocytopenia are typical. Patients with ALPS are at increased risk for developing B-cell and T-cell lymphomas as a result of the marked lymphoproliferation. In a recent study of the natural history of ALPS performed at the National Institutes of Health, 12% of the cohort developed either Hodgkin or non-Hodgkin lymphoma.[114,115]

The management of ALPS focuses on 3 main aspects of the syndrome: controlling the cytopenias, preventing infection, and malignancy surveillance. In addition, spleen guards should be worn to protect against rupture, and splenectomy should be avoided.[116]

Clinical laboratory findings

The unique laboratory finding, which is required for an ALPS diagnosis, is increased CD3+ $\alpha\beta$ CD4-CD8-double negative T-lymphocyte levels (>1.5% of total lymphocytes or >2.5% of CD3+ lymphocytes). Total lymphocyte counts are also normal or increased.[114,115] Serum vitamin B_{12} levels are increased in ALPS and have proved to be a reliable biomarker for lymphoproliferation. Patients with ALPS often have increased serum immunoglobulin levels (namely IgG, IgA, and IgM).[114] Anemia, neutropenia, or thrombocytopenia are common as a result of the autoimmunity associated with the syndrome. Autoantibodies are frequently positive, including rheumatoid factor, direct antiglobulin test, anticardiolipin antibody, antithyroid antibodies, and antinuclear antibodies.

Approximately 25% of patients with ALPS have peripheral eosinophila (>750 cells/μL).[114,115] The cause of the eosinophilia is likely a result of Th2 skewing that produces an increase in IL-5. Fas-mediated apoptosis of eosinophils (as assessed in vitro) is impaired in patients with ALPS, with and without eosinophilia, suggesting that this is not the cause of the observed eosinophilia.[117] Patients with eosinophilic ALPS also have more profound cytopenias and are at significantly increased risk for death as a result of infectious complications from their immunosuppression.[117]

Genetics and pathogenesis

Most ALPS cases are caused by heterozygous mutations in the FAS gene, which encodes the tumor necrosis factor (TNF) receptor superfamily-6 protein (TNFRSF6; Fas). Somatic or germline mutations in FAS-ligand, FAS-associated death domain, caspase 8, and caspase 10 have also been identified to cause ALPS. These mutations lead to defective lymphocyte apoptosis and thus lymphoproliferation.[114,118] An ALPS-like phenotype can also be caused by germline gain-of-function STAT3 mutations.[119]

Immunodysregulation, Polyendocrinopathy, Enteropathy, X-Linked Syndrome

Clinical features, infections, and management

Patients with immunodysregulation, polyendocrinopathy, enteropathy, X-linked syndrome (IPEX) frequently present with eosinophilia and severe atopy.[120] In addition, the classic triad of enteropathy, endocrinopathy, and dermatitis is observed.[121] Most commonly, these patients present with early onset severe and watery diarrhea, type 1 diabetes mellitus, and failure to thrive.[122] Endoscopic biopsies of the gastrointestinal tract show villous blunting and lymphocytic infiltration, similar to that described in celiac disease and graft-versus-host disease.[123] The dermatitis resembles that of eczema and may vary in severity. Patients with IPEX have frequent autoimmunity, recurrent infections largely from immunosuppression, and may have food allergy.[122,124]

Clinical laboratory findings

Many of these patients have increased serum IgE levels, increased serum IgA levels, peripheral eosinophilia, and normal T-lymphocyte and B-lymphocyte subsets; however, they lack the essential CD4+CD25+ FOXP3+ regulatory T lymphocytes. Regulatory T lymphocytes have been shown to secrete IL-10 and transforming growth factor β (TGF-β), and lead to suppression of serum IgE.[125] Presumably the deficiency in regulatory T lymphocytes contributes to the increased IgE levels.

Genetics and pathogenesis

Mutations in both the coding and noncoding regions of FOXP3 have been identified in most patients with IPEX. FOXP3 encodes the protein scurfin, a transcription factor that is the master regulator in the development and functioning of regulatory T lymphocytes.[126,127] Mice lacking FOXP3 (scurfy mice) share many characteristics of patients with IPEX.[126] The lack of regulatory T lymphocytes leads to the loss of peripheral tolerance and marked cytokine overproduction in effector T lymphocytes.

In addition to sequencing, flow cytometry is often used as a clinical tool to evaluate FOXP3 protein expression in suspected cases of IPEX.[122] IPEX-like phenotypes including eosinophilia can also be seen in patients with CD25 deficiency and gain-of-function mutations in STAT1 or STAT3.[119,128,129]

Loeys-Dietz Syndrome

Clinical features, infections, and management
Loeys-Dietz syndrome (LDS) is a connective tissue disorder with multisystem involvement, a large segment of which develops significant atopy, and eosinophilia. There is a great deal of clinical overlap between AD-HIES and LDS. Musculoskeletal abnormalities are variable and can include craniosynostosis, retained primary dentition, facial asymmetry, pectus deformity, scoliosis, flat feet, and joint hyperextensibility. In addition, patients may have a high arched or cleft palate, an abnormal uvula, and hypertelorism. Their skin is classically thin and translucent, and easy bruising and poor wound healing are not uncommon.[130,131] Vascular anomalies are a prominent feature of LDS. Diffuse arterial abnormalities, such as aneurysms and tortuosity, put patients at great risk for dissection or hemorrhages.[130,132]

Patients with LDS have an exaggerated allergic phenotype, which can include asthma, food allergy, atopic dermatitis, and allergic rhinitis. Gastrointestinal complaints, such as chronic abdominal pain, poor growth, constipation, and vomiting, are common among patients with LDS. Eosinophilic gastrointestinal disease (eg, eosinophilic esophagitis, colitis, or gastritis) is often diagnosed pathologically. Targeted elimination diets seem to be beneficial in reducing clinical symptoms.[131,133]

Clinical laboratory findings
Increased serum IgE and absolute eosinophil counts are prevalent laboratory findings in patients with LDS. These findings may be in part caused by the Th2 skewing that is apparent in this population. The Th2 cytokine production is associated with an increased CD4+CD25+ FOXP3+ regulatory T-lymphocyte population, which abnormally produces Th2 cytokines.[133]

Genetics and pathogenesis
Four genetic mutations have been identified in LDS. These mutations include heterozygous mutations in TGFBR1, TGFBR2, SMAD3, and TGFB2. Each mutation results in altered TGF-β signaling, yielding abnormal collagen and connective tissue growth, and effects on lymphocyte differentiation.[130–133] Despite the genetic and phenotypic variation seen in the LDS types, medical management is similar.[131]

DERMATOLOGIC SYNDROMES WITH IMMUNODYSREGULATION ASSOCIATED WITH EOSINOPHILIA
Comel-Netherton Syndrome

Clinical features, infections, and management
Comel-Netherton syndrome is a dermatologic condition associated with an exaggerated allergic phenotype, including severe atopic dermatitis, allergic rhinitis, peripheral eosinophilia, and increased serum IgE levels. The hallmark clinical features of Comel-Netherton syndrome are severe congenital ichthyosis and the pathognomonic bamboo hairs, known as trichorrexis invaginata. The extent of skin involvement varies and may include an erythroderma or migrating and scaly plaques.[134–136] The skin

lesions are usually pruritic secondary to the profound skin barrier defect and enhanced inflammation. S aureus skin infections are frequent. Additional findings associated with Comel-Netherton syndrome include failure to thrive, sparse or absent hair, eyebrows and eye lashes at birth, and chronic diarrhea.[135,136]

Mortality is highest in the neonatal period from sepsis, dehydration, or malnutrition.[135] Management is aimed at systemic and cutaneous symptom management. Emollients are essential for their skin, and adequate nutrition and hydration is critical. Intravenous immunoglobulin and anti-TNF-α monoclonal antibodies have been effective in reducing skin inflammation.[136,137]

Clinical laboratory findings
Increased serum IgE levels and absolute eosinophil counts are common, and lymphocyte phenotyping may show increased NK cells and decreased switched and unswitched memory B cells found.[135,136,138] Poor NK-cell cytotoxicity has also been identified.[136] Histopathology of skin biopsy shows epidermal hyperplasia, minimal granular layer, and typically, stratum corneum detachment.[135]

Genetics and pathogenesis
Comel-Netherton syndrome stems from loss-of-function mutations in SPINK5, which encodes the serine protease inhibitor LEKTI.[135,139,140] LEKTI is expressed in both the epithelia and the thymus. Murine models have shown that LEKTI deficiency leads to unopposed kallikrein-related peptidase activity, causing impaired epidermal differentiation, defective cornification, and poor skin barrier formation.[135,141,142]

Severe Dermatitis, Multiple Allergies, and Metabolic Wasting Syndrome

Clinical features, infections, and management
Severe dermatitis, multiple allergies, and metabolic wasting (SAM) syndrome closely resembles Comel-Netherton syndrome, with congenital ichthyosis, erythroderma, severe atopic dermatitis, peripheral eosinophilia, and increased serum IgE levels. The dermatitis has been described as papular, scaly, and with plaque formation. Like Comel-Netherton syndrome, hair is absent or sparse.[142,143] Unique to SAM syndrome is the early and severe development of food allergies and prominent metabolic wasting. Malabsorption and failure to thrive are also common, and eosinophilic esophagitis was identified in 1 patient. Recurrent infections, developmental delay, and minor cardiac defects, such as ventricular septal defects, have also been described.[142,143]

Clinical laboratory findings
Increased serum IgE levels and absolute eosinophil counts are found in SAM syndrome. Keratinocytes from those with SAM syndrome showed upregulation of proinflammatory cytokine genes, such as IL5, which likely contributes to the eosinophilia. Other laboratory immune defects have not been described. Skin biopsy pathology shows abnormally formed desmosomes and loss of cell-cell adhesion.[143]

Genetics and pathogenesis
Homozygous loss-of-function mutations in DSG-1 were identified in 2 consanguineous families with SAM syndrome.[143] As with the other desmogleins, DSG-1 plays a crucial role in cell-cell adhesion in keratinocytes, as well as in myocardial cells.[144] DSG-1 deficiency leads to absent cell-cell adhesion and abnormally formed epidermal desmosomes.[143] Without adequate cell-cell adhesion, the epidermal barrier dysfunction results.

SUMMARY

The differential diagnosis of eosinophilia is broad and includes disorders of immune deficiency or dysfunction, especially those with prominent atopy as a clinical manifestation. There is a great deal of overlap in many of these disorders, and thus, a thorough clinical and laboratory evaluation is warranted.

REFERENCES

1. Fulkerson PC, Schollaert KL, Bouffi C, et al. IL-5 triggers a cooperative cytokine network that promotes eosinophil precursor maturation. J Immunol 2014;193(8): 4043–52.
2. Davis SD, Schaller J, Wedgwood RJ. Job's syndrome. Recurrent, "cold", staphylococcal abscesses. Lancet 1966;1(7445):1013–5.
3. Buckley RW, Wray BB, Belmaker EZ. Extreme hyperimmunoglobulinemia E and undue susceptibility to infection. Pediatrics 1972;49:59–70.
4. Chamlin SL, McCalmont TH, Cunningham BB, et al. Cutaneous manifestations of hyper-IgE syndrome in infants and children. J Pediatr 2002; 141(4):572–5.
5. Eberting CL, Davis J, Puck JM, et al. Dermatitis and the newborn rash of hyper-IgE syndrome. Arch Dermatol 2004;140(9):1119–25.
6. Chu EY, Freeman AF, Jing H, et al. Cutaneous manifestations of DOCK8 deficiency syndrome. Arch Dermatol 2012;148(1):79–84.
7. Kong HH, Oh J, Deming C, et al. Temporal shifts in the skin microbiome associated with disease flares and treatment in children with atopic dermatitis. Genome Res 2012;22(5):850–9.
8. Grimbacher B, Holland SM, Gallin JI, et al. Hyper-IgE syndrome with recurrent infections–an autosomal dominant multisystem disorder. N Engl J Med 1999; 340(9):692–702.
9. Freeman AF, Davis J, Anderson VL, et al. *Pneumocystis jiroveci* infection in patients with hyper-immunoglobulin E syndrome. Pediatrics 2006;118(4): e1271–5.
10. Freeman AF, Domingo DL, Holland SM. Hyper IgE (Job's) syndrome: a primary immune deficiency with oral manifestations. Oral Dis 2009;15(1):2–7.
11. Freeman AF, Kleiner DE, Nadiminti H, et al. Causes of death in hyper-IgE syndrome. J Allergy Clin Immunol 2007;119(5):1234–40.
12. Sowerwine KJ, Holland SM, Freeman AF. Hyper-IgE syndrome update. Ann N Y Acad Sci 2012;1250:25–32.
13. Freeman AF, Holland SM. Clinical manifestations of hyper IgE syndromes. Dis Markers 2010;29(3–4):123–30.
14. Siegel AM, Heimall J, Freeman AF, et al. A critical role for STAT3 transcription factor signaling in the development and maintenance of human T cell memory. Immunity 2011;35(5):806–18.
15. Siegel AM, Stone KD, Cruse G, et al. Diminished allergic disease in patients with STAT3 mutations reveals a role for STAT3 signaling in mast cell degranulation. J Allergy Clin Immunol 2013;132(6):1388–96.
16. Borges WG, Hensley T, Carey JC, et al. The face of Job. J Pediatr 1998;133(2): 303–5.
17. Smithwick EM, Finelt M, Pahwa S, et al. Cranial synostosis in Job's syndrome. Lancet 1978;1(8068):826.

18. Liacouras CA, Furuta GT, Hirano I, et al. Eosinophilic esophagitis: updated consensus recommendations for children and adults. J Allergy Clin Immunol 2011;128(1):3–20 e6 [quiz: 21–2].

19. Leonard GD, Posadas E, Herrmann PC, et al. Non-Hodgkin's lymphoma in Job's syndrome: a case report and literature review. Leuk Lymphoma 2004;45(12):2521–5.

20. Gennery AR, Flood TJ, Abinun M, et al. Bone marrow transplantation does not correct the hyper IgE syndrome. Bone Marrow Transplant 2000;25(12):1303–5.

21. Goussetis E, Peristeri I, Kitra V, et al. Successful long-term immunologic reconstitution by allogeneic hematopoietic stem cell transplantation cures patients with autosomal dominant hyper-IgE syndrome. J Allergy Clin Immunol 2010;126(2):392–4.

22. Nester TA, Wagnon AH, Reilly WF, et al. Effects of allogeneic peripheral stem cell transplantation in a patient with job syndrome of hyperimmunoglobulinemia E and recurrent infections. Am J Med 1998;105(2):162–4.

23. Holland SM, DeLeo FR, Elloumi HZ, et al. STAT3 mutations in the hyper-IgE syndrome. N Engl J Med 2007;357(16):1608–19.

24. Speckmann C, Enders A, Woellner C, et al. Reduced memory B cells in patients with hyper IgE syndrome. Clin Immunol 2008;129(3):448–54.

25. Minegishi Y, Saito M, Tsuchiya S, et al. Dominant-negative mutations in the DNA-binding domain of STAT3 cause hyper-IgE syndrome. Nature 2007;448(7157):1058–62.

26. Ihle JN, Kerr IM. Jaks and Stats in signaling by the cytokine receptor superfamily. Trends Genet 1995;11(2):69–74.

27. Schindler C, Darnell JE Jr. Transcriptional responses to polypeptide ligands: the JAK-STAT pathway. Annu Rev Biochem 1995;64:621–51.

28. Hsu AP, Sowerwine KJ, Lawrence MG, et al. Intermediate phenotypes in patients with autosomal dominant hyper-IgE syndrome caused by somatic mosaicism. J Allergy Clin Immunol 2013;131(6):1586–93.

29. Milner JD, Brenchley JM, Laurence A, et al. Impaired T(H)17 cell differentiation in subjects with autosomal dominant hyper-IgE syndrome. Nature 2008;452(7188):773–6.

30. Renner ED, Rylaarsdam S, Anover-Sombke S, et al. Novel signal transducer and activator of transcription 3 (STAT3) mutations, reduced T(H)17 cell numbers, and variably defective STAT3 phosphorylation in hyper-IgE syndrome. J Allergy Clin Immunol 2008;122(1):181–7.

31. Schimke LF, Sawalle-Belohradsky J, Roesler J, et al. Diagnostic approach to the hyper-IgE syndromes: immunologic and clinical key findings to differentiate hyper-IgE syndromes from atopic dermatitis. J Allergy Clin Immunol 2010;126(3):611–7.e1.

32. Cho JS, Pietras EM, Garcia NC, et al. IL-17 is essential for host defense against cutaneous Staphylococcus aureus infection in mice. J Clin Invest 2010;120(5):1762–73.

33. Happel KI, Dubin PJ, Zheng M, et al. Divergent roles of IL-23 and IL-12 in host defense against Klebsiella pneumoniae. J Exp Med 2005;202(6):761–9.

34. Huang W, Na L, Fidel PL, et al. Requirement of interleukin-17A for systemic anti-Candida albicans host defense in mice. J Infect Dis 2004;190(3):624–31.

35. Kisand K, Bøe Wolff AS, Podkrajsek KT, et al. Chronic mucocutaneous candidiasis in APECED or thymoma patients correlates with autoimmunity to Th17-associated cytokines. J Exp Med 2010;207(2):299–308.

36. Puel A, Döffinger R, Natividad A, et al. Autoantibodies against IL-17A, IL-17F, and IL-22 in patients with chronic mucocutaneous candidiasis and autoimmune polyendocrine syndrome type I. J Exp Med 2010;207(2):291–7.
37. Puel A, Picard C, Cypowyj S, et al. Inborn errors of mucocutaneous immunity to *Candida albicans* in humans: a role for IL-17 cytokines? Curr Opin Immunol 2010;22(4):467–74.
38. Heimall J, Davis J, Shaw PA, et al. Paucity of genotype-phenotype correlations in STAT3 mutation positive hyper IgE syndrome (HIES). Clin Immunol 2011; 139(1):75–84.
39. Renner ED, Puck JM, Holland SM, et al. Autosomal recessive hyperimmunoglobulin E syndrome: a distinct disease entity. J Pediatr 2004;144(1):93–9.
40. Zhang Q, Davis JC, Lamborn IT, et al. Combined immunodeficiency associated with DOCK8 mutations. N Engl J Med 2009;361(21):2046–55.
41. Su HC. Dedicator of cytokinesis 8 (DOCK8) deficiency. Curr Opin Allergy Clin Immunol 2010;10(6):515–20.
42. Al-Herz W, Ragupathy R, Massaad MJ, et al. Clinical, immunologic and genetic profiles of DOCK8-deficient patients in Kuwait. Clin Immunol 2012;143(3):266–72.
43. Engelhardt KR, McGhee S, Winkler S, et al. Large deletions and point mutations involving the dedicator of cytokinesis 8 (DOCK8) in the autosomal-recessive form of hyper-IgE syndrome. J Allergy Clin Immunol 2009;124(6):1289–1302 e4.
44. Zhang Q, Davis JC, Dove CG, et al. Genetic, clinical, and laboratory markers for DOCK8 immunodeficiency syndrome. Dis Markers 2010;29(3–4):131–9.
45. Aydin SE, Kilic SS, Aytekin C, et al. DOCK8 deficiency: clinical and immunological phenotype and treatment options–a review of 136 patients. J Clin Immunol 2015;35(2):189–98.
46. Ozcan E, Notarangelo LD, Geha RS. Primary immune deficiencies with aberrant IgE production. J Allergy Clin Immunol 2008;122(6):1054–62 [quiz: 1063–4].
47. Leiding JW, Holland SM. Warts and all: human papillomavirus in primary immunodeficiencies. J Allergy Clin Immunol 2012;130(5):1030–48.
48. Alsum Z, Hawwari A, Alsmadi O, et al. Clinical, immunological and molecular characterization of DOCK8 and DOCK8-like deficient patients: single center experience of twenty-five patients. J Clin Immunol 2013;33(1):55–67.
49. Al-Mousa H, Hawwari A, Alsum Z. In DOCK8 deficiency donor cell engraftment post-genoidentical hematopoietic stem cell transplantation is possible without conditioning. J Allergy Clin Immunol 2013;131(4):1244–5.
50. Barlogis V, Galambrun C, Chambost H, et al. Successful allogeneic hematopoietic stem cell transplantation for DOCK8 deficiency. J Allergy Clin Immunol 2011;128(2):420–2.e2.
51. Bittner TC, Pannicke U, Renner ED, et al. Successful long-term correction of autosomal recessive hyper-IgE syndrome due to DOCK8 deficiency by hematopoietic stem cell transplantation. Klin Padiatr 2010;222(6):351–5.
52. Boztug H, Karitnig-Weiß C, Ausserer B, et al. Clinical and immunological correction of DOCK8 deficiency by allogeneic hematopoietic stem cell transplantation following a reduced toxicity conditioning regimen. Pediatr Hematol Oncol 2012; 29(7):585–94.
53. Gatz SA, Benninghoff U, Schütz C, et al. Curative treatment of autosomal-recessive hyper-IgE syndrome by hematopoietic cell transplantation. Bone Marrow Transplant 2011;46(4):552–6.
54. Ghosh S, Schuster FR, Fuchs I, et al. Treosulfan-based conditioning in DOCK8 deficiency: complete lympho-hematopoietic reconstitution with minimal toxicity. Clin Immunol 2012;145(3):259–61.

55. McDonald DR, Massaad MJ, Johnston A, et al. Successful engraftment of donor marrow after allogeneic hematopoietic cell transplantation in autosomal-recessive hyper-IgE syndrome caused by dedicator of cytokinesis 8 deficiency. J Allergy Clin Immunol 2010;126(6):1304–5.e3.
56. Metin A, Tavil B, Azık F, et al. Successful bone marrow transplantation for DOCK8 deficient hyper IgE syndrome. Pediatr Transplant 2012;16(4):398–9.
57. Cuellar-Rodriguez J, Freeman AF, Grossman J, et al. Matched related and unrelated donor hematopoietic stem cell transplantation for DOCK8 deficiency. Biol Blood Marrow Transplant 2015;21(6):1037–45.
58. Yong PF, Freeman AF, Engelhardt KR, et al. An update on the hyper-IgE syndromes. Arthritis Res Ther 2012;14(6):228.
59. Ramirez-Fort MK, Au SC, Javed SA, et al. Management of cutaneous human papillomavirus infection: pharmacotherapies. Curr Probl Dermatol 2014;45:175–85.
60. Pai SY, de Boer H, Massaad MJ, et al. Flow cytometry diagnosis of dedicator of cytokinesis 8 (DOCK8) deficiency. J Allergy Clin Immunol 2014;134(1):221–3.
61. Jing H, Zhang Q, Zhang Y, et al. Somatic reversion in dedicator of cytokinesis 8 immunodeficiency modulates disease phenotype. J Allergy Clin Immunol 2014; 133(6):1667–75.
62. Yang J, Zhang Z, Roe SM, et al. Activation of Rho GTPases by DOCK exchange factors is mediated by a nucleotide sensor. Science 2009;325(5946):1398–402.
63. Etienne-Manneville S, Hall A. Rho GTPases in cell biology. Nature 2002; 420(6916):629–35.
64. Hall A. Rho GTPases and the actin cytoskeleton. Science 1998;279(5350): 509–14.
65. Harada Y, Tanaka Y, Terasawa M, et al. DOCK8 is a Cdc42 activator critical for interstitial dendritic cell migration during immune responses. Blood 2012; 119(19):4451–61.
66. Lambe T, Crawford G, Johnson AL, et al. DOCK8 is essential for T-cell survival and the maintenance of CD8+ T-cell memory. Eur J Immunol 2011;41(12): 3423–35.
67. Hay BN, Martin JE, Karp B, et al. Familial immunodeficiency with cutaneous vasculitis, myoclonus, and cognitive impairment. Am J Med Genet A 2004; 125A(2):145–51.
68. Zhang Y, Yu X, Ichikawa M, et al. Autosomal recessive phosphoglucomutase 3 (PGM3) mutations link glycosylation defects to atopy, immune deficiency, autoimmunity, and neurocognitive impairment. J Allergy Clin Immunol 2014;133(5): 1400–9.e5.
69. Sassi A, Lazaroski S, Wu G, et al. Hypomorphic homozygous mutations in phosphoglucomutase 3 (PGM3) impair immunity and increase serum IgE levels. J Allergy Clin Immunol 2014;133(5):1410–9.e13.
70. Stray-Pedersen A, Backe PH, Sorte HS, et al. PGM3 mutations cause a congenital disorder of glycosylation with severe immunodeficiency and skeletal dysplasia. Am J Hum Genet 2014;95(1):96–107.
71. Tegtmeyer LC, Rust S, van Scherpenzeel M, et al. Multiple phenotypes in phosphoglucomutase 1 deficiency. N Engl J Med 2014;370(6):533–42.
72. Greig KT, Antonchuk J, Metcalf D, et al. Agm1/Pgm3-mediated sugar nucleotide synthesis is essential for hematopoiesis and development. Mol Cell Biol 2007; 27(16):5849–59.
73. Berglund G, Finnström O, Johansson SG, et al. Wiskott-Aldrich syndrome. A study of 6 cases with determination of the immunoglobulins A, D, G, M and ND. Acta Paediatr Scand 1968;57(2):89–97.

74. Snover DC, Frizzera G, Spector BD, et al. Wiskott-Aldrich syndrome: histopathologic findings in the lymph nodes and spleens of 15 patients. Hum Pathol 1981; 12(9):821–31.

75. Aldrich RA, Steinberg AG, Campbell DC. Pedigree demonstrating a sex-linked recessive condition characterized by draining ears, eczematoid dermatitis and bloody diarrhea. Pediatrics 1954;13(2):133–9.

76. Sullivan KE, Mullen CA, Blaese RM, et al. A multiinstitutional survey of the Wiskott-Aldrich syndrome. J Pediatr 1994;125(6 Pt 1):876–85.

77. Ochs HD, Filipovich AH, Veys P, et al. Wiskott-Aldrich syndrome: diagnosis, clinical and laboratory manifestations, and treatment. Biol Blood Marrow Transplant 2009;15(1 Suppl):84–90.

78. Mahlaoui N, Pellier I, Mignot C, et al. Characteristics and outcome of early-onset, severe forms of Wiskott-Aldrich syndrome. Blood 2013;121(9):1510–6.

79. Pellier I, Dupuis Girod S, Loisel D, et al. Occurrence of aortic aneurysms in 5 cases of Wiskott-Aldrich syndrome. Pediatrics 2011;127(2):e498–504.

80. Litzman J, Jones A, Hann I, et al. Intravenous immunoglobulin, splenectomy, and antibiotic prophylaxis in Wiskott-Aldrich syndrome. Arch Dis Child 1996; 75(5):436–9.

81. Mathew P, Conley ME. Effect of intravenous gammaglobulin (IVIG) on the platelet count in patients with Wiskott-Aldrich syndrome. Pediatr Allergy Immunol 1995;6(2):91–4.

82. Buchbinder D, Nugent DJ, Fillipovich AH. Wiskott-Aldrich syndrome: diagnosis, current management, and emerging treatments. Appl Clin Genet 2014;7:55–66.

83. Worth AJ, Booth C, Veys P. Stem cell transplantation for primary immune deficiency. Curr Opin Hematol 2013;20(6):501–8.

84. Al-Herz W, Bousfiha A, Casanova JL, et al. Primary immunodeficiency diseases: an update on the classification from the International Union of Immunological Societies expert committee for primary immunodeficiency. Front Immunol 2014;5:162.

85. Notarangelo LD, Ochs HD. Wiskott-Aldrich syndrome: a model for defective actin reorganization, cell trafficking and synapse formation. Curr Opin Immunol 2003;15(5):585–91.

86. Orange JS, Ramesh N, Remold-O'Donnell E, et al. Wiskott-Aldrich syndrome protein is required for NK cell cytotoxicity and colocalizes with actin to NK cell-activating immunologic synapses. Proc Natl Acad Sci U S A 2002;99(17): 11351–6.

87. Matalon O, Reicher B, Barda-Saad M. Wiskott-Aldrich syndrome protein–dynamic regulation of actin homeostasis: from activation through function and signal termination in T lymphocytes. Immunol Rev 2013;256(1):10–29.

88. Massaad MJ, Ramesh N, Geha RS. Wiskott-Aldrich syndrome: a comprehensive review. Ann N Y Acad Sci 2013;1285:26–43.

89. Hirschhorn R, Candotti F. Immunodeficiency due to defects of purine metabolism. In: Ochs HD, Smith CIE, Puck JM, editors. Primary immunodeficiency diseases. Oxford (United Kingdom): Oxford University Press; 2006. p. 169–96.

90. Felgentreff K, Perez-Becker R, Speckmann C, et al. Clinical and immunological manifestations of patients with atypical severe combined immunodeficiency. Clin Immunol 2011;141(1):73–82.

91. Sauer AV, Brigida I, Carriglio N, et al. Autoimmune dysregulation and purine metabolism in adenosine deaminase deficiency. Front Immunol 2012;3:265.

92. Lawrence MG, Brigida I, Carriglio N, et al. Elevated IgE and atopy in patients treated for early-onset ADA-SCID. J Allergy Clin Immunol 2013;132(6):1444–6.

93. Cederbaum SD, Kaitila I, Rimoin DL, et al. The chondro-osseous dysplasia of adenosine deaminase deficiency with severe combined immunodeficiency. J Pediatr 1976;89(5):737–42.

94. Hirschhorn R, Paageorgiou PS, Kesarwala HH, et al. Amerioration of neurologic abnormalities after "enzyme replacement" in adenosine deaminase deficiency. N Engl J Med 1980;303(7):377–80.

95. Rogers MH, Lwin R, Fairbanks L, et al. Cognitive and behavioral abnormalities in adenosine deaminase deficient severe combined immunodeficiency. J Pediatr 2001;139(1):44–50.

96. Buckley RH, Schiff RI, Schiff SE, et al. Human severe combined immunodeficiency: genetic, phenotypic, and functional diversity in one hundred eight infants. J Pediatr 1997;130(3):378–87.

97. Gaspar HB, Aiuti A, Porta F, et al. How I treat ADA deficiency. Blood 2009; 114(17):3524–32.

98. Santisteban I, Arredondo-Vega FX, Kelly S, et al. Novel splicing, missense, and deletion mutations in seven adenosine deaminase-deficient patients with late/delayed onset of combined immunodeficiency disease. Contribution of genotype to phenotype. J Clin Invest 1993;92(5):2291–302.

99. Kwan A, Abraham RS, Currier R, et al. Newborn screening for severe combined immunodeficiency in 11 screening programs in the United States. JAMA 2014; 312(7):729–38.

100. Puck JM. Laboratory technology for population-based screening for severe combined immunodeficiency in neonates: the winner is T-cell receptor excision circles. J Allergy Clin Immunol 2012;129(3):607–16.

101. Hershfield MS. Genotype is an important determinant of phenotype in adenosine deaminase deficiency. Curr Opin Immunol 2003;15(5):571–7.

102. Gangi-Peterson L, Sorscher DH, Reynolds JW, et al. Nucleotide pool imbalance and adenosine deaminase deficiency induce alterations of N-region insertions during V(D)J recombination. J Clin Invest 1999;103(6):833–41.

103. Hershfield MS, Mitchell BS. Immunodeficiency diseases caused by adenosine deaminase deficiency and purine nucleoside phosphorylase deficiency. In: Scriver CR, Beaudet AL, Sly WS, et al, editors. The metabolic and molecular basis of inherited disease. 7th edition. New York: McGraw-Hill; 1995. p. 1725–68.

104. Villa A, Notarangelo LD, Roifman CM. Omenn syndrome: inflammation in leaky severe combined immunodeficiency. J Allergy Clin Immunol 2008;122(6): 1082–6.

105. Aleman K, Noordzij JG, de Groot R, et al. Reviewing Omenn syndrome. Eur J Pediatr 2001;160(12):718–25.

106. Pai SY, Logan BR, Griffith LM, et al. Transplantation outcomes for severe combined immunodeficiency, 2000-2009. N Engl J Med 2014;371(5):434–46.

107. Siala N, Azzabi O, Kebaier H, et al. Omenn syndrome: two case reports. Acta Dermatovenerol Croat 2013;21(4):259–62.

108. Gennery AR, Hodges E, Williams AP, et al. Omenn's syndrome occurring in patients without mutations in recombination activating genes. Clin Immunol 2005; 116(3):246–56.

109. Shearer WT, Dunn E, Notarangelo LD, et al. Establishing diagnostic criteria for severe combined immunodeficiency disease (SCID), leaky SCID, and Omenn syndrome: the Primary Immune Deficiency Treatment Consortium experience. J Allergy Clin Immunol 2014;133(4):1092–8.

110. Tasher D, Dalal I. The genetic basis of severe combined immunodeficiency and its variants. Appl Clin Genet 2012;5:67–80.

111. Markert ML, Devlin BH, Alexieff MJ, et al. Review of 54 patients with complete DiGeorge anomaly enrolled in protocols for thymus transplantation: outcome of 44 consecutive transplants. Blood 2007;109(10):4539–47.

112. Pierdominici M, Mazzetta F, Caprini E, et al. Biased T-cell receptor repertoires in patients with chromosome 22q11.2 deletion syndrome (DiGeorge syndrome/velocardiofacial syndrome). Clin Exp Immunol 2003;132(2):323–31.

113. Vu QV, Wada T, Toma T, et al. Clinical and immunophenotypic features of atypical complete DiGeorge syndrome. Pediatr Int 2013;55(1):2–6.

114. Price S, Shaw PA, Seitz A, et al. Natural history of autoimmune lymphoproliferative syndrome associated with FAS gene mutations. Blood 2014;123(13):1989–99.

115. Sneller MC, Wang J, Dale JK, et al. Clinical, immunologic, and genetic features of an autoimmune lymphoproliferative syndrome associated with abnormal lymphocyte apoptosis. Blood 1997;89(4):1341–8.

116. Rao VK, Oliveira JB. How I treat autoimmune lymphoproliferative syndrome. Blood 2011;118(22):5741–51.

117. Kim YJ, Dale JK, Noel P, et al. Eosinophilia is associated with a higher mortality rate among patients with autoimmune lymphoproliferative syndrome. Am J Hematol 2007;82(7):615–24.

118. Neven B, Magerus-Chatinet A, Florkin B, et al. A survey of 90 patients with autoimmune lymphoproliferative syndrome related to TNFRSF6 mutation. Blood 2011;118(18):4798–807.

119. Milner JD, Vogel TP, Forbes L, et al. Early-onset lymphoproliferation and autoimmunity caused by germline STAT3 gain-of-function mutations. Blood 2015; 125(4):591–9.

120. Ochs HD, Ziegler SF, Torgerson TR. FOXP3 acts as a rheostat of the immune response. Immunol Rev 2005;203:156–64.

121. Powell BR, Buist NR, Stenzel P. An X-linked syndrome of diarrhea, polyendocrinopathy, and fatal infection in infancy. J Pediatr 1982;100(5):731–7.

122. d'Hennezel E, Bin Dhuban K, Torgerson T, et al. The immunogenetics of immune dysregulation, polyendocrinopathy, enteropathy, X linked (IPEX) syndrome. J Med Genet 2012;49(5):291–302.

123. Patey-Mariaud de Serre N, Canioni D, Ganousse S, et al. Digestive histopathological presentation of IPEX syndrome. Mod Pathol 2009;22(1):95–102.

124. Gambineri E, Perroni L, Passerini L, et al. Clinical and molecular profile of a new series of patients with immune dysregulation, polyendocrinopathy, enteropathy, X-linked syndrome: inconsistent correlation between forkhead box protein 3 expression and disease severity. J Allergy Clin Immunol 2008;122(6): 1105–1112 e1.

125. Akdis M, Blaser K, Akdis CA. T regulatory cells in allergy: novel concepts in the pathogenesis, prevention, and treatment of allergic diseases. J Allergy Clin Immunol 2005;116(5):961–8 [quiz: 969].

126. Bennett CL, Christie J, Ramsdell F, et al. The immune dysregulation, polyendocrinopathy, enteropathy, X-linked syndrome (IPEX) is caused by mutations of FOXP3. Nat Genet 2001;27(1):20–1.

127. Wildin RS, Smyk-Pearson S, Filipovich AH. Clinical and molecular features of the immunodysregulation, polyendocrinopathy, enteropathy, X linked (IPEX) syndrome. J Med Genet 2002;39(8):537–45.

128. Caudy AA, Reddy ST, Chatila T, et al. CD25 deficiency causes an immune dysregulation, polyendocrinopathy, enteropathy, X-linked-like syndrome, and defective IL-10 expression from CD4 lymphocytes. J Allergy Clin Immunol 2007;119(2):482–7.

129. Uzel G, Sampaio EP, Lawrence MG, et al. Dominant gain-of-function STAT1 mutations in FOXP3 wild-type immune dysregulation-polyendocrinopathy-enteropathy-X-linked-like syndrome. J Allergy Clin Immunol 2013;131(6): 1611–23.
130. Loeys BL, Chen J, Neptune ER, et al. A syndrome of altered cardiovascular, craniofacial, neurocognitive and skeletal development caused by mutations in TGFBR1 or TGFBR2. Nat Genet 2005;37(3):275–81.
131. MacCarrick G, Black JH 3rd, Bowdin S, et al. Loeys-Dietz syndrome: a primer for diagnosis and management. Genet Med 2014;16(8):576–87.
132. Loeys BL, Schwarze U, Holm T, et al. Aneurysm syndromes caused by mutations in the TGF-beta receptor. N Engl J Med 2006;355(8):788–98.
133. Frischmeyer-Guerrerio PA, Guerrerio AL, Oswald G, et al. TGFbeta receptor mutations impose a strong predisposition for human allergic disease. Sci Transl Med 2013;5(195):195ra94.
134. Burk C, Hu S, Lee C, et al. Netherton syndrome and trichorrhexis invaginata-a novel diagnostic approach. Pediatr Dermatol 2008;25(2):287–8.
135. Hovnanian A. Netherton syndrome: skin inflammation and allergy by loss of protease inhibition. Cell Tissue Res 2013;351(2):289–300.
136. Renner ED, Hartl D, Rylaarsdam S, et al. Comel-Netherton syndrome defined as primary immunodeficiency. J Allergy Clin Immunol 2009;124(3):536–43.
137. Fontao L, Laffitte E, Briot A, et al. Infliximab infusions for Netherton syndrome: sustained clinical improvement correlates with a reduction of thymic stromal lymphopoietin levels in the skin. J Invest Dermatol 2011;131(9):1947–50.
138. Sun JD, Linden KG. Netherton syndrome: a case report and review of the literature. Int J Dermatol 2006;45(6):693–7.
139. Chavanas S, Bodemer C, Rochat A, et al. Mutations in SPINK5, encoding a serine protease inhibitor, cause Netherton syndrome. Nat Genet 2000;25(2): 141–2.
140. Raghunath M, Tontsidou L, Oji V, et al. SPINK5 and Netherton syndrome: novel mutations, demonstration of missing LEKTI, and differential expression of transglutaminases. J Invest Dermatol 2004;123(3):474–83.
141. Furio L, Hovnanian A. Netherton syndrome: defective kallikrein inhibition in the skin leads to skin inflammation and allergy. Biol Chem 2014;395(9):945–58.
142. Samuelov L, Sprecher E. Peeling off the genetics of atopic dermatitis-like congenital disorders. J Allergy Clin Immunol 2014;134(4):808–15.
143. Samuelov L, Sarig O, Harmon RM, et al. Desmoglein 1 deficiency results in severe dermatitis, multiple allergies and metabolic wasting. Nat Genet 2013; 45(10):1244–8.
144. Amagai M, Stanley JR. Desmoglein as a target in skin disease and beyond. J Invest Dermatol 2012;132(3 Pt 2):776–84.

Eosinophilia in Dermatologic Disorders

Elisabeth de Graauw, MD[a,b], Helmut Beltraminelli, MD[a],
Hans-Uwe Simon, MD[b], Dagmar Simon, MD[a,*]

KEYWORDS

- Eosinophils • Atopic dermatitis • Drug hypersensitivity reaction
- Cutaneous lymphoma • Eosinophilic dermatitis • Hypereosinophilic syndromes

KEY POINTS

- Cutaneous eosinophil infiltration is observed in a broad spectrum of dermatologic disorders including allergic, autoimmune, infectious, and neoplastic diseases and can be associated with blood eosinophilia.
- The clinical presentation of eosinophilic dermatoses varies considerably, but pruritus is a common symptom.
- The diagnosis of eosinophilic dermatoses is usually based on histology, unless clinical signs and symptoms are unmistakable.
- The accumulation of eosinophils in the skin is reactive in most cases owing to the production of eosinophilopoietic cytokines by T cells or tumor/lymphoma cells.
- A potential pathogenic role of eosinophils in skin diseases has been attributed to host defense, immunoregulation, and fibrosis.

DERMATOLOGIC DISORDERS WITH EOSINOPHILIA

The presence of eosinophils in the skin is common in a broad spectrum of cutaneous disorders. To note, the skin lacks eosinophils under physiologic conditions. The clinical presentations of eosinophilic skin diseases are highly variable and include eczematous, papular, urticarial, bullous, nodular, and fibrotic lesions. Pruritus is a unique and striking feature of all of them, although not pathognomonic. In some patients presenting with itchy skin lesions, the disease can easily be diagnosed considering the patient history, age, clinical findings and distribution, for example, atopic dermatitis (AD),

The authors have nothing to disclose.
[a] Department of Dermatology, Inselspital, Freiburgstrasse, Bern CH-3010, Switzerland;
[b] Institute of Pharmacology, University of Bern, Inselspital, Bern CH-3010, Switzerland
* Corresponding author. Department of Dermatology, Inselspital, Bern University Hospital, Bern CH-3010, Switzerland.
E-mail address: dagmar.simon@insel.ch

insect bites, larva migrans infection, and drug reactions. Moreover, inflammatory skin lesions are the most common clinical manifestation of hypereosinophilic syndromes (HES),[1,2] To confirm or make the correct diagnosis, biopsies from active skin lesions have to be taken for histologic, immunohistochemical, and immunofluorescence investigations, and in some cases polymerase chain reaction analysis to check for clonality of infiltrating cells. Eosinophils can easily be identified by hematoxylin and eosin staining in skin biopsies. Their numbers, localization, and degranulation, as well as tissue damage, might provide diagnostic clues for the dermatopathologist; for example, flame figures in Wells' syndrome, V-shaped eosinophilic infiltrate in arthropod reactions, and eosinophil lining and blister formation at the dermal–epidermal junction in bullous pemphigoid (BP). The eosinophilia can be restricted to the skin, but may be accompanied by blood eosinophilia, for example, in AD, BP and cutaneous T-cell lymphoma (CTCL), and involve other organs as well, such as in a drug reaction with eosinophilia and systemic symptoms (DRESS). Associated blood eosinophilia may be as high greater than 1.5×10^6/L, as in HES.

PATHOGENIC MECHANISMS MEDIATED BY EOSINOPHILS

Although eosinophils are encountered in many skin diseases, their functional role in the pathogenesis remains largely unclear. There is evidence that eosinophils might contribute to pathogen defense, regulate inflammatory responses, and induce fibrosis/remodeling.[3,4] According to their cytokine expression, functionally different subpopulations seem to exist: eosinophils that potentially regulate inflammatory responses and/or fibrosis.[5] Moreover, the cytokine pattern of eosinophils is distinct in allergic reactive, infectious, and autoimmune diseases, as well as in lymphomas/tumors.[5] Eosinophils have been demonstrated to form extracellular DNA traps (EET) in the skin and thus may play a role in host defense.[3,6] Thymic stromal lymphopoietin, a cytokine expressed by epithelial cells, for example, in AD and BP, stimulates eosinophils to release EETs that are able to kill bacteria.[7] Other mechanisms by which eosinophils may release granule proteins are degranulation and cytolysis.[8,9] In flame figures, granule protein deposition coating collagen fibers can be detected, suggesting a role of eosinophils in tissue damage.[10] Interestingly, tissue damage mediated by major basic protein seems to be limited by extracellular aggregation generating large, nontoxic amyloid plaques.[11] In eczematous lesions, a correlation between eosinophils expressing matrix metalloproteinase-9 with interleukin (IL)-17$^+$ T cells and remodeling has been reported.[12] Moreover, eosinophils might be involved in causing pruritus, because they can affect skin nerves directly.[13]

CLINICAL PRESENTATIONS OF DERMATOSES WITH EOSINOPHILIA
Eczematous Pattern

Atopic dermatitis
AD is a chronic inflammatory skin disease based on a genetic predisposition. The prevalence is as high as 20% in children and 10% in adults. Typically, AD presents with pruritus and excoriated eczematous skin lesions on the face, neck, and extensor sites of the extremities in infants, and subsequent lichenification at the flexural folds in children and adults (**Fig. 1A**). The pathogenesis is complex, including an impaired skin barrier function that promotes adaptive immune responses to environmental allergens, together with inadequate innate immune responses to microbes followed by colonization of *Staphylococcus aureus* and viral infections.[14] The diagnosis of AD is based on the clinical signs rather than diagnostic procedures, which may identify triggers. Approximately 80% of AD patients have increased total and specific

A Atopic dermatitis **B** Drug hypersensitivity reaction

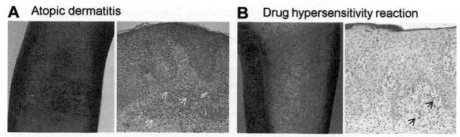

Fig. 1. Clinical presentations and histology of atopic dermatitis and drug hypersensitivity reaction. (*A*) Lichenification of eczematous lesions in arm fold. Spongiosis and perivascular lymphocytic infiltrate and eosinophils (*arrows*). (*B*) Maculopapular exanthema. Dense dermal infiltrate of lymphocytes and eosinophils (*arrows*) (hematoxylin-eosin, original magnification [*A*] ×100; [*B*] ×200).

immunoglobulin (Ig)E to environmental allergens. AD is the first manifestation of atopy preceding allergic rhinitis and bronchial asthma in most patients.

Tissue eosinophilia is a typical finding of AD, often associated with increased blood eosinophil levels and correlating with disease severity.[15] In the skin, eosinophils as part of the perivascular inflammatory infiltrate as well as extracellular granule protein deposits have been identified.[8,11] So far, the role of eosinophils in the pathogenesis of AD remains uncertain. It seems possible that eosinophils contribute to host defense against invading microbes through the defective skin barrier by generating EET, regulating the immune response, and/or remodeling.[5,7,12]

The treatment of AD aims to restore the barrier function, for example, by emollients, reduction of inflammation with topical corticosteroids and calcineurin inhibitors, or systemic immunomodulating agents, and avoidance of trigger factors. Successful therapy of acute AD is accompanied by a decrease of eosinophils in blood and skin.[16,17]

Contact dermatitis

Contact dermatitis (CD), either irritant (ICD) or allergic (ACD), is caused by exogenous triggers and thus manifests at exposure sites, often the hands. ACD develops as a consequence of contact hypersensitivity, usually to low-molecular-weight allergens (haptens), and involves innate and adaptive, predominantly T helper 1 immune responses, in both the sensitization and elicitation phases.[18] In ICD, an exposure to chemicals, wet and/or mechanical work causes damage of the epidermis resulting in a proinflammatory cytokine release by keratinocytes and inflammation.[18] Thus, ICD might pave the way for the development of ACD. The patient's history and clinical signs of acute and/or chronic eczematous lesions are usually diagnostic for CD and biopsies are done for differential diagnosis. Histologic examination shows an inflammatory infiltrate containing eosinophils in the upper dermis and epidermal spongiosis following distinct time courses in ACD and ICD.[12] Eosinophils producing reactive oxygen species were reported to play a role in the development of ICD.[19] Moreover, the numbers of eosinophils correlated with T cells expressing IL-17 and IL-22 known to promote eosinophil recruitment and profibrotic mediator production, suggesting a role in remodeling of eczema.[12] In terms of treatment, avoidance of the triggers is most important. To identify responsible contact allergens, patch tests should be performed.

Scabies and cutaneous larva migrans

Worldwide, secondary eosinophilia is most frequently caused by parasitic diseases, including scabies and larva migrans. Both scabies and hookworm-related cutaneous larva migrans are common in many developing countries and characterized by severe itching.[20–23] In scabies, a papular rash is observed. The presence of a linear serpiginous track moving forward in the skin is typical for larva migrans (**Fig. 2**). Eosinophils and T cells predominate in the infiltrates of scabies and larva migrans infected skin. The diagnosis is based on clinical signs and exposure as well as dermatoscopic and microscopic identification of scabies mites. Scabies can be treated with topicals (eg, permethrin 5%) or with systemic ivermectin (200 µg/kg in a single dose).[24] Cutaneous larva migrans is treated typically with single-dose oral albendazole or ivermectin or the topical application of thiabendazole.[22]

Primary cutaneous T-cell lymphoma

Mycosis fungoides (MF) and Sezary syndrome (SS) are epidermotropic forms of CTCL characterized by cutaneous infiltration of malignant, clonally expanded T cells.[25] Clinical signs of MF are well-defined, often pruritic erythematous patches in non–sun-exposed areas that may evolve to infiltrated plaques and tumors (**Fig. 5A**).[26] SS presents with an erythroderma, severe pruritus, atypical T cells in the peripheral blood, and lymphadenopathy.[26] Recently, it has been demonstrated that the malignant cells resemble central memory T cells in SS, and effector memory T cells in MF. These observations are consistent with clinical behavior and responsiveness to therapy as well as comparative genomic hybridization and gene expression profiling data.[27] MF and SS have been associated with a T helper 2 cytokine milieu including IL-5 leading to eosinophilia in skin and peripheral blood.

Lymphocytic variant of hypereosinophilic syndromes

Patients with hypereosinophilia owing to T cells with an aberrant immunophenotype present with severe pruritus and often widespread erythematous to erythrodermic skin lesions.[28,29] The aberrant T cells frequently produce IL-5 and/or IL-3 and stimulate the production and accumulation of eosinophils. Skin histology reveals perivascular infiltrates and exocytosis of lymphocytes and eosinophils.[29]

Langerhans cell histiocytosis

Langerhans cell histiocytosis is a rare disease mainly affecting children and manifests as either restricted (single-system) or extensive (multisystem) type.[30] On the skin, scaly, erythematous, seborrhea-like brown to red papules can be observed. The infiltrate of Langerhans cells (LC) that can be identified immunohistochemically by their expression of CD1a and/or CD207, is admixed with various numbers of macrophages, multinucleated giant cells, T cells, and eosinophils. LC were reported to cause eosinophilia either directly by expressing chemokine (c-c motif) ligand (CCL)5 or indirectly by recruiting T cells that produce IL-5.[30]

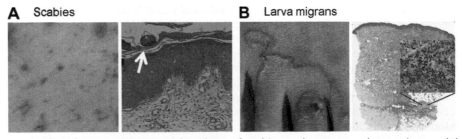

A Scabies   **B** Larva migrans

Fig. 2. Clinical presentations and histology of scabies and cutaneous larva migrans. (A) Erythematous excoriated papular and linear lesions. Mites in the horny layer (*arrow*). (B) Creeping eruption associated with larva migrans. Dense infiltrate of eosinophils in deep dermis and subcutaneous fat (hematoxylin-eosin, original magnification [A] ×100; [B] ×10, insert ×100).

Maculopapular Exanthema

Drug hypersensitivity reactions

Drug hypersensitivity reactions (DHR) are adverse drug reactions to pharmaceutical formulations that clinically resemble allergy, and are dose independent, unpredictable, noxious, and unintended (type B).[31] According to the onset of symptoms, DHR have been classified in immediate and nonimmediate or delayed reactions. In delayed DHR, most commonly the skin is affected and mainly presents with maculopapular rashes (see **Fig. 1**B), but also as delayed urticaria, fixed drug eruption, symmetric drug-related intertriginous and flexural exanthema, acute generalized exanthematous pustulosis, toxic epidermal necrolysis, or vasculitis.[31] It has been hypothesized that drugs directly or after processing by dendritic cells activate T cells that produce cytokines and cytotoxins resulting in tissue damage and an inflammatory response.[31] Eosinophils can be found among inflammatory cells in the skin and often peripheral blood eosinophil levels are increased.

Drug reaction with eosinophilia and systemic symptoms

An erythematous morbilliform rash in association with systemic organ involvement, such as hematologic, hepatic, renal, pulmonary, cardiac, neurologic, gastrointestinal, or endocrine abnormalities, is the most commonly encountered cutaneous finding of DRESS.[32] Eosinophils releasing toxic granule proteins have been implicated in causing tissue damage and thus organ failure.[33,34] Aromatic anticonvulsants and sulfonamides are the most frequent causes of DRESS occurring 2 to 6 weeks after initiation of therapy.[32] In addition to a certain genetic disposition (HLA haplotypes), reactivation of herpesviruses, and immunosuppression play a role in the pathogenesis of DRESS.[32] Leukocytosis and hypereosinophilia, as well as increased liver enzymes, urea nitrogen, and creatinine blood levels, are typical findings.[32] The culprit drug has to be withdrawn immediately. In addition therapy with corticosteroids, supportive care measures should be initiated.

Urticarial Pattern

Urticaria

Urticaria is a common, mast cell–driven disease presenting with wheals, angioedema, or both (**Fig. 3**A).[35] Acute urticaria is often associated with upper respiratory infections, drugs, or IgE-mediated reactions, and spontaneously regresses within 6 weeks. The pathogenesis of chronic spontaneous urticaria is not understood completely. Mast cell activation might be triggered by infections, allergic and pseudoallergic reactions,

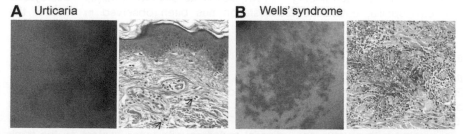

A Urticaria   **B** Wells' syndrome

Fig. 3. Clinical presentations and histology of urticaria and Wells' syndrome (eosinophilic dermatitis). (A) Wheals on the trunk, usually persisting less than 24 hours. In the dermis, edema and perivascular mixed infiltrate intermingled with eosinophils (arrows). (B) Persisting urticarial lesions. Flame figure and interstitial infiltration of eosinophils in the dermis (hematoxylin-eosin, original magnification [A] ×200; [B] ×40).

drugs, or autoimmune responses. For inducible forms of urticaria, the triggers, for example, heat, cold, pressure, and ultraviolet light, can easily be identified. Eosinophils are part of the mixed inflammatory infiltrate in an edematous dermis. By releasing tissue factor and inducing an increase of vascular permeability resulting in edema, eosinophils have been assumed to directly contribute to the development of wheals.[36]

Eosinophilic cellulitis (Wells' syndrome)

Episodes of pruritic dermatitis, persistent urticarial lesions, painful edematous swellings, and occasionally blisters are the clinical manifestations of Wells' syndrome (see **Fig. 3B**). A skin biopsy shows a dense eosinophilic infiltration of the dermis, degranulation, and flame figures.[37] Wells' syndrome has been classified as an organ restricted eosinophilic disorder among HESs.[38]

Episodic angioedema with eosinophilia (Gleich's syndrome)

Among the HES, this rare disease has been classified as undefined, episodic variant. In 1984, Gleich and colleagues[39] reported 4 patients with recurrent attacks of angioedema, urticaria, and fever, transient increase of body weight of up to 18%, and increased leukocyte counts without any inner organ dysfunction that could be controlled by corticosteroids. Recently, a multilineage cell cycling in association with the presence of aberrant and/or clonal T-cell populations has been reported in episodic angioedema with eosinophilia.[40] In skin biopsies, increased numbers of eosinophils and mast cells were observed during attacks, suggesting a role for both cell types in the pathogenesis of angioedema.[40]

Pregnancy-related diseases

Atopic eruption (including eczema, prurigo, papular dermatitis, and pruritic folliculitis of pregnancy) and polymorphic eruption (including pruritic urticarial, toxic erythema, toxemic rash, and late-onset prurigo of pregnancy) are the most common dermatoses of pregnancy distinguished from pemphigoid gestationis and intrahepatic cholestasis of pregnancy by morphology, onset, and (immune-)histologic findings.[40] All of them are accompanied by severe pruritus. Prominent tissue eosinophilia was observed in prurigo, polymorphic eruption, and eczema of pregnancy.[41]

Cutaneous mastocytosis

Cutaneous mastocytosis, also referred to as urticaria pigmentosa, is a rare disease that may be limited to the skin, but can be a manifestation of indolent, smoldering, and aggressive systemic mastocytosis.[42] Histopathologically, cutaneous mastocytosis is characterized by aggregates of mast cells in the dermis, whereas eosinophil infiltration is an uncommon finding.[43] In KIT D816V-associated systemic mastocytosis with eosinophilia, cutaneous manifestation has been observed in 58% of the patients.[44]

Blisters and Pustules

Bullous pemphigoid

BP, the most common autoimmune subepidermal blistering disease, is characterized by tissue-bound and circulating antibodies to the hemidesmosomal antigens BP180 (BPAG2, type XVII collagen) and BP230 (BPAG1).[45–47] Patients, typically in their late 70s, present with pruritus and urticarial erythema with tense blisters on the trunk and extremities (**Fig. 4A**).[46–48] Blood eosinophilia and dermal infiltrates consisting predominantly of eosinophils are observed in the majority of BP patients.[41–44] Using direct immunofluorescence techniques, deposition of IgG and/or C3, and in some cases IgE, along the basement membrane zone can be found.[47,48] In blister fluid and lesional

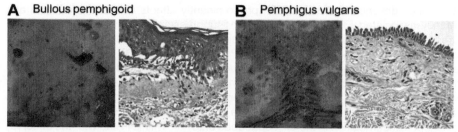

Fig. 4. Clinical presentations and histology of autoimmune blistering diseases: bullous pemphigoid and pemphigus vulgaris. (*A*) Erythematous lesions with dense blisters and erosions. Subepidermal blister and eosinophils in dermis and blister. (*B*) Eroded blisters and crusted lesions on erythematous base. Suprabasal acantholysis, mild dermal infiltrate, and scattered eosinophils (hematoxylin-eosin, original magnification [*A*] ×200; [*B*] ×200).

skin, several proteolytic enzymes are detected, including plasmin, matrix metalloproteinase-9, and neutrophil elastase, which are strongly expressed by neutrophils and eosinophils.[47,48] Increased levels of the cytokine IL-5 and the CCL 11 (eotaxin-1) and CCL5, important for eosinophil activation and attraction, have been detected in blister fluids.[46,47] Because of the potential side effects of systemic corticosteroids currently used for first-line treatment, novel therapeutic options, such as, inhibitory monoclonal antibodies directed against IL-5 and eotaxin, are of increasing interest.[45,48] Promising results have been reported with rituximab, a potent B-cell–depleting monoclonal antibody.[45,49]

Pemphigus group
Other autoimmune bullous diseases associated with eosinophil infiltration in the skin are those assigned to the pemphigus group. They are characterized by intraepithelial acantholysis owing to autoantibodies against cell–cell cohesion proteins resulting in blister formation and erosions in pemphigus vulgaris, and papillomatous oozing vegetations of large skin folds and erosions of the oral mucosa as in pemphigus vegetans (see **Fig. 4B**).[50,51] Eosinophil exocytosis and eosinophil abscesses have been reported to be common histopathologics findings in pemphigus vegetans.[51]

Incontinentia pigmenti
Incontinentia pigmenti is an X-linked dominant multisystem disease affecting ectodermal tissues caused by mutations of the *NEMO* gene. The first vesicobullous stage is characterized by acanthosis, keratinocyte necrosis, epidermal spongiosis, and eosinophil accumulation, and is followed by the verrucous, hyperpigmented, and hypopigmented stages.[52] IL-1 production by mutant keratinocytes gives rise to tumor necrosis factor-α synthesis by neighboring wild-type cells that in turn induce death and clearance of the mutant cells.[53] The expression of eotaxin by keratinocytes correlated with epidermal eosinophil infiltration; however, their pathogenic role has not been defined to date.[52]

Eosinophilic pustular folliculitis
Eosinophilic pustular folliculitis (EPF) is an inflammatory skin disease characterized by papulopustular eruptions forming annular plaques. Biopsies show spongiosis of hair follicle epithelium with infiltration of eosinophils and lymphocytes, forming eosinophilic follicular pustules that are a typical diagnostic feature.[54–56] In addition to classical EPF, mainly found in Japan, infancy-associated EPF and immunosuppression-associated EPF in the setting of human immunodeficiency virus infection and malignancies

have been described. Classical EPF predominantly affects the face and trunk, and infancy-associated EPF the scalp. Immunosuppression-associated EPF lacks face predilection and annular arrangement of lesions.[54,56] Eosinophilia and increased levels of IgE can be observed in EPF patients.[54] Eotaxin-1 (CCL11), a potent eosinophil attractant, and T helper 2 type cytokines such as IL-13, IL-4, and IL-5, are considered important in the eosinophil recruitment and activation in human immunodeficiency virus-associated EPF.[55] Recently, it has been shown that prostaglandin D2 stimulates sebocytes to produce eotaxin-3 (CCL26), a chemoattractant for eosinophils, inducing eosinophil accumulation in the pilosebaceous unit.[55,56] This is in line with the observation that inhibitors of cyclooxygenases involved in prostaglandin synthesis are effective in treating EPF.[55]

Nodular Lesions

Prurigo nodularis
Symmetrically distributed, firm, hyperkeratotic nodular lesions on the extensor surfaces of the extremities induced by extreme chronic pruritus and permanent scratching are the hallmarks of prurigo nodularis (PN), mainly affecting middle-aged woman.[57] The histologic analysis of PN lesions revealed an eosinophil infiltration in approximately 50%.[57] How eosinophils are involved in the pathogenesis of PN, possibly by inducing pruritus and/or stimulating fibrosis, remains to be elucidated.

Granuloma faciale
Granuloma faciale is a rare, benign inflammatory skin disease presenting with persistent red-brown plaques and nodules on the face that grow slowly.[58] Extrafacial lesions may occur.[54] To rule out other diagnoses, such as, lupus pernio, lupus vulgaris, lymphoma, discoid lupus erythematosus, and infections, a biopsy has to be taken. Interestingly, there are no granulomas but rather an eosinophil and neutrophil predominant infiltrate and small vessel vasculitis can be observed in the dermis with a typical grenz zone.[58] A local IL-5 production by T cells most likely contributes to eosinophil infiltration.[59]

Eosinophilic granulomatosis with polyangiitis (Churg-Strauss syndrome)
Palpable purpura and nodules that may undergo necrotic ulceration located on the limbs and scalp are prominent skin manifestations of the vasculitic phase of EGPA.[60] In the pathogenesis, both T helper 2 responses followed by ANCA production and eosinophil activation, as well T helper 1/T helper 17–mediated granuloma formation and vasculitis are thought to play a role in tissue damage.[60] In the eosinophilic phase, an extravascular tissue infiltration by eosinophils of virtually any organ, in particular lung, heart, and the gastrointestinal tract, has been observed. Eosinophilic infiltration and fibrinoid necrosis of small to medium-sized vessel walls are characteristic of the vasculitis phase affecting mainly the nervous system, kidneys, and skin.[60]

Angiolymphoid hyperplasia with eosinophilia and Kimura's disease
Angiolymphoid hyperplasia with eosinophilia (ALHE) is a rare disease presenting with unilateral erythematous papules and nodules predominantly in middle-aged woman.[61] Histologic examination shows an increased number of blood vessels with proliferation of endothelial cells possessing pathognomonic cytoplasmic vacuoles and a diffuse lymphocytic infiltrate with eosinophils. Kimura's disease (KD) is a benign reactive lymphoid proliferation, characterized by deep subcutaneous and intramuscular swellings and regional lymphadenopathy predominantly seen in young Asian men.[61] ALHE shares similarities with KD lesions predominantly in the head–neck region, benign and recurrent disease course, and eosinophil-rich lymphoid hyperplasia.[61] In contrast with

AHLE, KD is associated typically with peripheral blood eosinophilia, increased serum IgE levels, and lymphadenopathy. Although the cause of both ALHE and KD is not known, the localization of lesions, lymphoid infiltration, and the presence of eosinophils are suggestive of a reactive reaction possibly to an infectious agent.[61]

Primary cutaneous CD30[+] lymphoproliferative disorders: lymphomatoid papulosis and primary cutaneous anaplastic large-cell lymphoma

Characteristically, lymphomatoid papulosis (LYP) follows a chronic disease course with recurrent development of papulonodular lesions that undergo spontaneous regression after weeks or months (see **Fig. 5**B).[62] Primary cutaneous anaplastic large-cell lymphoma (PCALCL) comes with solitary or grouped, rapidly growing and ulcerating, large tumors or thick plaques.[62] The histology shows large pleomorphic and anaplastic tumor cells intermingled with small lymphocytes, eosinophils, and histiocytes. CD30[+] lymphomatoid papulosis has an excellent prognosis. Because the risk to develop second cutaneous or nodal lymphoid malignancies is increased, staging is recommended if clinical examination or laboratory tests are suggestive of extracutaneous disease. For treatment of PCALCL, surgical excision or radiotherapy has been recommended. For LYP, a wait-and-see strategy is suggested; otherwise, ultraviolet light therapy, methotrexate, topical steroids and immunomodulators, and retinoids have been recommended.[62]

Cutaneous B-cell lymphomas

To diagnose and classify cutaneous B-cell lymphoma (CBCL) and distinguish them from secondary skin involvement by a systemic lymphoma, a careful morphologic and immunohistochemical analysis and staging are required.[63] According to the cells of origin, CBCL are classified in primary cutaneous follicle-center lymphoma (PCFCL), primary cutaneous diffuse large B-cell lymphoma, leg type (PCDLBCL, LT), and primary cutaneous marginal zone lymphoma (PCMZL). They present with solitary patches and tumors of the trunk and head–neck area in PCFCL, rapidly growing tumors on the legs in PCDLBCL, and multifocal patches, plaques or nodules on trunk and arms in PCMZL.[63] It has been demonstrated that an aberrant expression of the B-cell lymphoma-6 transcriptional repressor protein via regulation of the transcription factor GATA-3 promotes a T helper 2–type inflammation that subsequently might trigger eosinophilia.[64]

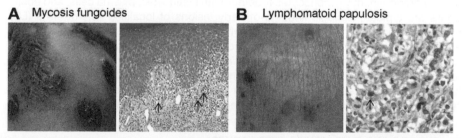

A Mycosis fungoides   **B** Lymphomatoid papulosis

Fig. 5. Clinical presentations and histology of nodular lesions in mycosis fungoides, a cutaneous T-cell lymphoma, and lymphomatoid papulosis, a primary cutaneous CD30[+] lymphoproliferative disorder. (*A*) Patches and nodular lesions. Dense infiltrate of lymphocytes and some eosinophils (*arrows*) in the dermis with exocytosis of lymphocytes. (*B*) Papular and nodular erythematous-brownish lesions. Mixed cellular infiltrate of large atypical cells with few admixed small lymphocytes, eosinophils (*arrow*), neutrophils, and histiocytes (hematoxylin-eosin, original magnification [*A*] ×100; [*B*] ×400).

Hodgkin's lymphoma

Cutaneous specific manifestations of Hodgkin's lymphoma (HL) clinically present as reddish-brown papules, plaques, nodules, and ulcerated tumors sharing the same histologic findings with the nodal counterpart.[65] Hodgkin/Reed Sternberg tumor cells were shown to induce tumor necrosis factor-α–mediated eotaxin production by fibroblasts and thus contribute to the recruitment of eosinophils.[66] There is increasing evidence that the microenvironment, including eosinophils and their products, promote tumor progression in HL.[67]

Eosinophilic dermatosis of hematologic malignancies

Eosinophilic dermatosis presenting with pruritic, indurated erythematous papules and nodules, and in some cases vesicles and bullae resembling insect bites, on face, trunk and extremities has been reported as a nonspecific cutaneous reaction in patients with hematologic malignancies, mainly chronic lymphocytic leukemia.[68] Eosinophil infiltration has been observed interstitially in the dermis as well as in the epidermis and subcutis.

Cutaneous features of hypereosinophilic syndromes

The most common manifestations of HESs are dermatologic findings (37%).[1,2] Splinter hemorrhages and nail fold infarcts owing to thromboembolism can be the first signs of HESs associated with endomyocardial involvement.[2] In patients with myeloproliferative HESs, severe mucosal ulceration has been observed.[2]

Fibrosis

Eosinophilic fasciitis

Painful erythematous swelling followed by induration and thickening of the skin associated with blood eosinophilia, hypergammaglobulinemia, and an increased erythrocyte sedimentation rate are suggestive of eosinophilic fasciitis (EF), a rare connective tissue disease of unknown etiology. The diagnosis is based on the histolopathology of a deep biopsy. By releasing toxic granule proteins as well as profibrotic mediators, eg, metalloproteinases and tumor growth factor-β, infiltrating eosinophils in the fascia seem to play a direct role in the pathogenesis of EF.[69] Furthermore, increased levels of IL-5 have been observed in patients with EF.[70]

Localized scleroderma

Thickening of collagen bundles as well as a dense perivascular and periadnexal infiltrate of predominantly lymphocytes together with histiocytes, plasma cells, and eosinophils are typical histologic findings of early lesions of localized scleroderma (LS). Morphea is the most common subtype of LS presenting with oval-shaped lesions with a whitish and sclerotic center surrounded by a lilac ring.[71] Various triggers, such as, drugs, mechanical trauma, *Borrelia* infection, have been discussed as initiators of LS; however, their causative role remains unclear.[71] Morphea-like skin lesions have been reported in eosinophilia myalgia syndrome and toxic oil syndrome characterized by blood hypereosinophilia, disabling myalgias, and multiorgan dysfunction.[72]

DIAGNOSTIC AND THERAPEUTIC APPROACHES

Dermatologic disorders with eosinophilia usually present with pruritus, but variable morphologies as described often preclude determination of an exact diagnosis. Cutaneous and/or peripheral blood eosinophilia are confirmed by histology of a skin biopsy and differential blood cell count, respectively (**Fig. 6**). In the first instance, common eosinophilic dermatoses should be considered, such as AD, autoimmune blistering

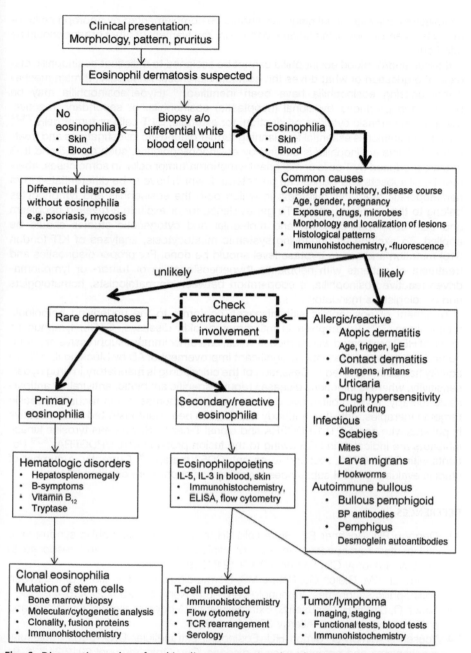

Fig. 6. Diagnostic workup for skin diseases associated with eosinophilia. ELISA, enzyme-linked immunosorbent assay; IgE, immunoglobulin E; IL, interleukin; TCR, T-cell receptor.

diseases, and drug hypersensitivity reactions. To confirm or exclude those, additional serologic tests, immunohistochemical or immunofluorescence tests, and allergy workup have to be done. Furthermore, potential infections, for example, acquired while traveling, should be ruled out. In addition to the patient's history and clinical examination, the differential diagnosis should be complemented by appropriate laboratory tests and imaging. In addition to the skin, involvement of other organs should be ruled out.

If tissue and/or blood eosinophilia cannot be assigned to a distinct eosinophilic disease, the question of what drives the eosinophilia arises. Principally, 2 main mechanisms causing eosinophilia have been identified.[73] (Hyper)eosinophilia may be primary and produced by clonal (neoplastic) eosinophils, or secondary, reactive, owing to an extrinsic cytokine production, for example, by T cells or tumor cells.[73,74] This discrimination is essential for planning further diagnostic investigations and treatment. Reactive eosinophilia is caused by eosinophilopoietins, such as IL-5 and IL-3 that are produced by T cells or malignant lymphoma/tumor cells. In some cases, aberrant T-cell subsets and clones can be detected, which have to be differentiated from hematopoietic stem cell disorders in which both the eosinophils and lymphocytes belong to the neoplastic clone. To get evidence for or exclude a myeloid neoplasm and thus eosinophil clonality, and molecular and cytogenetic studies should be applied. To exclude an underlying systemic mastocytosis, analyses of KIT (codon 816) mutation and serum tryptase level should be done. For proper diagnostics and treatment of patients with neoplastic (hyper)eosinophilia or tumor- or lymphoma-driven reactive eosinophilia, a cooperation between dermatologists, hematologists and oncologists is mandatory.

Treatment of eosinophilic skin diseases conforms to the underlying pathologic mechanisms.[75–80] Eosinophilia in inflammatory skin diseases, CTCL, lymphocytic forms of HES are treated with corticosteroids, and other immunosuppressive or immunomodulating drugs. Recently, a significant improvement of AD by blocking IL-4/IL-13 activity has been reported.[77] Cessation of the culprit drug is mandatory in drug hypersensitivity, whereas infectious diseases require specific antibiotic, antiviral, or antiparasitic therapy. Myeloproliferative disorders and lymphomas are in focus of specific targeted therapies. Anti–IL-5 antibody therapy has been demonstrated to be effective in patients with non-FIP1L1/PDGFRA and clonal T-cell HES, whereas tyrosine kinase inhibitors are indicated in HES owing to the fusion protein FIP1L1/PDGFRA.[78,79] Patients with SS, a CTCL, respond to an anti-CD52 therapy.[80] Currently, a number of studies evaluating novel substances targeting eosinophils are ongoing.[76]

REFERENCES

1. Ogbogu PU, Bochner BS, Butterfield JH, et al. Hypereosinophilic syndrome: a multicenter, retrospective analysis of clinical characteristics and response to therapy. J Allergy Clin Immunol 2009;124:1319–25.
2. Leiferman KM, Gleich GJ, Peters MS. Dermatologic manifestations of the hypereosinophilic syndromes. Immunol Allergy Clin North Am 2007;27:415–41.
3. Simon D, Simon HU, Yousefi S. Extracellular DNA traps in allergic, infectious, and autoimmune diseases. Allergy 2013;68:409–16.
4. Yousefi S, Simon D, Simon HU. Eosinophil extracellular DNA traps: molecular mechanisms and potential roles in disease. Curr Opin Immunol 2012;24:736–9.
5. Roth N, Städler S, Lemann M, et al. Distinct eosinophil cytokine expression patterns in skin diseases - the possible existence of functionally different eosinophil subpopulations. Allergy 2011;66:1477–86.
6. Simon D, Hoesli S, Roth N, et al. Eosinophil extracellular DNA traps in skin diseases. J Allergy Clin Immunol 2011;127:194–9.
7. Morshed M, Yousefi S, Stöckle C, et al. Thymic stromal lymphopoietin stimulates the formation of eosinophil extracellular traps. Allergy 2012;67:1127–37.

8. Leiferman KM, Ackerman SJ, Sampson HA, et al. Dermal deposition of eosinophil-granule major basic protein in atopic dermatitis. Comparison with onchocerciasis. N Engl J Med 1985;313:282–5.
9. Cheng JF, Ott NL, Peterson EA, et al. Dermal eosinophils in atopic dermatitis undergo cytolytic degeneration. J Allergy Clin Immunol 1997;99:683–92.
10. Peters MS, Schroeter AL, Gleich GJ. Immunofluorescence identification of eosinophil granule major basic protein in the flame figures of Wells' syndrome. Br J Dermatol 1983;109:141–8.
11. Soragni A, Yousefi S, Stoeckle C, et al. Toxicity of eosinophil MBP is repressed by intracellular crystallization and promoted by extracellular aggregation. Mol Cell 2015;57(6):1011–21.
12. Simon D, Aeberhard C, Erdemoglu Y, et al. Th17 cells and tissue remodeling in atopic and contact dermatitis. Allergy 2014;69:125–31.
13. Foster EL, Simpson EL, Fredrikson LJ, et al. Eosinophils increase neuron branching in human and murine skin and in vitro. PLoS One 2011;6:22029.
14. Schneider L, Tilles S, Lio P, et al. Atopic dermatitis: a practice parameter update 2012. J Allergy Clin Immunol 2013;131:295–9.
15. Kiehl P, Falkenberg K, Vogelbruch M, et al. Tissue eosinophilia in acute and chronic atopic dermatitis: a morphometric approach using quantitative image analysis of immunostaining. Br J Dermatol 2001;145:720–9.
16. Simon D, Vassina E, Yousefi S, et al. Reduced dermal infiltration of cytokine-expressing inflammatory cells in atopic dermatitis after short-term topical tacrolimus treatment. J Allergy Clin Immunol 2004;114:887–95.
17. Simon D, Hösli S, Kostylina G, et al. Anti-CD20 (rituximab) treatment improves atopic eczema. J Allergy Clin Immunol 2008;121:122–8.
18. Martin SF, Esser PR, Weber FC, et al. Mechanisms of chemical-induced innate immunity in allergic contact dermatitis. Allergy 2011;66:1152–63.
19. Nakashima C, Otsuka A, Kitoh A, et al. Basophils regulate the recruitment of eosinophils in a murine model of irritant contact dermatitis. J Allergy Clin Immunol 2014;134:100–7.
20. Wozel G. Eosinophile Dermatosen. Hautarzt 2007;58:347–60.
21. Walton SF, Oprescu FI. Immunology of scabies and translational outcomes: identifying the missing links. Curr Opin Infect Dis 2013;26:116–22.
22. Heukelbach J, Feldmeier H. Epidemiological and clinical characteristics of hookworm-related cutaneous larva migrans. Lancet Infect Dis 2008;8:302–9.
23. Veraldi S, Persico MC, Francia C, et al. Chronic hookworm-related cutaneous larva migrans. Int J Infect Dis 2013;17:277–9.
24. Gilmore SJ. Control Strategies for Endemic Childhood Scabies. PLoS One 2011; 6:15990.
25. Ionescu MA, Rivet J, Daneshpouy M, et al. In situ eosinophil activation in 26 primary cutaneous T-cell lymphomas with blood eosinophilia. J Am Acad Dermatol 2005;52:32–94.
26. Jawed SI, Myskowski PL, Horwitz S, et al. Primary cutaneous T-cell lymphoma (mycosis fungoides and Sézary syndrome): part I. J Am Acad Dermatol 2014;70:205.
27. Wilcox RA. Cutaneous T-cell lymphoma: 2014 update on diagnosis, risk-stratification, and management. Am J Hematol 2014;89:837–51.
28. Simon HU, Plötz SG, Dummer R, et al. Abnormal clones of T cells producing interleukin-5 in idiopathic eosinophilia. N Engl J Med 1999;341:1112–20.
29. Simon HU, Plötz SG, Simon D, et al. Clinical and immunological features of patients with interleukin-5-producing T cell clones and eosinophilia. Int Arch Allergy Immunol 2001;124:242–5.

30. Egeler RM, van Halteren AG, Hogendoorn PC, et al. Langerhans cell histiocytosis: fascinating dynamics of the dendritic cell-macrophage lineage. Immunol Rev 2010;234:213–32.
31. Demoly P, Adkinson NF, Brockow K, et al. International consensus on drug allergy. Allergy 2014;69:420–37.
32. Husain Z, Reddy BY, Schwartz RA. DRESS syndrome: part II. management and therapeutics. J Am Acad Dermatol 2013;68:709.
33. Acharya KR, Ackerman SJ. Eosinophil granule proteins: form and function. J Biol Chem 2014;289:17406–15.
34. Arsenovic N, Sheehan L, Clark D, et al. Fatal carbamazepine induced fulminant eosinophilic (hypersensitivity) myocarditis: emphasis on anatomical and histological characteristics, mechanisms and genetics of drug hypersensitivity and differential diagnosis. J Forensic Leg Med 2010;17:57–61.
35. Zuberbier T, Aberer W, Asero R, et al. The EAACI/GA2LEN/EDF/WAO Guideline for the definition, classification, diagnosis, and management of urticaria: the 2013 revision and update. Allergy 2014;69:868–87.
36. Cugno M, Marzano AV, Asero R, et al. Activation of blood coagulation in chronic urticaria: pathophysiological and clinical implications. Intern Emerg Med 2010;5: 97–101.
37. Moossavi M, Mehregan DR. Wells' syndrome: a clinical and histopathologic review of seven cases. Int J Dermatol 2003;42:62–7.
38. Simon HU, Rothenberg ME, Bochner BS, et al. Refining the definition of hypereosinophilic syndrome. J Allergy Clin Immunol 2010;126:45–9.
39. Gleich GJ, Schroeter AL, Marcoux JP, et al. Episodic angioedema associated with eosinophilia. N Engl J Med 1984;310:1621–6.
40. Khoury P, Herold J, Alpaugh A, et al. Episodic angioedema with eosinophilia (Gleich's syndrome) is a multilineage cell cycling disorder. Haematologica 2015;100(3):300–7.
41. Ambros-Rudolph CM, Müllegger RR, Vaughan-Jones SA, et al. The specific dermatoses of pregnancy revisited and reclassified: results of a retrospective two-center study on 505 pregnant patients. J Am Acad Dermatol 2006;54:395–404.
42. Valent P, Escribano L, Broesby-Olsen S, et al. Proposed diagnostic algorithm for patients with suspected mastocytosis: a proposal of the European Competence Network on Mastocytosis. Allergy 2014;69:1267–74.
43. Ishida M, Iwai M, Kagotani A, et al. Cutaneous mastocytosis with abundant eosinophilic infiltration: a case report with review of the literature. Int J Clin Exp Pathol 2014;7:2695–7.
44. Maric I, Robyn J, Metcalfe DD, et al. KIT D816V-associated systemic mastocytosis with eosinophilia and FIP1L1/PDGFRA-associated chronic eosinophilic leukemia are distinct entities. J Allergy Clin Immunol 2007;120:680–7.
45. Daniel BS, Murrell DF, Borradori L. Bullous pemphigoid: therapeutic algorithm and practical management. Expert Opin Orphan Drugs 2013;1:405–12.
46. Schmidt E, Zillikens D. Pemphigoid diseases. Lancet 2013;381:320–32.
47. Di Zenzo G, della Torre R, Zambruno G, et al. Bullous pemphigoid: from the clinic to the bench. Clin Dermatol 2012;30:3–16.
48. Nishie W. Update on the pathogenesis of bullous pemphigoid: an autoantibody-mediated blistering disease targeting collagen XVII. J Dermatol Sci 2014;73: 179–86.
49. Ronaghy A, Streilein RD, Hall RP. Rituximab decreases without preference all subclasses of IgG anti-BP180 autoantibodies in refractory bullous pemphigoid (BP). J Dermatol Sci 2014;74:93–4.

50. Ruocco V, Ruocco E, Lo Schiavo A, et al. Pemphigus: etiology, pathogenesis, and inducing or triggering factors: facts and controversies. Clin Dermatol 2013;31: 374–81.
51. Zaraa I, Sellami A, Bouguerra C, et al. Pemphigus vegetans: a clinical, histological, immunopathological and prognostic study. J Eur Acad Dermatol Venereol 2011;25:1160–7.
52. Jean-Baptiste S, O'Toole EA, Chen M, et al. Expression of eotaxin, an eosinophil-selective chemokine, parallels eosinophil accumulation in the vesiculobullous stage of incontinentia pigmenti. Clin Exp Immunol 2002;127: 470–8.
53. Conte MI, Pescatore A, Paciolla M, et al. Insight into IKBKG/NEMO locus: report of new mutations and complex genomic rearrangements leading to incontinentia pigmenti disease. Hum Mutat 2014;35:165–77.
54. Nervi SJ, Schwartz RA, Dmochowski M. Eosinophilic pustular folliculitis: a 40 year retrospect. J Am Acad Dermatol 2006;55:285–9.
55. Katoh M, Nomura T, Miyachi Y, et al. Eosinophilic pustular folliculitis: a review of the Japanese published works. J Dermatol 2013;40:15–20.
56. Fujiyama T, Tokura Y. Clinical and histopathological differential diagnosis of eosinophilic pustular folliculitis. J Dermatol 2013;40:419–23.
57. Weigelt N, Metze D, Ständer S. Prurigo nodularis: systematic analysis of 58 histological criteria in 136 patients. J Cutan Pathol 2010;37:578–86.
58. Simpson RC, Crichlow S, Harman KE. Pigmented facial plaques. Granuloma faciale (GF). Clin Exp Dermatol 2010;35:805–6.
59. Gauger A, Ronet C, Schnopp C, et al. High local interleukin 5 production in granuloma faciale (eosinophilicum): role of clonally expanded skin-specific CD4+ cells. Br J Dermatol 2005;153:454–7.
60. Greco A, Rizzo MI, De Virgilio A, et al. Churg-Strauss syndrome. Autoimmun Rev 2015;14(4):341–8.
61. Buder K, Ruppert S, Trautmann A, et al. Angiolymphoid hyperplasia with eosinophilia and Kimura's disease - a clinical and histopathological comparison. J Dtsch Dermatol Ges 2014;12:224–8.
62. Kempf W, Pfaltz K, Vermeer MH, et al. EORTC, ISCL, and USCLC consensus recommendations for the treatment of primary cutaneous CD30-positive lymphoproliferative disorders: lymphomatoid papulosis and primary cutaneous anaplastic large-cell lymphoma. Blood 2011;118:4024–35.
63. Wilcox RA. Cutaneous B-cell lymphomas: 2015 update on diagnosis, risk-stratification, and management. Am J Hematol 2015;90:73–6.
64. Kusam S, Toney LM, Sato H, et al. Inhibition of Th2 differentiation and GATA-3 expression by BCL-6. J Immunol 2003;170:2435–41.
65. Cerroni L, Beham-Schmid C, Kerl H. Cutaneous Hodgkin's disease: an immunohistochemical analysis. J Cutan Pathol 1995;22:229–35.
66. Jundt F, Anagnostopoulos I, Bommert K, et al. Hodgkin/Reed-Sternberg cells induce fibroblasts to secrete eotaxin, a potent chemoattractant for T cells and eosinophils. Blood 1999;94:2065–71.
67. Aldinucci D, Gloghini A, Pinto A, et al. The classical Hodgkin's lymphoma microenvironment and its role in promoting tumour growth and immune escape. J Pathol 2010;221:248–63.
68. Farber MJ, La Forgia S, Sahu J, et al. Eosinophilic dermatosis of hematologic malignancy. J Cutan Pathol 2012;39:690–5.
69. Pinal-Fernandez I, Selva-O'Callaghan A, Grau JM. Diagnosis and classification of eosinophilic fasciitis. Autoimmun Rev 2014;13:379–82.

70. French LE, Dziadzio L, Kelly EA, et al. Cytokine abnormalities in a patient with eosinophilic fasciitis. Ann Allergy Asthma Immunol 2003;90:452–5.
71. Kreuter A. Localized scleroderma. Dermatol Ther 2012;25:135–47.
72. Hertzman PA, Blevins WL, Mayer J, et al. Association of the eosinophilia-myalgia syndrome with the ingestion of tryptophan. N Engl J Med 1990;322:869–73.
73. Simon D, Simon HU. Eosinophilic disorders. J Allergy Clin Immunol 2007;119: 1291–300.
74. Valent P, Klion AD, Rosenwasser LJ, et al. ICON: eosinophil disorders. World Allergy Organ J 2012;5:174–81.
75. Wechsler ME, Fulkerson PC, Bochner BS, et al. Novel targeted therapies for eosinophilic disorders. J Allergy Clin Immunol 2012;130:563–71.
76. Radonjic-Hoesli S, Valent P, Klion AD, et al. Novel targeted therapies for eosinophil-associated diseases and allergy. Annu Rev Pharmacol Toxicol 2015; 55:633–56.
77. Beck LA, Thaçi D, Hamilton JD, et al. Dupilumab treatment in adults with moderate-to-severe atopic dermatitis. N Engl J Med 2014;371:130–9.
78. Plötz SG, Simon HU, Darsow U, et al. Use of an anti-interleukin-5 antibody in the hypereosinophilic syndrome with eosinophilic dermatitis. N Engl J Med 2003;349: 2334–9.
79. Klion AD, Noel P, Akin C, et al. Elevated serum tryptase levels identify a subset of patients with a myeloproliferative variant of idiopathic hypereosinophilic syndrome associated with tissue fibrosis, poor prognosis, and imatinib responsiveness. Blood 2003;101:4660–6.
80. de Masson A, Guitera P, Brice P, et al. Long-term efficacy and safety of alemtuzumab in advanced primary cutaneous T-cell lymphomas. Br J Dermatol 2014; 170:720–4.

Management of Hypereosinophilic Syndromes

Florence Roufosse, MD, PhD

KEYWORDS

- Idiopathic hypereosinophilic syndrome
- *FIP1L1-PDGFRA*–associated myeloid neoplasm
- Lymphocytic variant hypereosinophilic syndrome • Corticosteroid
- Imatinib mesylate • Hydroxyurea • Interferon-α • Targeted therapy

KEY POINTS

- Clinical manifestations in a patient with persistent hypereosinophilia may be related to underlying disease, organ damage and dysfunction provoked by eosinophils, or both. Pathologic assessment is key to establishing a direct role for eosinophils in signs and symptoms, thereby defining a hypereosinophilic syndrome.
- Most patients presenting with hypereosinophilia have an underlying disease or condition driving polyclonal eosinophil expansion. Many of these conditions are treatable, and the causal relationship with hypereosinophilia is confirmed when posttreatment eosinophil counts return to normal. Corticosteroid treatment often effectively reduces eosinophil counts if the response to specific treatment is delayed or the underlying disease is untreatable.
- Clonal hypereosinophilia is infrequent but must be identified, because prognosis is poor in the absence of therapy with the tyrosine kinase inhibitor imatinib mesylate (for *FIP1L1-PDGFRA*–positive patients), cytoreductive agents, or allogeneic stem cell transplantation.
- Idiopathic hypereosinophilic syndrome qualifies patients with persistent unexplained hypereosinophilia associated with eosinophil-mediated damage. Most patients respond to first-line corticosteroid treatment, but use of second-line agents (most commonly hydroxyurea and interferon-α) is often necessary to reduce the toxicity of long-term maintenance therapy.

INTRODUCTION

Hypereosinophilia (HE) is not uncommon, and may be discovered in a variety of settings, from the asymptomatic patient undergoing a routine checkup in the general

Disclosure Statement: F. Roufosse has received consultancy fees from GlaxoSmithKline.
Department of Internal Medicine, Hôpital Erasme, Institute for Medical Immunology, Université Libre de Bruxelles, 808 Route de Lennik, Brussels 1070, Belgium
E-mail address: florence.roufosse@erasme.ulb.ac.be

Immunol Allergy Clin N Am 35 (2015) 561–575
http://dx.doi.org/10.1016/j.iac.2015.05.006   immunology.theclinics.com

practitioner's office to the patient with acute life-threatening eosinophil-mediated end-organ damage in the intensive care unit. Between these extremes, the most frequent situation is that of a symptomatic patient with signs and symptoms of organ and system involvement (eg, respiratory, cardiovascular, digestive, neurologic, cutaneous) presenting to the relevant specialist. The tasks of the physician are to determine whether the HE itself is contributing to damage and disease manifestations (thereby defining a hypereosinophilic syndrome [HES]), identify the cause of the patient's HE if possible, and finally treat the cause, deleterious hypereosinophilic state, or both.

This article proposes a practical approach to these different facets of HES management and has been designed to address questions encountered in routine practice. Most of what follows concerns the typical symptomatic hypereosinophilic patient whose life is not in immediate danger, allowing for stepwise investigations followed by initiation of adapted therapy. Management of patients with acute life-threatening disease is different, initially focusing on rapid therapeutic control of eosinophilia, and is addressed in **Table 1**. The etiologic workup of persistent HE is covered by Ogbogu and Curtis, and novel therapies for eosinophilic disorders are addressed by Bochner, both elsewhere in this issue. Furthermore, several recent reviews discuss HES management with a more classic layout,[1–4] and complement the content of this article.

ASSESSMENT FOR THE PRESENCE OF EOSINOPHIL-MEDIATED COMPLICATIONS

Activated eosinophils are prone to infiltrate various tissues and release a wide array of mediators, inducing organ or system damage and dysfunction, as developed in detail by Weller and Akuthota elsewhere in this issue. According to the currently accepted definition, diagnosis of a HES can be proposed in the presence of documented persistent HE (ie, in routine practice: [1] blood eosinophil count greater than 1.5×10^9/L on at least 2 occasions, ideally at minimum 1 month apart, and/or [2] tissue eosinophilia that is considered excessive by the pathologist) and organ damage or dysfunction attributable to tissue eosinophils.[5] The major difference from previous definitions is that identification of an underlying disease responsible for HE (eg, lymphoma, parasitic infection) is no longer incompatible with a diagnosis of HES, reflecting that the deleterious effects of eosinophils on tissue may be indistinguishable, whatever the cause of HE. Indeed, an important defining feature that has been maintained over time pertains to the direct and predominant involvement of eosinophils in organ damage.

When a symptomatic patient is found to have HE, signs and symptoms may be due to an underlying disease, eosinophils, or both. Establishing that eosinophils are responsible for clinical manifestations is important in guiding therapeutic decisions, and requires a thorough and systematic evaluation that can be conducted in the outpatient clinic in most cases. Hospitalization is indicated in the presence of life-threatening complications, or if the patient is acutely ill.

A careful clinical examination and routine blood testing are crucial first steps toward the identification of signs, symptoms, and markers of organ damage and dysfunction. Findings will guide additional studies, including radiologic and isotopic imaging, endoscopies, and biopsies (see Ref.[4] and article by Weller and Akuthota elsewhere in this issue).

Pathologic Assessment for Hypereosinophilic Syndrome

Establishing that eosinophils contribute to disease mostly relies on the ability to demonstrate their presence in damaged tissues, and all efforts should be made to do so. Biopsies and fluid sampling for cytology (eg, pleural fluid, bronchoalveolar

Table 1
General management of hypereosinophilic syndrome and treatment of acute life-threatening presentations

Condition	Recommendation	Comments
General measures		
Management of specific manifestations of eosinophil-mediated damage		
• Intravascular/cardiac thrombus	• Heparin, warfarin, thrombectomy	
• Embolic stroke, acute arterial occlusion	• Fibrinolysis	
• Heart failure	• ACE inhibitor, diuretic	
• Structural cardiac damage (fibrosis)	• Surgery: Valve repair or replacement, thrombectomy, endocardectomy, transplantation	• Eosinophilia should be controlled
Prevention/treatment of complications of long-term corticosteroid treatment		
• Osteoporosis	• Calcium, vitamin D supplementation, biphosphonates	• Bone density scan at baseline
• Hypertension	• Antihypertensive(s)	
• Diabetes	• Antidiabetic(s)	
• Gastritis, peptic ulcer	• Proton pump inhibitor	
Acute presentation with life-threatening hypereosinophilic syndrome		
• Urgent evaluation and treatment	• Hospitalisation, intensive care unit	• Stop all unnecessary medications (drug allergy, DRESS)
• Initial rapid evaluation	• Blood sampling	• CBC+differential, blood smear, routine chemistry, troponin, vitamin B12, tryptase, IgE, IgG, IgM, ANCA, FISH/PCR for FIP1L1-PDGFRA, T cell phenotyping, TCR rearrangement studies
	• Thoracic (abdominal) imaging (radiograph, CT)	
	• Echocardiogram	
	• Bone marrow smear/biopsy	• If tests suggest possible MP disease or lymphoma
• Hemodynamic instability, hypoxia	• Inotropic support, medical treatment for heart failure, mechanical ventilation	
• Risk of prior exposure to S. Stercoralis	• Ivermectin 200 microg/kg 2 d	• Draw blood for serology (larvae in stools, BALF)
Eosinophil-lowering therapy		
• First-line	• Prednisone 15 mg/kg IV	• Check for response within 4–6 h
• CS-resistance and MP features	• Imatinib mesylate 400–600 mg	• With 1 mg/kg PDN; response within days
• Very marked HE (eg, >100 G/L)	• Vincristine 1–2 mg/m² IV	• Few reports, mostly children; response within hours
• No response to above	• Initiate second-line agents for HES	• See **Table 2**, idiopathic HES; eventually combination therapy
	• HLA typing	• For future ASCT

Abbreviations: ACE, angiotensin-converting enzyme; ANCA, anti-neutrophil cytoplasmic antibodies; ASCT, allogeneic stem cell transplantation; BALF, bronchoalveolar fluid; CBC, complete blood count; CS, corticosteroid; CT, computed tomography; DRESS, drug reaction with eosinophilia and systemic symptoms; FISH, fluorescent in situ hybridization; HE, hypereosinophilia; HES, hypereosinophilic syndrome; HLA, human leukocyte antigen; Ig, immunoglobulin; IV, intravenous; MP, myeloproliferative; PCR, polymerase chain reaction; PDN, prednisone; Rx, treatment; TCR, T-cell receptor.

lavage, stools, ascites, urine, cerebrospinal fluid, synovial fluid) should be guided by clinical manifestations and by results of blood tests and imaging studies. The presence of eosinophils or Charcot-Leyden crystals is revealed by appropriate staining (hematoxylin-eosin, May-Grunwald-Giemsa, Wright-Giemsa). Readily accessible sites for biopsy include skin and soft tissue (eg, fascia, muscle), lungs, and the upper and lower digestive tract. Liver, kidney, peripheral nerve, and heart can also be biopsied, whereas sites less amenable to pathologic assessment include the brain, most of the small intestine, and large vessels. Hence, in a patient with multiple systemic manifestations, biopsies should first be attempted at the most accessible and safest sites.

Shortcomings of Pathology in the Evaluation of the Hypereosinophilic Patient

Biopsies for HES diagnosis may be disappointing, because of either sampling error or extensive eosinophil degranulation. For example, eosinophils infiltrating the deeper layers of the intestinal wall (submucosa, muscularis propria or serosa), will not be detected in superficial biopsies.[6,7] Deeper (or surgical) biopsies may be more rewarding, but generally, medical imaging will show a thickened and contrast-enhanced intestinal wall; ascites may suggest serosal involvement. In a hypereosinophilic patient with abdominal complaints, these indirect signs may be considered sufficient evidence of eosinophil-mediated digestive involvement.

In other instances, eosinophils that were indeed present in a biopsied tissue may have largely degranulated before the procedure, leaving behind rare intact cells in the presence of extracellular granule proteins that escape detection by routine stains. Positive immunohistologic staining for eosinophil cationic protein (ECP), major basic protein (MBP),[8,9] or eosinophil protein X (EPX),[10] conducted by expert hands and interpreted carefully, may be sufficient to conclude that a patient has HES. However, to date it remains unknown as to how long these products remain detectable or whether their presence can be held responsible for ongoing damage, namely in a treated patient with normal blood eosinophil counts.

On the other hand, eosinophils may indeed be detected in biopsies within mixed inflammatory infiltrates, but their contribution to damage remains uncertain. For example, in bullous pemphigoid (BP), the major pathogenic mechanism consists in binding of autoantibodies to basal epidermal cells. Whether nearby eosinophils truly contribute to local damage through their procoagulant properties remains speculative.[11] Similarly, in eosinophilic granulomatosis with polyangiitis (EGPA), it is not clear whether necrotizing vasculitis is a direct consequence of the eosinophilia that can be observed within vessel walls or is related to antineutrophil cytoplasmic antibodies.[12] By contrast, eosinophils clearly play a role in the pulmonary infiltrates and eosinophilic cardiomyopathy that complicate the course of this disease.

Evaluation of Eosinophil-Mediated Damage Using Methods Other than Histology

It is noteworthy that, for certain eosinophil-mediated complications, highly specific abnormalities shown by imaging studies may be considered sufficient evidence for HES. Combined endothelial toxicity and procoagulant effects of activated eosinophils are responsible for characteristic damage involving the heart, brain, and blood vessels.[13] Endomyocardial fibrosis, mitral valve entrapment and regurgitation, and intraventricular (often apical) thrombus formation detected by an echocardiogram or cardiac MRI generally obviate an endomyocardial biopsy in a hypereosinophilic patient.[14] The presence of multiple bilateral ischemic brain lesions in watershed areas (best appreciated using diffusion-weighted imaging combined with MRI)[15] or thrombosis of large vessels[16,17] is also characteristic.

Are There Surrogate or Predictive Markers for Eosinophil-Mediated Damage?

It must be underlined that eosinophils are not necessarily deleterious, and it is well known that the extent and severity of organ damage are not correlated with the degree of HE. Thorough evaluation of a hypereosinophilic patient may indeed fail to show the slightest indication that eosinophils are causing damage.

To spare patients the inconvenience of invasive investigations, efforts have been made to identify markers that reliably reflect or predict eosinophil-mediated complications. A recent study has shown that expression of the activation markers CD25, CD69, and HLA-DR by eosinophils, and serum levels of eotaxin and various cytokines (interleukin [IL]-5, IL-9, IL-13, IL-17) are comparable in symptomatic patients with HES and in asymptomatic patients with persistent unexplained and uncomplicated HE (hypereosinophilia of undetermined significance, or HE_{US}).[18] Serum levels of eosinophil degranulation products may be more promising markers to distinguish quiescent from activated eosinophils.[19] Serum cationic proteins seem to correlate with disease severity in HES, but their quantification is challenging and unavailable in routine practice settings. Development of more reliable methods for simultaneous measurement of ECP, MBP, EPX, and eosinophil-derived neurotoxin is in progress.[20]

DIAGNOSTIC EVALUATION OF HYPEREOSINOPHILIA

The search for an underlying cause of HE, developed in detail by Ogbogu and Curtis elsewhere in this issue, is conducted simultaneously with assessment for eosinophil-mediated damage. In most patients, an underlying disease or condition (eg, drug allergy, parasitic infections, or cancer) Is found after clinical examination and a limited series of relatively routine investigations. When these first-line investigations are negative, further testing is warranted. Diagnostic evaluation of HE is therefore conducted in a stepwise manner, first ruling out more common causes, then pursuing with more elaborate second-line tests to detect rare but specific treatable conditions such as FIP1L1-PDGFRA–associated myeloid neoplasms. The requirement for bone marrow biopsy with cytogenetic testing is guided by results of first-line investigations. Indications include the presence of myeloproliferative features or T-cell abnormalities (clonality, aberrant phenotype), to rule out a (chronic) myeloid neoplasm or T-cell lymphoma.

Establishing a Link Between a Given Condition or Disease and Hypereosinophilia

Identification of certain causes of HE is straightforward and can be achieved rapidly and unequivocally. For example, the presence of numerous Strongyloides stercoralis larvae in stools from a patient who has traveled to an endemic area and has typical digestive, respiratory, and cutaneous complaints indicates an active parasitic infection causing HE. This finding should put an end to diagnostic evaluations and prompt anthelminthic therapy with subsequent evaluation for therapeutic success. Likewise, detection of a CHIC2 deletion by fluorescent in situ hybridization and/or a FIP1L1-PDGFRA fusion by polymerase chain reaction in blood or bone marrow of a hypereosinophilic patient is sufficient for diagnosis of myeloid neoplasm and initiation of imatinib mesylate (IM) before irreversible damage occurs.

In other situations, the cause of HE can be inferred from a characteristic clinical presentation with a high degree of certainty. Development of a generalized rash associated with fever and elevated liver enzymes in a patient who has recently initiated anticonvulsant therapy is more than likely to represent drug reaction with eosinophilia and systemic symptoms (DRESS) syndrome.[21] Five to 8 weeks after the incident, a positive lymphocyte transformation test in the presence of the drug in soluble form will help identify the offending agent in most cases.[22,23]

In many instances, however, etiologic workup leads the clinician to hypothesize that a given condition could be driving HE, and proving this assumption may take some time. Trichinellosis, for example, may present with largely nonspecific clinical manifestations, and resolve spontaneously over a variable period of time. A positive serology does not necessarily indicate an active infection, but in the absence of an alternative diagnosis for a symptomatic hypereosinophilic patient, treatment for trichinellosis should be administered, with subsequent evaluation to ensure that eosinophils have dropped durably and symptoms have disappeared. The time frame for normalization of eosinophil counts remains undefined, but may be months to years. Similarly, in patients with drug allergy, it may take weeks or months for HE to regress after drug withdrawal.

In conditions where HE is an uncommon complication, the clinician should also refrain from drawing hasty conclusions. For example, the discovery of lung cancer during etiologic workup may or may not be related to HE. The presence of abundant eosinophils within the tumor biopsy may suggest a causal role, which will only be confirmed if curative surgery[24] or successful chemotherapy/radiotherapy is followed by normalization of eosinophil counts (or if normal counts are maintained in a patient who received prior corticosteroid treatment). Investigating the production of eosinophilopoietic/eosinophilotactic factors, such as IL-5 or granulocyte-macrophage colony stimulating factor by tumor cells, is not feasible in routine practice.[24]

An increasingly common diagnostic shortcut is taken when abnormal T-cell phenotyping and T-cell receptor (TCR) gene rearrangement studies are misinterpreted, leading to the erroneous diagnosis of lymphocytic variant HES (L-HES).[25,26] First, T-cell lymphoma should be suspected and investigated thoroughly in these circumstances. Second, the relevance of abnormal phenotypes should be explored with the help of clinicians and biologists with expertise. Only the CD3$^-$CD4$^+$ T-cell subset has repeatedly been shown to overproduce IL-5 in vitro, clearly establishing a direct role in eosinophil expansion.[27] For other phenotypes (eg, CD3$^+$CD4$^+$CD7$^-$, CD3$^+$TCRα/β^+CD4$^-$CD8$^-$), or in the presence of an isolated clonal TCR gene rearrangement pattern, production of eosinophilopoietic cytokines should be demonstrated before concluding that the patient has L-HES.

TREATMENT OF HYPEREOSINOPHILIC SYNDROMES ASSOCIATED WITH A KNOWN UNDERLYING CONDITION

In most situations where HE is reactive (secondary) and judged deleterious, systemic corticosteroid therapy represents the most effective and rapid means of reducing eosinophils. By contrast, primary HE that can accompany various myeloid neoplasms (including *FIP1L1-PDGFRA*–associated disease) is typically corticosteroid resistant, and treatment should target the underlying hematologic disorder or cytogenetic abnormality.

Decision on Whether to Treat the Underlying Condition, the Hypereosinophilia, or Both

Once a disease causing HE has been identified and a role for eosinophils in at least part of the clinical manifestations has been established, the most appropriate therapeutic strategy must be adopted. In practice, eradicating HE by treating the underlying condition is a logical, but not always applicable, strategy. Indeed, the condition itself may or may not warrant treatment; if treated, a response may be observed more or less rapidly, if at all. Furthermore, HE per se may or may not jeopardize the function of target organs in the short term; in the latter case, signs and symptoms may or may not be tolerable. Sometimes, the therapeutic agent(s) used to treat the underlying disease may also be effective in reducing eosinophilia. Whether to specifically treat HE in a specific situation is guided by these considerations, as illustrated in the following paragraphs describing the approach to selected clinical conditions.

Situations whereby the underlying condition is the major focus of treatment include most infections (eg, helminth infection, scabies) and cancer. Successful treatment using agents that have no direct effect on eosinophils typically results in resolution of HE and accompanying HES.[24] If treatment fails (eg, metastatic lung cancer refractory to chemotherapy), management of the HES with corticosteroids may improve the patient's quality of life.[28]

The approach to drug allergy depends on the clinical presentation and the complexity of comorbidities and their treatment. Patients with severe, potentially life-threatening complications of HE, such as DRESS syndrome, cardiomyopathy, or pulmonary hypersensitivity, should be hospitalized for surveillance and treatment. Certain drugs are more likely culprits than others (eg, antiepileptics, sulfonamides, allopurinol, clozapine), and should be withdrawn in all cases. Systemic corticosteroid treatment may accelerate eosinophil apoptosis and clearance from target organs, although this strategy may increase the risk of infectious complications.[29] For less severe drug reactions in patients on multiple medications, there is time for sequential withdrawal and/or replacement by compounds with different chemical compositions while verifying the impact on blood eosinophil levels. The use of drugs considered essential to the well-being of a patient and causing asymptomatic HE may eventually be pursued, provided eosinophil-mediated complications are monitored.

Other instances in which it is justified to withhold therapy directed against the condition causing HE include disorders for which treatment has an unacceptable risk/benefit balance or is nonexistent. For example, Wells syndrome with marked eosinophilia and flame figures in a skin biopsy was the presenting feature of nodal B-cell lymphocytic lymphoma in an elderly patient.[30] Because of her age and the indolent nature of the hematologic disease, lymphoma was not treated, and her debilitating eosinophil-mediated cutaneous condition responded well to oral corticosteroids. Another more complex example is that of a young patient with congenital CARD9 deficiency complicated by invasive *Trichophyton rubrum* infection, who developed marked and persistent HE as the infection progressed, with abundant subcutaneous eosinophilic infiltrates and marked pruritus (Roufosse F, unpublished observation, 2013). Elevated eosinophil counts were observed in 9 of 10 patients with CARD9 mutations and dermatophytosis, including this patient,[31] suggesting that eosinophil expansion may result from deficient CARD9 signaling or a T-helper 2 polarized immune response to fungal invasion. No treatment is currently available for this congenital immunodeficiency, and the benefits of treating HE must be weighed carefully against the risk of further impairing the immune response.

Finally, certain autoimmune or T-cell–driven disorders associated with HE require immunosuppressive or cytotoxic therapy that also targets eosinophils. Examples include T-cell lymphoma, BP, inflammatory bowel disease, and graft-versus-host disease. Recurrence of HE may herald a disease flare. Management of EGPA has been reviewed recently[32] and is not covered herein.

Specific Management of Myeloid Neoplasms

Most cases of myeloid neoplasm are associated with the *FIP1L1-PDGFRA* fusion gene. Because this represents a particularly aggressive form of chronic HE, with high rates of morbidity and mortality,[33] treatment is mandatory, regardless of the clinical presentation. The tyrosine kinase inhibitor (TKI) IM is approved by the Food and Drug Administration for this indication, and is used as first-line treatment because practically all patients respond[34] (**Table 2**). Eosinophil counts typically drop within

Table 2
Management of hypereosinophilic syndrome (HES) variants

Condition	Recommendation	Comments
Eosinophil-lowering therapy		
Idiopathic HES		
• Initial therapy	• PDN 1 mg/kg/d	• Dose can be lower if symptoms mild; RR 85%
• Second-line agents (for CS-resistant patients or those with unacceptable CS-toxicity)	• Hydroxyurea, up to 2 g/d	• Response within 2 wk; taper to lower maintenance dose
	• IFNα, 1–2 10⁶ U/2d; then increase to 10–14 10⁶ U/wk	• Progressive dosing to reduce flu-like symptoms; side effects often dose-limiting; Pegylated-IFN possible option
	• Imatinib mesylate 400–800 mg/d	• Most effective in CS-refractory patients and/or with MP features
	• Mepolizumab 750 mg IV monthly[b]	• RR 84% if CS-responsive; not commercialised (compassionate use)
	• Alemtuzumab 30 mg IV or sc, 3/wk	• Only for very severe cases; induces marked immunosuppression
	• Other agents	• Case reports: CSA, MTX, CTX, ARA-C, 2CDA, VCR, fludarabine
• Treatment-refractory severe HES	• ASCT	• Only curative treatment for HES
FIP1L1-PDGFRA+ CEL		
• Initial therapy	• Imatinib mesylate 100–400 mg/d	• Eosinophil counts decrease within days in almost all cases
		• Goal: molecular remission (within weeks to months)
• Cardiac involvement present	• PDN 0.5–1 mg/kg/d for first 1–2 wk	• To prevent acute heart failure
• Maintenance	• Imatinib mesylate 100 mg/d	• Lower dosing may be effective (100 mg/wk)
• Imatinib-resistance (primary or secondary)	• Expert referral, HLA-typing	• High morbidity/mortality; at risk for blastic transformation
	• Alternative TKI, ASCT	• Durable response to TKI unlikely

Lymphocytic variant HES

Initial therapy	• PDN 0.5–1 mg/kg/d then taper	• High RR (90%); maintenance often 10–25 mg/d
	• IFNα: see idiopathic HES	• High RR (87%); acts on eosinophils and pathogenic T cells
Second-line agents	• CSA 2–5 mg/kg/d	• Adapt dose to trough (response rate may be >50%)
	• Mepolizumab 750 mg IV monthly[b]	• RR equivalent to idiopathic HES
Progression to T cell lymphoma	• (R-)CHOP, ASCT	• Poor response to classical chemotherapy

Follow-Up[a]

Idiopathic HES	3–4 mo	Monitoring of disease activity[c] and iatrogenic complications
	6 mo	Once disease has been stabilised with Rx for 18–24 mo
FIP1L1-PDGFRA+ myeloid neoplasm	3 mo	See above + Cytogenetic remission (FISH or PCR)
	6 mo	Once cytogenetic remission has been maintained 18–24 mo
Lymphocytic variant HES	3–4 mo	See above + T cell phenotyping, abs T cell counts; FDG-PET if new or evolving lymph node enlargement[d]
	6 mo	

Abbreviations: 2CDA, cladribine; ARA-C, cytarabine; ASCT, allogeneic stem cell transplantation; CEL, chronic eosinophilic leukemia; CS, corticosteroid; CSA, cyclosporin A; CTX, cyclophosphamide; FDG, ^{18}F-fluorodeoxyglucose; FISH, fluorescent in situ hybridization; IFN-α, interferon-α; MP, myeloproliferative; MTX, methotrexate; PCR, polymerase chain reaction; PDN, prednisone; (R-)CHOP, (rituximab-) cyclophosphamide-hydroxydaunorubicin-vincristine-prednisone; RR, response rate; TKI, tyrosine kinase inhibitor; VCR, vincristine.

[a] Patient must first be stabilised with treatment; during this period and depending on the presentation, the interval between visits is shorter (daily, weekly, monthly).

[b] Recent studies in asthma show efficacy of sub-cutaneous and lower dosing regimens.

[c] Eosinophil counts, chemistry for relevant target organs (troponin, liver enzymes), physical examination, and eventual functional/imaging studies as appropriate.

[d] Increased hypermetabolism of lymph nodes, spleen may suggest progression to lymphoma.

days, and clinical manifestations of reversible damage regress, but disappearance of the *FIP1L1-PDGFRA* fusion gene (ie, the goal of therapy) typically takes longer.[34] Remission can then be maintained with a lower dose[34,35] with regular monitoring for molecular relapse. Tolerance is generally excellent, and patients are often maintained in molecular remission for years with continuous treatment. Recent data show that some patients remain in remission even after prolonged interruption of IM,[34] suggesting they may be cured.

Rare cases of *FIP1L1-PDGFRA*–associated myeloid neoplasm with primary or secondary resistance to IM have been reported, and switching to other TKIs (nilotinib, ponatinib, sorafenib) should be attempted, although chances of success are lower.[1,36–38] Such patients should be referred to centers with expertise for allogeneic stem cell transplantation (ASCT).[39]

In a small proportion of patients with persistent HE, a chromosomal rearrangement other than the *FIP1L1-PDGFRA* fusion is identified or bone marrow blasts are increased (remaining <20%). These patients meet criteria for chronic eosinophilic leukemia (CEL),[5] and should also be referred for appropriate management. Patients with less common rearrangements involving *PDGFRA* or *PDGFRB* and various fusion partners may respond extremely well to IM.[40,41]

SPECIFIC MANAGEMENT OF LYMPHOCYTIC VARIANT HYPEREOSINOPHILIC SYNDROME

L-HES is an indolent and benign lymphoproliferative disorder that generally responds to oral corticosteroid therapy.[42] However, patients often require second-line agents for corticosteroid-sparing purposes (see **Table 2**). Interferon-α,[42] mepolizumab,[43] and cyclosporin A[42] are the most effective, and isolated responses to hydroxyurea and alemtuzumab have been reported. Modalities for administering these agents are discussed in the section on idiopathic HES.

It is essential that patients with L-HES be monitored for the development of peripheral T-cell lymphoma, as malignant progression may be observed, generally after several years of stable disease.[27,42] However, the existence of enlarged hypermetabolic lymph nodes should not be interpreted as evidence for malignancy, as this is relatively frequent in L-HES during the benign phase.[42] New or enlarged lymph nodes developing during treatment should be biopsied to detect lymphoma. Patients who do develop lymphoma generally fail to respond to conventional chemotherapy with CHOP (cyclophosphamide-hydroxydaunorubicin-vincristine-prednisone)-like regimens, but can be cured by ASCT.[44]

TREATMENT OF SYMPTOMATIC AND UNEXPLAINED HYPEREOSINOPHILIA

From a practical standpoint, when eosinophil-mediated organ damage or dysfunction occurs in the absence of a detectable cause or condition associated with HE (ie, idiopathic HES, including organ-restricted eosinophilic disorders), eosinophil-targeted treatment is justified to control symptoms, restore vital organ function, and prevent further deterioration with development of irreversible damage. Although controlling eosinophilia is the therapeutic end point, eosinophils need not necessarily be strictly maintained within the normal range, and the benefits of tighter eosinophil control must be weighed against iatrogenic complications of therapy. Indeed, idiopathic HES is a chronic inflammatory disease, and with the exception of ASCT none of the current treatment options are curative, so they must be administered on a long-term basis.

Several agents are available for treatment of idiopathic HES, as discussed here and in **Table 2**. To limit toxicity and improve tolerance, treatment should be tapered progressively to the lowest effective dose once remission is achieved. Disease activity may fluctuate spontaneously, so it is worthwhile to repeatedly attempt dose tapering after an initial failure to control disease with low-dose treatment. Combination therapy with 2 or more agents may allow further dose reductions and decrease toxicity. Notwithstanding these precautions, regular monitoring for treatment-induced toxicity is essential, with implementation of preventive and therapeutic measures as appropriate (see **Table 1**).

Corticosteroid Treatment

First-line treatment with an oral corticosteroid is effective in most cases.[45] Initial prednisone (PDN) dosing depends on the severity of clinical manifestations and is generally between 20 and 60 mg/d. Eosinophil counts may drop within hours, and when clinical remission is achieved treatment can be tapered progressively. Some patients with organ-restricted disease such as eosinophilic gastroenteritis, chronic eosinophilic pneumonia, or Wells syndrome experience prolonged remissions after corticosteroid withdrawal, whereas others flare within days or weeks and require prolonged maintenance treatment. Most patients with multisystem HES also require continuous treatment, with a median daily maintenance dose of PDN of 10 mg.[45]

In the absence of an initial response to corticosteroid, higher doses can be administered (eg, 15 mg/kg/d intravenously), but this approach is unlikely to produce a durable decrease in eosinophils, and a second-line agent should be considered without delay. Patients less likely to respond to corticosteroid include those with features of myeloproliferative disease (high serum vitamin B12 and/or tryptase levels, anemia, thrombocytopenia, circulating leukocyte precursors, organomegaly, bone marrow fibrosis).

Corticosteroid-Sparing Agents and Second-Line Treatment

Patients who fail to respond to corticosteroid or those who experience significant toxicity with maintenance treatment (PDN >10 mg/d) require second-line agents, most of which were inspired from the treatment of chronic myeloproliferative neoplasms (see **Table 2**).

The most commonly used and least expensive agent for idiopathic HES is hydroxyurea. A prospective study showed that initial combination therapy with relatively high doses of PDN (1 mg/kg) and hydroxyurea (2 g) controlled disease in 15 of 15 patients; remission was maintained with hydroxyurea alone (0.5–1 g/d) after progressive tapering of both compounds.[46]

Interferon-α is a more expensive and less well tolerated alternative for patients who do not respond to corticosteroids and hydroxyurea. Roughly half of patients with HES respond, but treatment is often interrupted because of poor tolerance.[45] Besides flu-like symptoms, side effects that should be monitored include depression, hepatotoxicity, autoimmunity, and thyroid gland dysfunction. Pegylated interferon may have equivalent efficacy and be better tolerated, and has been used both as switch-over treatment from nonpegylated forms of interferon-α and as initial treatment.[47]

IM is a second-line alternative for corticosteroid-refractory patients and those with features of chronic myeloproliferative disease.[48] Although rare cases have been reported with a dramatic and rapid response, most patients with idiopathic HES fail to respond at all, and those who do generally require higher doses[49] (and more time) to respond than those with *FIP1L1-PDGFRA*–positive disease. Dose-related side effects include rash, cytopenias, fluid retention, and hepatotoxicity. The very few data available for other TKIs is not promising.[50]

Case reports mention use of various immunosuppressive and cytotoxic agents (see **Table 2**) to treat idiopathic HES, with variable results. One study showed a high response rate to the monoclonal anti-CD52 antibody, alemtuzumab, in 10 of 12 patients with severe refractory disease (9 idiopathic HES, 3 CEL with abnormal cytogenetics), but treatment had to be repeated and was associated with opportunistic infections and secondary malignancy.[51]

Novel monoclonal antibodies directed against IL-5, such as mepolizumab,[52] or its receptors, such as benralizumab, are extremely promising for idiopathic HES, as developed by Bochner elsewhere in this issue, but are not yet approved for use other than in the setting of investigational trials.

Finally, ASCT is an option for patients with treatment-refractory and life-threatening HES. Reduced intensity conditioning regimens have been administered successfully to patients with significant disease-related morbidity.[53]

SUMMARY AND FUTURE CONSIDERATIONS

With the recognition more than 40 years ago that chronic HE could be deleterious and the subsequent identification of pathogenic mechanisms underlying HE in specific disease variants, management of patients has improved significantly, resulting in less morbidity and better survival. However, because most available therapeutic agents for HES deplete eosinophils through nonspecific mechanisms, long-term iatrogenic toxicity and treatment-refractory disease remain subjects of concern. This situation reflects gaps in our current understanding of pathogenesis in most cases, most obviously for idiopathic HES but also for L-HES, in which the underlying T-cell disorder remains poorly characterized.

Future developments toward tailored therapy and better patient outcome include (1) identification of biomarkers that would reliably distinguish harmful from innocuous eosinophils, to avoid overtreating some patients; (2) identification of biomarkers that reflect ongoing eosinophil-mediated damage, to adapt treatment to disease activity; (3) wider access to more targeted eosinophil-specific agents currently in development for asthma, such as anti–IL-5 (receptor) antibodies, and others (see article by Bochner elsewhere in this issue); and (4) further understanding of molecular mechanisms and perturbed signaling pathways driving eosinophilia, for the development of therapy targeting upstream triggers of disease.

REFERENCES

1. Cogan E, Roufosse F. Clinical management of the hypereosinophilic syndromes. Expert Rev Hematol 2012;5(3):275–89.
2. Simon HU, Klion A. Therapeutic approaches to patients with hypereosinophilic syndromes. Semin Hematol 2012;49(2):160–70.
3. Klion A. Hypereosinophilic syndrome: current approach to diagnosis and treatment. Annu Rev Med 2009;60:293–306.
4. Klion A. How I treat hypereosinophilic syndromes. Blood 2015. [Epub ahead of print].
5. Valent P, Klion AD, Horny HP, et al. Contemporary consensus proposal on criteria and classification of eosinophilic disorders and related syndromes. J Allergy Clin Immunol 2012;130(3):607–12.
6. Mungan Z, Attila T, Kapran Y, et al. Eosinophilic jejunitis presenting as intractable abdominal pain. Case Rep Gastroenterol 2014;8(3):377–80.
7. Talley NJ, Shorter RG, Phillips SF, et al. Eosinophilic gastroenteritis: a clinicopathological study of patients with disease of the mucosa, muscle layer, and subserosal tissues. Gut 1990;31(1):54–8.

8. Cantarini L, Volpi N, Carbotti P, et al. Eosinophilia-associated muscle disorders: an immunohistological study with tissue localisation of major basic protein in distinct clinicopathological forms. J Clin Pathol 2009;62(5):442–7.
9. Wright BL, Leiferman KM, Gleich GJ. Eosinophil granule protein localization in eosinophilic endomyocardial disease. N Engl J Med 2011;365(2):187–8.
10. Nair P, Ochkur SI, Protheroe C, et al. The identification of eosinophilic gastroenteritis in prednisone-dependent eosinophilic bronchitis and asthma. Allergy Asthma Clin Immunol 2011;7(1):4.
11. Marzano AV, Tedeschi A, Berti E, et al. Activation of coagulation in bullous pemphigoid and other eosinophil-related inflammatory skin diseases. Clin Exp Immunol 2011;165(1):44–50.
12. Khoury P, Grayson PC, Klion AD. Eosinophils in vasculitis: characteristics and roles in pathogenesis. Nat Rev Rheumatol 2014;10(8):474–83.
13. Roufosse F. L4. Eosinophils: how they contribute to endothelial damage and dysfunction. Presse Med 2013;42(4 Pt 2):503–7.
14. Kleinfeldt T, Nienaber CA, Kische S, et al. Cardiac manifestation of the hypereosinophilic syndrome: new insights. Clin Res Cardiol 2010;99(7):419–27.
15. Grigoryan M, Geisler SD, St Louis EK, et al. Cerebral arteriolar thromboembolism in idiopathic hypereosinophilic syndrome. Arch Neurol 2009;66(4):528–31.
16. Todd S, Hemmaway C, Nagy Z. Catastrophic thrombosis in idiopathic hypereosinophilic syndrome. Br J Haematol 2014;165(4):425.
17. Ponsky TA, Brody F, Giordano J, et al. Brachial artery occlusion secondary to hypereosinophilic syndrome. J Vasc Surg 2005;42(4):796–9.
18. Chen YY, Khoury P, Ware JM, et al. Marked and persistent eosinophilia in the absence of clinical manifestations. J Allergy Clin Immunol 2014;133(4):1195–202.
19. Confalonieri M, Tacconi F, De Amici M, et al. Benign idiopathic hypereosinophilia: a feeble masquerader or a smouldering form of the hypereosinophilic syndrome? Haematologica 1995;80(1):50–3.
20. Makiya MA, Herrick JA, Khoury P, et al. Development of a suspension array assay in multiplex for the simultaneous measurement of serum levels of four eosinophil granule proteins. J Immunol Methods 2014;411:11–22.
21. Husain Z, Reddy BY, Schwartz RA. DRESS syndrome: part I. Clinical perspectives. J Am Acad Dermatol 2013;68(5):693.e1–14.
22. Jurado-Palomo J, Cabanas R, Prior N, et al. Use of the lymphocyte transformation test in the diagnosis of DRESS syndrome induced by ceftriaxone and piperacillin-tazobactam: two case reports. J Investig Allergol Clin Immunol 2010;20(5):433–6.
23. Kano Y, Hirahara K, Mitsuyama Y, et al. Utility of the lymphocyte transformation test in the diagnosis of drug sensitivity: dependence on its timing and the type of drug eruption. Allergy 2007;62(12):1439–44.
24. Pandit R, Scholnik A, Wulfekuhler L, et al. Non-small-cell lung cancer associated with excessive eosinophilia and secretion of interleukin-5 as a paraneoplastic syndrome. Am J Hematol 2007;82(3):234–7.
25. Christoforidou A, Kotsianidis I, Margaritis D, et al. Long-term remission of lymphocytic hypereosinophilic syndrome with imatinib mesylate. Am J Hematol 2012;87(1):131–2.
26. d'Elbee JM, Parrens M, Mercie P, et al. Hypereosinophilic syndrome—lymphocytic variant transforming into peripheral T-cell lymphoma with severe oral manifestations. Oral Surg Oral Med Oral Pathol Oral Radiol 2013;116(3):e185–90.
27. Roufosse F, Cogan E, Goldman M. Lymphocytic variant hypereosinophilic syndromes. Immunol Allergy Clin North Am 2007;27(3):389–413.

28. Lo CH, Jen YM, Tsai WC, et al. Rapidly evolving asymptomatic eosinophilia in a patient with lung adenocarcinoma causes cognitive disturbance and respiratory insufficiency: case report. Oncol Lett 2013;5(2):495–8.
29. Funck-Brentano E, Duong TA, Bouvresse S, et al. Therapeutic management of DRESS: a retrospective study of 38 cases. J Am Acad Dermatol 2015;72(2): 246–52.
30. Spinelli M, Frigerio E, Cozzi A, et al. Bullous Wells' syndrome associated with non-Hodgkin's lymphocytic lymphoma. Acta Derm Venereol 2008;88(5):530–1.
31. Lanternier F, Pathan S, Vincent QB, et al. Deep dermatophytosis and inherited CARD9 deficiency. N Engl J Med 2013;369(18):1704–14.
32. Greco A, Rizzo MI, De Virgilio A, et al. Churg-Strauss syndrome. Autoimmun Rev 2015;14(4):341–8.
33. Vandenberghe P, Wlodarska I, Michaux L, et al. Clinical and molecular features of FIP1L1-PDFGRA (+) chronic eosinophilic leukemias. Leukemia 2004;18(4):734–42.
34. Legrand F, Renneville A, Macintyre E, et al. The spectrum of FIP1L1-PDGFRA-associated chronic eosinophilic leukemia: new insights based on a survey of 44 cases. Medicine 2013;92(5):e1–9.
35. Helbig G, Moskwa A, Hus M, et al. Durable remission after treatment with very low doses of imatinib for FIP1L1-PDGFRalpha-positive chronic eosinophilic leukaemia. Cancer Chemother Pharmacol 2011;67(4):967–9.
36. Savage N, George TI, Gotlib J. Myeloid neoplasms associated with eosinophilia and rearrangement of PDGFRA, PDGFRB, and FGFR1: a review. Int J Lab Hematol 2013;35(5):491–500.
37. Metzgeroth G, Erben P, Martin H, et al. Limited clinical activity of nilotinib and sorafenib in FIP1L1-PDGFRA positive chronic eosinophilic leukemia with imatinib-resistant T674I mutation. Leukemia 2012;26(1):162–4.
38. Al-Riyami AZ, Hudoba M, Young S, et al. Sorafenib is effective for imatinib-resistant FIP1L1/PDGFRA T674I mutation-positive acute myeloid leukemia with eosinophilia. Leuk Lymphoma 2013;54(8):1788–90.
39. Halaburda K, Prejzner W, Szatkowski D, et al. Allogeneic bone marrow transplantation for hypereosinophilic syndrome: long-term follow-up with eradication of FIP1L1-PDGFRA fusion transcript. Bone Marrow Transpl 2006;38(4):319–20.
40. Curtis CE, Grand FH, Musto P, et al. Two novel imatinib-responsive PDGFRA fusion genes in chronic eosinophilic leukaemia. Br J Haematol 2007;138(1): 77–81.
41. Cheah CY, Burbury K, Apperley JF, et al. Patients with myeloid malignancies bearing PDGFRB fusion genes achieve durable long-term remissions with imatinib. Blood 2014;123(23):3574–7.
42. Lefevre G, Copin MC, Staumont-Salle D, et al. The lymphoid variant of hypereosinophilic syndrome: study of 21 patients with CD3-CD4+ aberrant T-cell phenotype. Medicine 2014;93(17):255–66.
43. Roufosse F, de Lavareille A, Schandene L, et al. Mepolizumab as a corticosteroid-sparing agent in lymphocytic variant hypereosinophilic syndrome. J Allergy Clin Immunol 2010;126(4):828–35.
44. Bergua JM, Prieto-Pliego E, Roman-Barbera A, et al. Resolution of left and right ventricular thrombosis secondary to hypereosinophilic syndrome (lymphoproliferative variant) with reduced intensity conditioning allogenic stem cell transplantation. Ann Hematol 2008;87(11):937–8.
45. Ogbogu PU, Bochner BS, Butterfield JH, et al. Hypereosinophilic syndrome: a multicenter, retrospective analysis of clinical characteristics and response to therapy. J Allergy Clin Immunol 2009;124(6):1319–25.

46. Dahabreh IJ, Giannouli S, Zoi C, et al. Management of hypereosinophilic syndrome: a prospective study in the era of molecular genetics. Medicine 2007; 86(6):344–54.
47. Butterfield JH, Weiler CR. Use of pegylated interferon in hypereosinophilic syndrome. Leuk Res 2012;36(2):192–7.
48. Cools J, DeAngelo DJ, Gotlib J, et al. A tyrosine kinase created by fusion of the PDGFRA and FIP1L1 genes as a therapeutic target of imatinib in idiopathic hypereosinophilic syndrome. N Engl J Med 2003;348(13):1201–14.
49. Butterfield JH. Success of short-term, higher-dose imatinib mesylate to induce clinical response in FIP1L1-PDGFRalpha-negative hypereosinophilic syndrome. Leuk Res 2009;33(8):1127–9.
50. Hochhaus A, le Coutre PD, Kantarjian HM, et al. Effect of the tyrosine kinase inhibitor nilotinib in patients with hypereosinophilic syndrome/chronic eosinophilic leukemia: analysis of the phase 2, open-label, single-arm A2101 study. J Cancer Res Clin Oncol 2013;139(12):1985–93.
51. Strati P, Cortes J, Faderl S, et al. Long-term follow-up of patients with hypereosinophilic syndrome treated with Alemtuzumab, an anti-CD52 antibody. Clin Lymphoma Myeloma Leuk 2013;13(3):287–91.
52. Rothenberg ME, Klion AD, Roufosse FE, et al. Treatment of patients with the hypereosinophilic syndrome with mepolizumab. N Engl J Med 2008;358(12): 1215–28.
53. Sauvage D, Roufosse F, Sanoussi I, et al. Treatment-refractory hypereosinophilic syndrome responding to fludarabine in a 12-year-old boy. Leuk Lymphoma 2015; 25:1–3.

Novel Therapies for Eosinophilic Disorders

Bruce S. Bochner, MD

KEYWORDS

- Eosinophil • Therapies • Antibodies • Targets • Pharmacology • Biomarkers

KEY POINTS

- A sizable unmet need exists for new, safe, selective, and effective treatments for eosinophil-associated diseases, such as hypereosinophilic syndrome, eosinophilic gastrointestinal disorders, nasal polyposis, and severe asthma.
- An improved panel of biomarkers to help guide diagnosis, treatment, and assessment of disease activity is also needed.
- An impressive array of novel therapeutic agents, including small molecules and biologics, that directly or indirectly target eosinophils and eosinophilic inflammation are undergoing controlled clinical trials, with many already showing promising results.
- A large list of additional eosinophil-related potential therapeutic targets remains to be pursued, including cell surface structures, soluble proteins that influence eosinophil biology, and eosinophil-derived mediators that have the potential to contribute adversely to disease pathophysiology.

INTRODUCTION

Eosinophilic disorders, also referred to as eosinophil-associated diseases, consist of a range of infrequent conditions affecting virtually any body compartment and organ.[1] The most commonly affected areas include the bone marrow, blood, mucosal surfaces, and skin, often with immense disease- and treatment-related morbidity,

Disclosure Statement: Dr Bochner's research efforts are supported by grants AI072265, AI097073 and HL107151 from the National Institutes of Health. He has current or recent consulting or scientific advisory board arrangements with, or has received honoraria from, Sanofi-Aventis, Pfizer, Svelte Medical Systems, Biogen Idec, TEVA, and Allakos, Inc. and owns stock in Allakos, Inc. and Glycomimetics, Inc. He receives publication-related royalty payments from Elsevier and UpToDate and is a coinventor on existing and pending Siglec-8-related patents and, thus, may be entitled to a share of future royalties received by Johns Hopkins University on the potential sales of such products. Dr B.S. Bochner is also a cofounder of Allakos, which makes him subject to certain restrictions under university policy. The terms of this arrangement are being managed by the Johns Hopkins University and Northwestern University in accordance with their conflict of interest policies.
Division of Allergy-Immunology, Department of Medicine, Northwestern University Feinberg School of Medicine, 240 East Huron Street, Room M-306, Chicago, IL 60611, USA
E-mail address: bruce.bochner@northwestern.edu

whereas involvement of other organs, such as the cardiovascular system, have a particularly prominent impact on disease mortality. Treatment efficacy based on results from controlled clinical trials is almost nonexistent. Instead, empirically derived standard-of-care disease management typically involves the off-label prescription of drugs whose use is more commonly associated with autoimmune diseases, leukemia, and lymphoma. A mainstay of initial treatment involves the use of glucocorticosteroids, which are usually, but not always, effective in controlling eosinophilia and end-organ damage but are fraught with undesirable side effects when used for long-term disease management. Even though steroid-sparing activity may not be a sufficient reason for drug approval,[2] both physicians and those afflicted with eosinophilic disorders yearn for the day when other more eosinophil-directed, disease-specific, and perhaps disease-modifying agents will be available.

Other articles in this issue of *Immunology and Allergy Clinics of North America* focus on the spectrum of eosinophil-associated diseases from diagnosis to treatment, so the purpose of this section is to provide a perspective on where the field stands when it comes to innovative new therapies for eosinophilic disorders, focusing mainly on those that are eosinophil specific or at least eosinophil selective. As will become clear, many such promising and exciting agents, including small molecules and biologics, are in various stages of clinical development, with some on the verge of approval by the Food and Drug Administration (FDA) in 2015 or soon thereafter.

As part of the discussion of eosinophil-selective therapies, the surface phenotype of the eosinophil is reviewed, in part to explain the current rationale behind drugs that directly target the eosinophil but also, it is hoped, to serve as a springboard for future ideas and efforts. Given that eosinophil activation and eosinophilic inflammation are often part of a spectrum involving a range of cells and mediators, novel therapies that indirectly target eosinophils by neutralizing eosinophil-related pathways is also covered. Finally, a discussion of future therapeutic considerations and unmet needs is included. For completeness, the reader is referred on to other recent excellent, relevant reviews on similar or overlapping topics.[3,4]

THE EOSINOPHIL SURFACE AS A TARGET

The eosinophil arises from precursors in the bone marrow, just like all other leukocytes.[5,6] Not surprisingly, this cell has its own unique set of intracellular signaling pathways that are necessary for specific differentiation into the eosinophil lineage.[7] Also not surprisingly, the mature eosinophil has its own specific characteristics, such as mediator release profiles, granule contents, tinctorial properties, and surface phenotype.[8–11] Surface phenotype is particularly relevant when it comes to consideration of developing eosinophil-targeting drugs (**Fig. 1**).[8,9,12–14] Until very recently, it was thought that there were no 100% purely eosinophil-specific cell surface proteins. With the discovery of epidermal growth factor–like module containing mucin-like hormone-like receptor 1 (EMR1, the human counterpart of F4/80 in the mouse), a member of the G protein–coupled epidermal growth factor-7-transmembrane family, this changed when it was reported that EMR1 is truly eosinophil specific (**Fig. 2**).[15] Expression was conserved in monkeys, and targeting with an afucosylated immunoglobulin G1 (IgG1) antibody that is particularly effective at engaging natural killer (NK) cell antibody-dependent cellular cytotoxicity (ADCC) resulted in selective eosinophil depletion in vitro and in vivo.[16] Thus, EMR1 antibody has potential as a possible future option for highly selective and specific targeting and depletion of eosinophils.

There are many cell surface proteins that are selectively, albeit not exclusively, expressed by eosinophils. Probably because of similarities in their hematopoietic

Chemokine, complement and other chemotactic factor receptors

CD35	CCR1
CD88	CCR2
C3aR	CCR3
PAFR	CCR6
LTB₄R	CCR8
CysLT1	CXCR1
CysLT2	CXCR2
fMLPR	CXCR3
Histamine	CXCR4
(H4 receptor)	CRTh2

Adhesion molecules

CD11a	CD44
CD11b	CD49d
CD11c	CD49f
CD15	CD62L
CD15s	CD147
CD18	CD162
CD29	CD174
αd integrin	CD321
β7 integrin	

Apoptosis, signaling and others

CD9	CD134	EMR1
CD12	CD137	Glucocorticoid
CD17	CD139	receptor
CD24	CD148	Siglec-8
CD28	CD151	Siglec-10
CD30	CD153	LIR1
CD37	CD154	LIR2
CD39	CD161	LIR3
CD40	CD165	LIR7
CD43	CD172a	TLR2
CD52	CD178	TLR3
CD53	CD226	TLR4
CD58	CD244	TLR8
CD60a	CD253	TLR9
CD63	CD261	TLR10
CD65	CD262	
CD66	CD263	**Enzymes**
CD69*	CD264	
CD71	CD265	CD10
CD80	CD295	CD13
CD81	CD298	CD45
CD82	CD300a	CD45RB
CD86*	CD300f	CD45RC
CD92	CD302	CD45RO
CD93	CD352	CD46
CD95	PIRA	CD55
CD97	PIRB	CD59
CD98	P2X	CD87
CD99	P2Y	CD156a
		PAR-2

Immunoglobulin receptors and related immunoglobulin family members

CD4	CD58
CD16*	CD66
CD31	CD84
CD32	CD85
CD33	CD89
CD47	CD100
CD48	CD101
CD50	CD112
CD54*	HLA class I
	HLA-DR*

Cytokine receptors

GM-CSF	IL-6
IFN-α	IL-9
IFN-γ	IL-13
Leukemia	IL-33
inhibitory factor	Stem cell
IL-3	factor
IL-4	TNFα
IL-5	TNFβ

Fig. 1. Surface molecules expressed by human eosinophils. There is some overlap among categories for some of these proteins. Common names for chemokine (CC and CXC) receptors, toll-like receptors (TLRs), and others were sometimes used instead of the CD names because of the greater use and familiarity among most readers of the former. The asterisk indicates activated eosinophils. C3aR, C3a receptor; CysLT, cysteinyl leukotriene receptor type; EMR1, epidermal growth factor–like module containing mucin-like hormone receptor-like 1; fMLPR, formyl-methionyl-leucyl-phenylalanine receptor; GM-CSF, granulocyte-macrophage colony-stimulating factor; IFN, interferon; IL, interleukin; LIR, leukocyte immunoglobulin-like receptor; LTB4R, leukotriene B4 receptor; P2X and P2Y, two types of purinergic receptors; PAFR, platelet activating factor receptor; PIR, paired immunoglobulin-like receptor; TNF, tumor necrosis factor. (Courtesy of Jacqueline Schaffer, MAMS, Chicago, IL.)

pathways, there is a subset of surface markers whose expression is shared among basophils and/or mast cells (see **Fig. 2**). Such examples include the heterodimeric receptor for interleukin 5 (IL-5) (CD125/CD131),[17] the type 3 CC chemokine receptor (CCR3, CD193),[18] and the sialic acid-binding immunoglobulin-like lectin inhibitory receptor Siglec-8.[19–21] Among these, biologics targeting IL-5 or its receptor and small molecules targeting CCR3 are in various stages of clinical trials, as discussed later. Another cell surface receptor expressed by eosinophils and a relatively small subset of other leukocytes includes the chemoattractant receptor expressed on type 2 helper T cells (CRTh2, also called DP2, the type 2 prostaglandin D2 receptor or CD294 found on eosinophils, basophils, mast cells, and Th2 lymphocytes), for which small molecule antagonists are advancing in the clinic (also see later discussion). Some receptors, such as Siglec-8,[22] Fas (CD95),[23] and others on eosinophils, can on engagement directly activate cell death.[24] Finally, the surface of the eosinophil is equipped with a broad range of other proteins, glycans, and lipids involved in cell signaling, migration, activation, and other biological processes (see **Fig. 1**) that are too numerous to review here in their entirety, yet each of which could potentially be targeted with varying degrees of eosinophil selectivity. Just like the trend in the cancer field of using tumor surface markers to facilitate delivery of toxic payloads

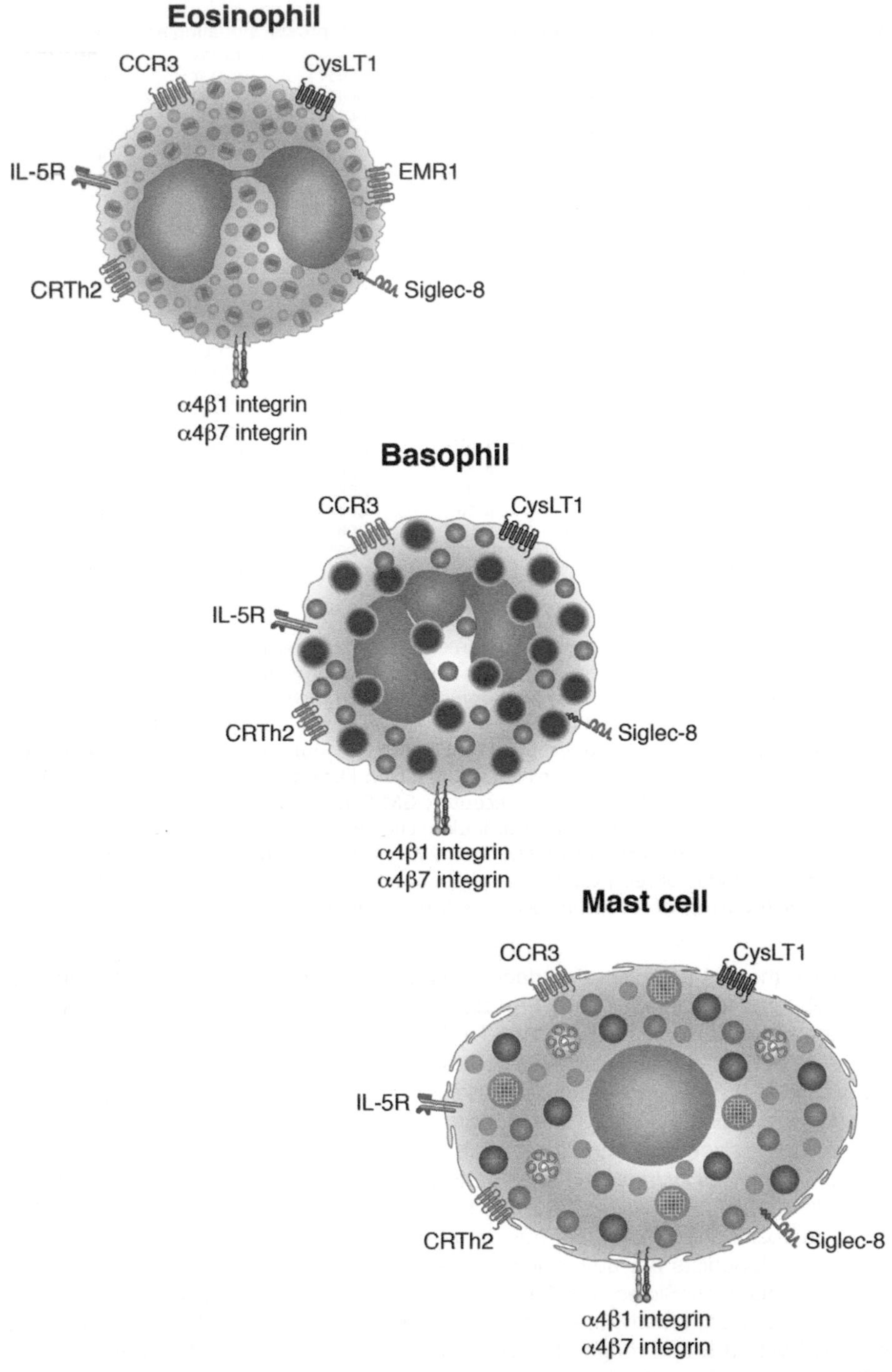

Eosinophil

Basophil

Mast cell

Fig. 2. Examples of surface receptors that are selectively expressed on human eosinophils and, therefore, of potential therapeutic relevance. Note that almost all of these are also expressed on basophils and mast cells. EMR1, epidermal growth factor–like module containing mucin-like hormone receptor-like 1; IL, interleukin. (*Courtesy of* Jacqueline Schaffer, MAMS, Chicago, IL.)

via antibody-drug conjugates, liposomes, or nanoparticles, such strategies might someday become available for eosinophil targeting by leveraging the eosinophil phenotype.

THE EOSINOPHIL INTERIOR AS A TARGET

Eosinophils possess several intracellular structures that provide opportunities for therapeutic targeting.[9] A prime example among these is the glucocorticoid receptor (GR), which can exist in different splice variants and isoforms.[25,26] In human eosinophils, the GR-α splice variant is present in particularly high copy number.[27] Furthermore, the proapoptotic GR-A isoform was 5-fold higher in eosinophils than in neutrophils, whereas the nonapoptotic GR-D isoform was 5-fold higher in neutrophils compared with eosinophils, making eosinophils particularly susceptible (and the neutrophil much less or nonsusceptible) to clinically beneficial effects of glucocorticoids, such as apoptosis.[28] It is clear that some patients with hypereosinophilic syndrome (HES) fail to respond to glucocorticoid therapy,[29] perhaps because of reduced GR expression[30] or perhaps because these cells are deficient in the steroid-sensitive GR isoform. Whether conditions exist to enhance the function or expression of the GR-A isoform in eosinophils, rendering them more sensitive to lower concentrations of steroids, is not yet known.

Eosinophils also possess several unique cytoplasmic granule proteins, such as eosinophil cationic protein (ECP), eosinophil-derived neurotoxin, and eosinophil peroxidase (EPX), that, once released, can have putative toxic effects on bystander cells. Previous studies using these granule proteins, or antagonists thereof, in animal models of eosinophilic inflammation showed promise,[31–33] raising the possibility that future therapies focusing on reducing or neutralizing eosinophil-derived substances, rather than eosinophils per se, might be of clinical benefit. A similar example of this would include therapies targeting sulfidopeptide leukotrienes, some of which are made and released in the form of leukotriene C4 (LTC$_4$) by activated eosinophils. It also underscores our lack of understanding of exactly how targeting eosinophils favorably impacts disease, a perfect example being why it is that the use of eosinophil-selective therapies reduce asthma exacerbations ([34,35] and see later discussion).

One other aspect worth mentioning in this section relates to genetic abnormalities associated with certain forms of eosinophilia. As a result of truly paradigm-changing findings, it is now known that at least some forms of HES are the result of chromosomal defects leading to clonal forms of disease, including eosinophilic leukemia. For example, the discovery that the tyrosine kinase inhibitor imatinib mesylate can reverse virtually all aspects of disease in patients with the Fip1-like 1 gene fused with the platelet-derived growth factor receptor α (FIP1L1-PDGFR) deletion mutation on chromosome 4, as well as some other patients with HES without this detectable mutation, suggests that molecular gain-of-function mutations are causal in a subset of eosinophilic disorders.[36–38]

APPROVED THERAPIES THAT ALSO TARGET EOSINOPHILS OR EOSINOPHIL-RELATED PATHWAYS

The current standards of care for the treatment of eosinophil-associated disorders, including HES, eosinophilic esophagitis (EoE), and others, are the subject of their own articles in this volume of Immunology and Allergy Clinics of North America, so they will only be mentioned in passing for completeness and for comparison with future therapies. As mentioned earlier, the current mainstay of the initial treatment of nearly all forms of eosinophilic disorders begins with glucocorticoids. For HES, when imatinib mesylate therapy is not indicated or effective, the most common agent to be added next to maintain disease control and facilitate oral steroid tapering or elimination is hydroxyurea. Although there are no controlled trials of this agent in HES, there are strong indications from the literature that it can be quite effective, presumably as a result of diminished hematopoiesis of many leukocyte types including eosinophils.[29] If still ineffective, hydroxyurea is most often replaced by parenteral administration of interferon-α.[39,40] Other immunosuppressive agents are sometimes tried, with only modest benefit at best.[29] For EoE, the mainstays of treatment include food-elimination diets, swallowed topical steroids, and mechanical dilation for severe strictures.[41]

When considering other potential therapies for eosinophilic disorders, opportunities may exist to try other agents approved for other clinical indications. For instance, therapies targeting surface structures (**Table 1**) whose expression is shared by differing subsets of cell types that include eosinophils, such as CD25 (daclizumab), CD33 (gemtuzumab), α4β1 integrin (CD49d/CD29, natalizumab), α4β7 integrin (vedolizumab), and CD52 (alemtuzumab), would also bind to eosinophils, offering opportunities for their potential use in eosinophil-associated diseases provided the cost and risk-benefit ratio favors such use. So far, it is known that natalizumab use increases blood eosinophil counts,[42,43] presumably by blocking leukocyte emigration from the circulation, whereas vedolizumab seems to lack this property.[44,45] The effects of blockade of vascular cell adhesion molecule 1 (VCAM-1, CD106) or mucosal addressin cell adhesion molecule 1 (MAdCAM-1), the ligands for α4β1 integrin and α4β7 integrin, in eosinophil-associated diseases, including eosinophilic gastrointestinal disorders have not been studied in humans. The use of alemtuzumab in advanced stages of HES or chronic eosinophilic leukemia has been reported in small numbers of patients, with some patients undergoing disease remission but not without drug-related toxicities.[46] Whether the potential beneficial effects of alemtuzumab were caused by direct targeting of eosinophils versus targeting of other cells cannot be determined.

NOVEL EOSINOPHIL-SELECTIVE THERAPIES BEING TESTED IN CLINICAL TRIALS

Currently, the eosinophil-selective therapies being tested in humans that are looking very promising include antibodies to IL-5 (mepolizumab [IgG1] and reslizumab [IgG4]) and the IL-5 receptor (benralizumab [afucosylated IgG1, formerly called MEDI-563]) (see **Table 1**). Each of these antibodies neutralizes IL-5 biology; but given the enhanced ADCC activity of the benralizumab formulation, it actively depletes IL-5 receptor-bearing cells, which includes eosinophils and basophils (see **Fig. 2**).[47,48]

Among these 3 biological agents, the most published information exists for mepolizumab. It has shown efficacy in controlled trials of eosinophilic asthma (eg, reduced exacerbations, improved lung function),[49-54] nasal polyposis (eg, reduced polyp size),[55] and in idiopathic and lymphocytic HES syndrome (eg, steroid-sparing effects).[56-58] These studies showed fairly consistent, prompt reductions (≥80% declines within days) in circulating eosinophil counts and partial (≈50%–60%) reductions in extravascular eosinophils in affected organs when studied.[59,60] It is also interesting to note that given the enrollment criteria of persistent eosinophilia in the mepolizumab asthma studies cited earlier, cohorts ended up being enriched to 10% to 35% with subjects that had concomitant nasal polyposis. One additional study with mepolizumab failed to find any changes in normal levels of cells, including mucosal eosinophils, in duodenal biopsies in subjects with EoE, despite finding a decrease in esophageal eosinophilia.[61] In open-label studies, efficacy was also seen in eosinophilic granulomatosis with polyangiitis[62-64] with a double-blind

Table 1
Examples of molecules being targeted with drugs (including biologics) to directly or indirectly affect human eosinophils

Strategy	Target	Drug	Cells Targeted Besides Eosinophils	Antieosinophil Effects In Vitro	Antieosinophil Effects In Vivo	Status
Cell surface protein	$\alpha 4\beta 1$, $\alpha 4\beta 7$ integrins	Natalizumab	T cells, B cells, NK cells, monocytes, basophils	Inhibits leukocyte adhesion to VCAM-1, MAdCAM-1, and fibronectin	Increases number of circulating eosinophils; inhibits their accumulation at sites of inflammation	Approved for relapsing, remitting multiple sclerosis (natalizumab [Tysabri])
	$\alpha 4\beta 7$ integrin	Vedolizumab	T cells, B cells, NK cells, monocytes, basophils	Inhibits leukocyte adhesion to MAdCAM-1	No effect on numbers of circulating eosinophils	Approved for inflammatory bowel disease (vedolizumab [Entyvio])
	$\beta 7$ integrins ($\alpha 4\beta 7$ and $\alpha E\beta 7$)	Etrolizumab	T cells, B cells, NK cells, monocytes, basophils	Inhibits leukocyte adhesion to MAdCAM-1 and E-cadherin	Unknown	Phase 3 for inflammatory bowel disease (Genentech)
	CCR3	GW766944 (small molecule)	Basophils and mast cells	Blocks chemokine-mediated migration	No significant effect on sputum or blood eosinophils	Phase 2 for asthma (GlaxoSmithKline)
	CD52	Alemtuzumab	Most leukocytes	Unknown	Depletes eosinophils	Approved for cancer (alemtuzumab [Campath])

(continued on next page)

Table 1
(continued)

Strategy	Target	Drug	Cells Targeted Besides Eosinophils	Antieosinophil Effects In Vitro	Antieosinophil Effects In Vivo	Status
	CD131 (common β-chain)	CSL311 monoclonal antibody	Cells expressing the common β chain for the IL-3, IL-5, and GM-CSF receptor	Unknown	Unknown	Phase 2 in asthmatic patients (CSL Limited)
	CRTh2	OC000459 (small molecule)	Basophils, mast cells, Th2 cells	Blocks PGD2 effects	Reduces numbers of tissue eosinophils	Various phases for asthma, EoE, atopic dermatitis (Oxagen, Atopix Therapeutics)
	EMR1	Afucosylated anti-EMR1 monoclonal antibody	None	Targets cells for ADCC	Depletes primate eosinophils	Preclinical (KaloBios)
	IL-4 receptor α chain	Dupilumab and AMG 317 monoclonal antibody	All IL-4 receptor α chain-bearing cells	Inhibits IL-4 and IL-13 biology	Dupilumab reduces numbers of airway eosinophils, but AMG317 did not	Phase 2–3 for atopic dermatitis and asthma (Regeneron, Amgen)
	IL-5 receptor	Benralizumab	Basophils and mast cells	Targets cells for ADCC	Eosinophil and basophil depleting	Phase 3 for eosinophilic asthma (AstraZeneca/Medimmune)
	Siglec-8	Siglec-8 monoclonal antibody	Basophils and mast cells	Engagement causes eosinophil death and inhibits mast cell degranulation	Unknown	Preclinical

Soluble mediator antagonist					
Eotaxin-1	Bertilimumab	Basophils and mast cells	Inhibits eotaxin-1-mediated eosinophil activation	Unknown	Various phases of development for ulcerative colitis and bullous pemphigoid (Immune Pharmaceuticals) Development discontinued
GM-CSF	KB003 monoclonal antibody	All GM-CSF receptor-bearing cells	Inhibits GM-CSF biology	Unknown	Development discontinued
IgE	Omalizumab	Basophils and mast cells	No direct effects	Reduces numbers of eosinophils at sites of allergic inflammation	Approved for asthma and urticaria (omalizumab [Xolair])
IL-4	Pitrakinra, altrakincept, and pascolizumab	Leukocytes and tissue-resident cells	No direct effects	Reduces numbers of eosinophils at sites of allergic inflammation	Development discontinued
IL-5	Mepolizumab, reslizumab	None	Inhibits IL-5 biology	Reduces bone marrow, circulating and tissue eosinophils	Phase 3 for eosinophilic asthma; some data in HES, eosinophilic granulomatosis and polyangiitis, EoE, atopic dermatitis, and chronic rhinosinusitis/nasal polyposis (GlaxoSmithKline, TEVA)

(continued on next page)

Table 1
(continued)

Strategy	Target	Drug	Cells Targeted Besides Eosinophils	Antieosinophil Effects In Vitro	Antieosinophil Effects In Vivo	Status
	IL-9	MEDI-528 monoclonal antibody	All IL-9 receptor-bearing cells	Inhibits IL-9 biology	No effect on blood eosinophil counts or asthma	Development discontinued
	IL-13	Tralokinumab, lebrikizumab, anrukinzumab, RPC4046, QAX576 monoclonal antibodies	All IL-13 receptor-bearing cells	Inhibits IL-13 biology	Reduces numbers of eosinophils in blood and at sites of allergic inflammation	Various phases for asthma and EoE (AstraZeneca/Medimmune, Genentech/Roche, Receptos)
	Sulfidopeptide leukotrienes	Montelukast, zileuton (small molecules)	Leukocytes and tissue-resident cells	Inhibits effects of LTC4, LTD4, and LTE4 on eosinophil activation and migration	Reduces numbers of eosinophils in blood and at sites of allergic inflammation	Approved for asthma (montelukast [Singulair]; zileuton [Zyflo CR]) and allergic rhinitis (montelukast [Singulair])
	TSLP	AMG 157 monoclonal antibody	Many leukocyte types	Inhibits TSLP biology	Reduces numbers of eosinophils in blood and at sites of allergic inflammation	Phase 2 for asthma (Amgen)
Others	CCR3 and CD131 (common β chain)	TPI ASM8, antisense oligonucleotides, inhaled	Basophils, mast cells, and others	Downregulates expression of CCR3 and CD131 common β chain transcripts	Reduces numbers of eosinophils in blood and at sites of allergic airways inflammation	Development discontinued
	FIP1L1-PDGFR deletion mutation	Imatinib and next-generation tyrosine kinase inhibitors	Any cell possessing this deletion mutation; also cells possessing the chromosomal translocation t(9;22)(q34;q11)	Inhibits gain-of-function activity	Normalizes numbers of bone marrow, circulating and tissue eosinophils	Approved for chronic myelogenous leukemia and HES (imatinib mesylate [Gleevec])

Food-elimination diets	Specific food avoidance	Unknown but likely mucosal and immunologic cells	No direct effects	Reduces numbers of eosinophils in blood and at sites of esophageal inflammation	Often prescribed for EoE and eosinophilic gastritis
Glucocorticoid steroid receptor	Glucocorticoids	Virtually all cells	Causes eosinophil death and reduces production of eosinophil-recruitment factors	Reduces bone marrow, circulating and tissue eosinophils	Many approved for oral, topical, and inhaled use; new formulations under development for specific use in EoE
Mitochondrial function	Dexpramipexole	Unknown	Unknown	Found incidentally in clinical trials of amyotrophic lateral sclerosis to gradually reduce blood eosinophil counts; mechanism unknown	Phase 2 for HES and chronic rhinosinusitis/nasal polyposis (Knopp Biosciences)
Interferon-α	Interferon alfa-2b (Intron A), peginterferon alfa-2a (Pegasys), peginterferon alfa-2b (Peg-Intron)	All interferon-α receptor-bearing cells	No direct effects	Reduces bone marrow, circulating and tissue eosinophils	Used to treat HES, mainly as a steroid-replacing agent
Ribonucleotide reductase	Hydroxyurea	Virtually all hematopoietic cells and some cancers	No direct effects	Reduces bone marrow, circulating and tissue eosinophils	Used off label for HES, mainly as a steroid-sparing or steroid-replacing agent

Abbreviations: PGD2, prostaglandin 2; TSLP, thymic stromal lymphopoietin.

placebo-controlled clinical trial underway. In an open-label study of EoE, reduced tissue eosinophils was seen with mepolizumab.[65] In controlled mepolizumab trials in EoE, reduced tissue eosinophils were also seen; but unfortunately there were no clear clinical benefits.[66]

There are fewer published clinical data available for reslizumab and benralizumab. Both have shown reductions in exacerbations in controlled trials of eosinophilic asthma[67–69] but not with benralizumab in chronic obstructive pulmonary disease (COPD).[70] Unique to benralizumab was a study showing that a single dose given in the emergency department for an acute exacerbation of asthma reduced exacerbation and hospitalization rates over the subsequent 3-month period by 50% to 60%.[71] Like with mepolizumab treatment of EoE, reslizumab reduced tissue eosinophils but without a concomitant improvement, compared with placebo, in symptoms.[72] All studies with either benralizumab or reslizumab showed prompt reductions ($\geq$80% declines within days and even more pronounced and prolonged with benralizumab) in circulating eosinophil counts and reductions in airway eosinophils and in esophageal biopsies.[72,73]

Other eosinophil-related receptors have been targeted in recent or ongoing clinical trials. Given the selective expression of CCR3, a G protein–coupled 7-spanner receptor, on eosinophils and its important role in eosinophil migration and accumulation suggested in preclinical models, it seemed likely that this receptor would be an obvious small molecule therapeutic target for eosinophil-associated disease.[18,74–77] So far, one such antagonist (GW766994) was tested in human asthma and was well tolerated; but despite effectively blocking CCR3 activity, it failed to have an effect on levels of eosinophils in blood or sputum, nor did it significantly impact lung function.[78] As of January 2015, no other studies with GW766994 were listed in clinicaltrials.gov, making it questionable as to whether additional indications or studies will be pursued. Another G protein–coupled 7-spanner receptor with a similar pattern of expression to CCR3 is CRTh2, also called DP2, a receptor for prostaglandin D2. So far, one oral small molecule antagonist (OC000459) showed modest efficacy in asthma[79,80] and in EoE.[81] As of January 2015, the only studies of this class of agents listed as active on clinicaltrials.gov involved a study with OC000459 in moderate to severe atopic dermatitis and another with AZD1981, a different small molecule CRTh2 antagonist being tested in chronic idiopathic urticaria.

Etrolizumab is a humanized monoclonal antibody that distinguishes itself from natalizumab and vedolizumab in that it uniquely recognizes $\alpha4\beta7$ integrin and $\alpha E\beta7$ integrin, the latter not expressed on eosinophils but recognizing E-cadherin. A recent phase 2 study in moderate to severe ulcerative colitis was positive, but there was no mention of effects on circulating numbers of eosinophils.[82] Additional studies in ulcerative colitis are ongoing. An antibody against CD131, the common β chain shared by the IL-3, IL-5, and granulocyte-macrophage colony-stimulating factor (GM-CSF) receptor, is in early clinical trials for asthma (see NCT01759849 on the clinicaltrials.gov Web site). Finally, dexpramipexole (KNS-760704) is an oral drug originally developed for the treatment of amyotrophic lateral sclerosis, but it failed in phase 3 studies.[83] During its development, subjects receiving this drug were coincidentally noted to have a gradual decline in blood eosinophil counts. As a result, it is now being tested in HES (see NCT02101138 on the clinicaltrials.gov Web site) and chronic sinusitis with nasal polyposis (see NCT02217332 on the clinicaltrials.gov Web site). The exact mechanism of action of this agent, including its antieosinophil properties, is unknown; but it is thought to alter mitochondrial function.

NOVEL THERAPIES THAT MAY INDIRECTLY AFFECT EOSINOPHILS THAT ARE BEING TESTED IN CLINICAL TRIALS

Agents Moving Forward

The cytokines IL-4 and IL-13 have several important biological properties relevant to eosinophilic inflammatory responses, including their ability to enhance eosinophil recruitment responses via induction of the adhesion molecule VCAM-1 and of CCR3-active chemokines.[84,85] The receptors for IL-4 and IL-13 are heterodimeric, sharing a common IL-4 receptor α chain (IL-4Rα1) while also using the common γc chain or IL-13 receptor α1 chains, respectively. Although eosinophils express the IL-13 receptor,[86] the clinically beneficial effects of antagonizing IL-13 in vivo are more likely to be caused by its effects on other cells, thereby secondarily improving eosinophilic inflammation. Several monoclonal antibodies that specifically block IL-13 biology are in clinical trials for either asthma, ulcerative colitis, or EoE and include lebrikizumab,[87–89] anrukinzumab,[90] tralokinumab,[91–93] GSK679586,[94,95] and RPC4046 (https://clinicaltrials.gov/ct2/show/NCT02098473). However, by targeting IL-4Rα1 instead, blockade of both IL-4 and IL-13 biology can be achieved, as was explored with monoclonal antibody AMG 317 in asthma[96] and, so far, more successfully in atopic dermatitis and asthma with dupilumab.[97,98] Also to be mentioned in this section is an antibody to thymic stromal lymphopoietin (TSLP), a highly proinflammatory and proallergic cytokine produced by tissue resident cells. In one proof-of-concept phase 2 study, the anti-TSLP antibody AMG 157 attenuated both the acute and late-phase airway allergic response as well as reduced blood and airway eosinophilia.[99] Finally, given the fact that eosinophils are highly susceptible to the proapoptotic effects of glucocorticoids, it was of interest that in a very similar phase 2 proof-of-concept study, AZD5423, an inhaled nonsteroidal agonist of the GR that, in theory, should have reduced side effects compared with glucocorticoids, significantly blocked the late-phase airway allergic response as well as reduced sputum eosinophilia.[100] Although showing extremely promising clinical benefits in early phase clinical trials, along with reductions in eosinophilic inflammation, none of these agents have been tested in HES; none show anywhere near the same magnitude and specificity of reductions in eosinophils as has been seen with IL-5 or IL-5 receptor-targeting drugs.

Agents Whose Development is Not Currently Moving Forward

Several other anticytokine and antichemokine therapies that either directly or indirectly target eosinophils have been tested, mainly in asthma, but have not fared as well, so they are only reviewed briefly. One set consists of agents targeting Th2 cytokines other than IL-5, namely, IL-4 and IL-9, with specific biologics. Agents whose development has been discontinued because of a lack of efficacy include pascolizumab (anti-IL-4 antibody), soluble IL-4 receptor (altrakincept), pitrakinra, a mutein of IL-4, and an anti-IL-9 antibody MEDI-528.[101,102] For MEDI-528 where it was reported, there was no effect on blood eosinophil counts. For antagonism of eotaxin-1, the antibody bertilimumab was developed and tested in allergic disorders about a decade ago but apparently without success because further testing for this indication was not pursued. It is currently about to begin testing in ulcerative colitis and bullous pemphigoid.[103] As of this writing, there are no known antibodies against eotaxin-2 or eotaxin-3 in clinical trials. If true, this would be unfortunate, especially given compelling data suggesting a prominent role for eotaxin-3 in the pathophysiology of EoE and eosinophilic gastritis.[104,105] KB003, an antibody to GM-CSF, a cytokine with overlapping biology to that of IL-5, was tested in a phase 2, double-blind, placebo controlled trial in asthmatic patients inadequately controlled with corticosteroids; according to a press release dated January 29, 2014 from KaloBios, the company developing this antibody, it failed to meet its end point of improved pulmonary function.[106] No data were released regarding any specific aspects of eosinophil biology, such as the effects on blood levels or airway eosinophilia; but it is known that infusion with GM-CSF causes eosinophilia,[107] and some patients with HES and exacerbations of chronic rhinosinusitis with nasal polyposis have elevated levels of GM-CSF in their blood.[108,109] Finally, development of TPI ASM8, a formulation of inhaled antisense oligonucleotides designed to reduce allergic inflammation by downregulating both CCR3 and the common β chain (CD125) of the IL-3, IL-5, and GM-CSF receptor, seems to have been discontinued but had shown some favorable impact on allergen-induced sputum eosinophilia in initial trials.[110–112]

FUTURE CONSIDERATIONS

Although many novel small molecule and biologic agents are advancing in clinical trials, there still are no FDA-approved drugs that would meet the criteria often referred to as personalized or precision medicine for eosinophil-associated diseases with one exception: imatinib mesylate for FIP1L1-PDGFR–associated proliferative disorders. Yet excitement is building with the reasonable anticipation that, within the next few years, agents that selectively or specifically target eosinophils (eg, those targeting IL-5 or its receptor) may actually become approved for clinical use. Because all of these agents are new, the excitement among physicians and patients who will finally gain access to these potential paradigm-changing treatments must be mitigated by what will still be unknown about these drugs. Questions that remain include their cost, safety and side effect profiles, longevity of responses, safety of discontinuation of therapy, and potential for the development of human-antihuman antibodies (HAHAs) against biologics. Overall, mepolizumab has a good safety profile, with rare infusion or injection reactions, insignificant rates of HAHA formation, and prolonged efficacy, even with reduced dosing intervals for maintenance therapy; but stoppage of treatment leads to disease recurrence, suggesting that this is not a disease-remitting agent.[62,64,113,114] Dosing intervals can be expanded without loss of efficacy; there has been no evidence of neutralizing HAHAs, but more information is needed for this and other agents. One report identified rebound blood eosinophilia following discontinuation of reslizumab.[115] In early studies of benralizumab, some cases of transient neutropenia were reported.[48] So far, it seems that one can maintain normal immune function with very low numbers of eosinophils or without eosinophils entirely.[116] We know virtually nothing about the combined use of multiple antieosinophil biologics in the same patient at the same time or if any of these treatments are disease modifying, meaning that they can be used for a defined period of time then stopped, with prolonged disease remission. Unfortunately, this does not seem to be the case for mepolizumab in asthma[114] or for imatinib mesylate and HES,[117] with disease recurrence seen following discontinuation of either treatment.[117] Sorely needed are ways of detecting organ-specific disease activity, such as the esophageal string test in EoE[118] and nuclear medicine–based scans of eosinophil trafficking and accumulation.[119–121] Reliable biomarkers of disease activity, remission, and drug responsiveness other than blood eosinophil counts, would improve disease management, including confidence and safety during tapering of treatment.[122,123] Examples of such biomarkers might include the presence of an activated eosinophil surface phenotype as detected by flow cytometry[124,125] and a variety of measurements in biological fluids, such as serum periostin in IL-13–driven asthma[126,127]; serum CCL17 in HES and atopic dermatitits[29,128]; serum levels of soluble receptors, such as for IL-5, EMR1, and

Siglec-8 in various forms of HES[16,123,129]; and detection of EPX in biological fluids.[130] Some studies suggest that elevated levels of IL-5 might be a feature of certain subsets of eosinophilic disorders[131,132] as well as responsiveness to anti–IL-5 treatment.[133] These approaches and others will require rigorous validation in controlled clinical trials before garnering confidence as clinically useful parameters in eosinophil-associated disease assessment and management.

SUMMARY

There is still much to be learned about eosinophil-associated diseases, in part because they tend to be uncommon disorders and in part because the best way to test mechanistic hypotheses in human diseases that lack a clear genetic origin is with pharmacology. Such types of unique and novel eosinophil-targeted treatments, including monoclonal antibodies, are finally in development, with many showing safety and efficacy. Although none are yet FDA approved, each offers promise as we strive to provide the best possible treatment of patients with eosinophilic disorders, including the ability to replace drugs with unacceptable side effects, especially when used chronically, with others of equal if not superior efficacy and reduced toxicity. Together with an improved panel of biomarkers to help guide diagnosis, treatment, and assessment of disease activity, we may soon see a remarkable new era of management of these difficult conditions.

REFERENCES

1. Bochner BS, Book W, Busse WW, et al. Workshop report from the National Institutes of Health Taskforce on the Research Needs of Eosinophil-Associated Diseases (TREAD). J Allergy Clin Immunol 2012;130:587–96.
2. Boucher RM, Gilbert-McClain L, Chowdhury B. Hypereosinophilic syndrome and mepolizumab. N Engl J Med 2008;358:2838–9 [author reply: 2839–40].
3. Radonjic-Hoesli S, Valent P, Klion AD, et al. Novel targeted therapies for eosinophil-associated diseases and allergy. Annu Rev Pharmacol Toxicol 2015; 55:633–56.
4. Fulkerson PC, Rothenberg ME. Targeting eosinophils in allergy, inflammation and beyond. Nat Rev Drug Discov 2013;12:117–29.
5. Iwasaki H, Mizuno S, Mayfield R, et al. Identification of eosinophil lineage-committed progenitors in the murine bone marrow. J Exp Med 2005;201:1891–7.
6. Gauvreau GM, Ellis AK, Denburg JA. Haemopoietic processes in allergic disease: eosinophil/basophil development. Clin Exp Allergy 2009;39:1297–306.
7. Ackerman SJ, Bochner BS. Mechanisms of eosinophilia in the pathogenesis of hypereosinophilic disorders. Immunol Allergy Clin North Am 2007;27:357–75.
8. Rothenberg ME, Hogan SP. The eosinophil. Annu Rev Immunol 2006;24:147–74.
9. Kita H, Bochner BS. Biology of eosinophils. In: Adkinson NF Jr, Bochner BS, Busse WW, et al, editors. Middleton's allergy principles and practice. 8th edition. Philadelphia: Elsevier Sanders; 2014. p. 265–79.
10. Lee JJ, Rosenberg HF, editors. Eosinophils in health and disease. Amsterdam: Elsevier; 2012.
11. Rosenberg HF, Dyer KD, Foster PS. Eosinophils: changing perspectives in health and disease. Nat Rev Immunol 2013;13:9–22.
12. von Gunten S, Ghanim V, Valent P, et al. Appendix A. CD molecules. In: Adkinson NF Jr, Bochner BS, Busse WW, et al, editors. Middleton's allergy principles and practice. 8th edition. Philadelphia: Elsevier Sanders; 2014. p. 1663–87.

13. Tachimoto H, Bochner BS. The surface phenotype of human eosinophils. Chem Immunol 2000;76:45–62.
14. Bochner BS. Verdict in the case of therapies versus eosinophils: the jury is still out. J Allergy Clin Immunol 2004;113:3–9.
15. Hamann J, Koning N, Pouwels W, et al. EMR1, the human homolog of F4/80, is an eosinophil-specific receptor. Eur J Immunol 2007;37:2797–802.
16. Legrand F, Tomasevic N, Simakova O, et al. The eosinophil surface receptor epidermal growth factor-like module containing mucin-like hormone receptor 1 (EMR1): a novel therapeutic target for eosinophilic disorders. J Allergy Clin Immunol 2014;133:1439–47.
17. Migita M, Yamaguchi N, Mita S, et al. Characterization of the human IL-5 receptors on eosinophils. Cell Immunol 1991;133:484–97.
18. Heath H, Qin SX, Rao P, et al. Chemokine receptor usage by human eosinophils - The importance of CCR3 demonstrated using an antagonistic monoclonal antibody. J Clin Invest 1997;99:178–84.
19. Kikly KK, Bochner BS, Freeman S, et al. Identification of SAF-2, a novel siglec expressed on eosinophils, mast cells and basophils. J Allergy Clin Immunol 2000;105:1093–100.
20. Bochner BS. Siglec-8 on human eosinophils and mast cells, and Siglec-F on murine eosinophils, are functionally related inhibitory receptors. Clin Exp Allergy 2009;39:317–24.
21. Kiwamoto T, Kawasaki N, Paulson JC, et al. Siglec-8 as a drugable target to treat eosinophil and mast cell-associated conditions. Pharmacol Ther 2012;135: 327–36.
22. Nutku E, Aizawa H, Hudson SA, et al. Ligation of Siglec-8: a selective mechanism for induction of human eosinophil apoptosis. Blood 2003;101:5014–20.
23. Matsumoto K, Schleimer RP, Saito H, et al. Induction of apoptosis in human eosinophils by anti-Fas antibody treatment in vitro. Blood 1995;86:1437–43.
24. Shen Z, Malter JS. Determinants of eosinophil survival and apoptotic cell death. Apoptosis 2015. http://dx.doi.org/10.1007/s10495-014-1072-2.
25. Bender IK, Cao Y, Lu NZ. Determinants of the heightened activity of glucocorticoid receptor translational isoforms. Mol Endocrinol 2013;27:1577–87.
26. Oakley RH, Cidlowski JA. The biology of the glucocorticoid receptor: new signaling mechanisms in health and disease. J Allergy Clin Immunol 2013; 132:1033–44.
27. Pujols L, Mullol J, Roca-Ferrer J, et al. Expression of glucocorticoid receptor alpha- and beta-isoforms in human cells and tissues. Am J Physiol Cell Physiol 2002;283:C1324–31.
28. Hsu J, Cao Y, Bender IK, et al. Glucocorticoid receptor translational isoforms contribute to distinct glucocorticoid responses of neutrophils and eosinophils [abstract]. J Allergy Clin Immunol 2012;129:AB62.
29. Ogbogu PU, Bochner BS, Butterfield JH, et al. Hypereosinophilic syndrome: a multicenter, retrospective analysis of clinical characteristics and response to therapy. J Allergy Clin Immunol 2009;124:1319–25.
30. Prin L, Lefebvre P, Gruart V, et al. Heterogeneity of human eosinophil glucocorticoid receptor expression in hypereosinophilic patients: absence of detectable receptor correlates with resistance to corticotherapy. Clin Exp Immunol 1989;78: 383–9.
31. Gundel RH, Letts LG, Gleich GJ. Human eosinophil major basic protein induces airway constriction and airway hyperresponsiveness in primates. J Clin Invest 1991;87:1470–3.

32. Uchida DA, Ackerman SJ, Coyle AJ, et al. The effect of human eosinophil granule major basic protein on airway responsiveness in the rat in vivo. Am Rev Respir Dis 1993;147:982–8.
33. Lefort J, Nahori MA, Ruffie C, et al. In vivo neutralization of eosinophil-derived major basic protein inhibits antigen-induced bronchial hyperreactivity in sensitized guinea pigs. J Clin Invest 1996;97:1117–21.
34. Wenzel SE. Eosinophils in asthma–closing the loop or opening the door? N Engl J Med 2009;360:1026–8.
35. Bochner BS, Gleich GJ. What targeting eosinophils has taught us about their role in diseases. J Allergy Clin Immunol 2010;126:16–25.
36. Cools J, DeAngelo DJ, Gotlib J, et al. A tyrosine kinase created by fusion of the PDGFRA and FIP1L1 genes as a therapeutic target of imatinib in idiopathic hypereosinophilic syndrome. N Engl J Med 2003;348:1201–14.
37. Klion AD, Noel P, Akin C, et al. Elevated serum tryptase levels identify a subset of patients with a myeloproliferative variant of idiopathic hypereosinophilic syndrome associated with tissue fibrosis, poor prognosis, and imatinib responsiveness. Blood 2003;101:4660–6.
38. Jain N, Cortes J, Quintas-Cardama A, et al. Imatinib has limited therapeutic activity for hypereosinophilic syndrome patients with unknown or negative PDGFRalpha mutation status. Leuk Res 2009;33:837–9.
39. Butterfield JH, Gleich GJ. Response of six patients with idiopathic hypereosinophilic syndrome to interferon-α. J Allergy Clin Immunol 1994;94:1318–26.
40. Butterfield JH. Treatment of hypereosinophilic syndromes with prednisone, hydroxyurea, and interferon. Immunol Allergy Clin North Am 2007;27:493–518.
41. Kern E, Hirano I. Emerging drugs for eosinophilic esophagitis. Expert Opin Emerg Drugs 2013;18:353–64.
42. Ghosh S, Goldin E, Gordon FH, et al. Natalizumab for active Crohn's disease. N Engl J Med 2003;348:24–32.
43. Miller DH, Khan OA, Sheremata WA, et al. A controlled trial of natalizumab for relapsing multiple sclerosis. N Engl J Med 2003;348:15–23.
44. Fedyk ER, Wyant T, Yang LL, et al. Exclusive antagonism of the $\alpha4\beta7$ integrin by vedolizumab confirms the gut-selectivity of this pathway In primates. Inflamm Bowel Dis 2012;18:2107–19.
45. Soler D, Chapman T, Yang LL, et al. The binding specificity and selective antagonism of vedolizumab, an anti-$\alpha4\beta7$ integrin therapeutic antibody in development for inflammatory bowel diseases. J Pharmacol Exp Ther 2009; 330:864–75.
46. Verstovsek S, Tefferi A, Kantarjian H, et al. Alemtuzumab therapy for hypereosinophilic syndrome and chronic eosinophilic leukemia. Clin Cancer Res 2009;15: 368–73.
47. Kolbeck R, Kozhich A, Koike M, et al. MEDI-563, a humanized anti-IL-5 receptor alpha mAb with enhanced antibody-dependent cell-mediated cytotoxicity function. J Allergy Clin Immunol 2010;125:1344–53.e2.
48. Busse WW, Katial R, Gossage D, et al. Safety profile, pharmacokinetics, and biologic activity of MEDI-563, an anti-IL-5 receptor alpha antibody, in a phase I study of subjects with mild asthma. J Allergy Clin Immunol 2010;125:1237–44.
49. Nair P, Pizzichini MM, Kjarsgaard M, et al. Mepolizumab for prednisone-dependent asthma with sputum eosinophilia. N Engl J Med 2009;360:985–93.
50. Pavord ID, Korn S, Howarth P, et al. Mepolizumab for severe eosinophilic asthma (DREAM): a multicentre, double-blind, placebo-controlled trial. Lancet 2012;380:651–9.

51. Ortega HG, Liu MC, Pavord ID, et al. Mepolizumab treatment in patients with severe eosinophilic asthma. N Engl J Med 2014;371:1198–207.
52. Liu Y, Zhang S, Li DW, et al. Efficacy of anti-interleukin-5 therapy with mepolizumab in patients with asthma: a meta-analysis of randomized placebo-controlled trials. PLoS One 2013;8:e59872.
53. Haldar P, Brightling CE, Hargadon B, et al. Mepolizumab and exacerbations of refractory eosinophilic asthma. N Engl J Med 2009;360:973–84.
54. Bel EH, Wenzel SE, Thompson PJ, et al. Oral glucocorticoid-sparing effect of mepolizumab in eosinophilic asthma. N Engl J Med 2014;371:1189–97.
55. Gevaert P, Van Bruaene N, Cattaert T, et al. Mepolizumab, a humanized anti-IL-5 mAb, as a treatment option for severe nasal polyposis. J Allergy Clin Immunol 2011;128:989–95.
56. Garrett JK, Jameson SC, Thomson B, et al. Anti-interleukin-5 (mepolizumab) therapy for hypereosinophilic syndromes. J Allergy Clin Immunol 2004;113:115–9.
57. Rothenberg ME, Klion AD, Roufosse FE, et al. Treatment of patients with the hypereosinophilic syndrome with mepolizumab. N Engl J Med 2008;358:1215–28.
58. Roufosse F, de Lavareille A, Schandene L, et al. Mepolizumab as a corticosteroid-sparing agent in lymphocytic variant hypereosinophilic syndrome. J Allergy Clin Immunol 2010;126:828–35.
59. Plotz SG, Simon HU, Darsow U, et al. Use of an anti-interleukin-5 antibody in the hypereosinophilic syndrome with eosinophilic dermatitis. N Engl J Med 2003; 349:2334–9.
60. Flood-Page P, Menzies-Gow A, Phipps S, et al. Anti-IL-5 treatment reduces deposition of ECM proteins in the bronchial subepithelial basement membrane of mild atopic asthmatics. J Clin Invest 2003;112:1029–36.
61. Conus S, Straumann A, Bettler E, et al. Mepolizumab does not alter levels of eosinophils, T cells, and mast cells in the duodenal mucosa in eosinophilic esophagitis. J Allergy Clin Immunol 2010;126:175–7.
62. Kim S, Marigowda G, Oren E, et al. Mepolizumab as a steroid-sparing treatment option in patients with Churg-Strauss syndrome. J Allergy Clin Immunol 2010; 125:1336–43.
63. Kahn JE, Grandpeix-Guyodo C, Marroun I, et al. Sustained response to mepolizumab in refractory Churg-Strauss syndrome. J Allergy Clin Immunol 2010;125: 267–70.
64. Herrmann K, Gross WL, Moosig F. Extended follow-up after stopping mepolizumab in relapsing/refractory Churg-Strauss syndrome. Clin Exp Rheumatol 2012; 30:S62–5.
65. Stein ML, Collins MH, Villanueva JM, et al. Anti-IL-5 (mepolizumab) therapy for eosinophilic esophagitis. J Allergy Clin Immunol 2006;118:1312–9.
66. Straumann A, Conus S, Grzonka P, et al. Anti-interleukin-5 antibody treatment (mepolizumab) in active eosinophilic oesophagitis: a randomised, placebo-controlled, double-blind trial. Gut 2010;59:21–30.
67. Castro M, Mathur S, Hargreave F, et al. Reslizumab for poorly controlled, eosinophilic asthma: a randomized, placebo-controlled study. Am J Respir Crit Care Med 2011;184:1125–32.
68. Castro M, Wenzel SE, Bleecker ER, et al. Benralizumab, an anti-interleukin 5 receptor alpha monoclonal antibody, versus placebo for uncontrolled eosinophilic asthma: a phase 2b randomised dose-ranging study. Lancet Respir Med 2014;2:879–90.
69. Castro M, Zangrilli J, Wechsler ME, et al. Reslizumab for inadequately controlled asthma with elevated blood eosinophil counts: results from two multicentre,

parallel, double-blind, randomised, placebo-controlled, phase 3 trials. Lancet Respir Med 2015;3:355–66.

70. Brightling CE, Bleecker ER, Panettieri RA Jr, et al. Benralizumab for chronic obstructive pulmonary disease and sputum eosinophilia: a randomised, double-blind, placebo-controlled, phase 2a study. Lancet Respir Med 2014;2: 891–901.

71. Nowak RM, Parker JM, Silverman RA, et al. A randomized trial of benralizumab, an antiinterleukin 5 receptor alpha monoclonal antibody, after acute asthma. Am J Emerg Med 2015;33:14–20.

72. Spergel JM, Rothenberg ME, Collins MH, et al. Reslizumab in children and adolescents with eosinophilic esophagitis: results of a double-blind, randomized, placebo-controlled trial. J Allergy Clin Immunol 2012;129:456–63, 463.e1–3.

73. Laviolette M, Gossage DL, Gauvreau G, et al. Effects of benralizumab on airway eosinophils in asthmatic patients with sputum eosinophilia. J Allergy Clin Immunol 2013;132:1086–96.e5.

74. Fulkerson PC, Fischetti CA, McBride ML, et al. A central regulatory role for eosinophils and the eotaxin/CCR3 axis in chronic experimental allergic airway inflammation. Proc Natl Acad Sci U S A 2006;103:16418–23.

75. Humbles AA, Lu B, Friend DS, et al. The murine CCR3 receptor regulates both the role of eosinophils and mast cells in allergen-induced airway inflammation and hyperresponsiveness. Proc Natl Acad Sci U S A 2002;99: 1479–84.

76. Ma W, Bryce PJ, Humbles AA, et al. CCR3 is essential for skin eosinophilia and airway hyperresponsiveness in a murine model of allergic skin inflammation. J Clin Invest 2002;109:621–8.

77. Wise EL, Duchesnes C, da Fonseca PC, et al. Small molecule receptor agonists and antagonists of CCR3 provide insight into mechanisms of chemokine receptor activation. J Biol Chem 2007;282:27935–43.

78. Neighbour H, Boulet LP, Lemiere C, et al. Safety and efficacy of an oral CCR3 antagonist in patients with asthma and eosinophilic bronchitis: a randomized, placebo-controlled clinical trial. Clin Exp Allergy 2014;44:508–16.

79. Barnes N, Pavord I, Chuchalin A, et al. A randomized, double-blind, placebo-controlled study of the CRTH2 antagonist OC000459 in moderate persistent asthma. Clin Exp Allergy 2012;42:38–48.

80. Singh D, Cadden P, Hunter M, et al. Inhibition of the asthmatic allergen challenge response by the CRTH2 antagonist OC000459. Eur Respir J 2013;41: 46–52.

81. Straumann A, Hoesli S, Bussmann C, et al. Anti-eosinophil activity and clinical efficacy of the CRTH2 antagonist OC000459 in eosinophilic esophagitis. Allergy 2013;68:375–85.

82. Vermeire S, O'Byrne S, Keir M, et al. Etrolizumab as induction therapy for ulcerative colitis: a randomised, controlled, phase 2 trial. Lancet 2014;384:309–18.

83. Cudkowicz ME, van den Berg LH, Shefner JM, et al. Dexpramipexole versus placebo for patients with amyotrophic lateral sclerosis (EMPOWER): a randomised, double-blind, phase 3 trial. Lancet Neurol 2013;12:1059–67.

84. Zimmermann N, Hershey GK, Foster PS, et al. Chemokines in asthma: cooperative interaction between chemokines and IL-13. J Allergy Clin Immunol 2003; 111:227–42.

85. Steinke JW, Rosenwasser LJ, Borish L. Cytokines in allergic inflammation. In: Adkinson NF Jr, Bochner BS, Busse WW, et al, editors. Middleton's allergy principles and practice. 8th edition. Philadelphia: Elsevier Sanders; 2014. p. 65–82.

86. Luttmann W, Knoechel B, Foerster M, et al. Activation of human eosinophils by IL-13. Induction of CD69 surface antigen, its relationship to messenger RNA expression, and promotion of cellular viability. J Immunol 1996;157:1678–83.
87. Corren J, Lemanske RF, Hanania NA, et al. Lebrikizumab treatment in adults with asthma. N Engl J Med 2011;365:1088–98.
88. Noonan M, Korenblat P, Mosesova S, et al. Dose-ranging study of lebrikizumab in asthmatic patients not receiving inhaled steroids. J Allergy Clin Immunol 2013;132:567–74.
89. Scheerens H, Arron JR, Zheng Y, et al. The effects of lebrikizumab in patients with mild asthma following whole lung allergen challenge. Clin Exp Allergy 2014;44:38–46.
90. Reinisch W, Panes J, Khurana S, et al. Anrukinzumab, an anti-interleukin 13 monoclonal antibody, in active UC: efficacy and safety from a phase IIa randomised multicentre study. Gut 2015;64:894–900.
91. Danese S, Rudzinski J, Brandt W, et al. Tralokinumab for moderate-to-severe UC: a randomised, double-blind, placebo-controlled, phase IIa study. Gut 2015;64(2):243–9.
92. Murray LA, Zhang H, Oak SR, et al. Targeting interleukin-13 with tralokinumab attenuates lung fibrosis and epithelial damage in a humanized SCID idiopathic pulmonary fibrosis model. Am J Respir Cell Mol Biol 2014;50:985–94.
93. Piper E, Brightling C, Niven R, et al. A phase II placebo-controlled study of tralokinumab in moderate-to-severe asthma. Eur Respir J 2013;41:330–8.
94. Hodsman P, Ashman C, Cahn A, et al. A phase 1, randomized, placebo-controlled, dose-escalation study of an anti-IL-13 monoclonal antibody in healthy subjects and mild asthmatics. Br J Clin Pharmacol 2013;75:118–28.
95. De Boever EH, Ashman C, Cahn AP, et al. Efficacy and safety of an anti-IL-13 mAb in patients with severe asthma: a randomized trial. J Allergy Clin Immunol 2014;133:989–96.
96. Corren J, Busse W, Meltzer EO, et al. A randomized, controlled, phase 2 study of AMG 317, an IL-4Rα antagonist, in patients with asthma. Am J Respir Crit Care Med 2010;181:788–96.
97. Wenzel S, Ford L, Pearlman D, et al. Dupilumab in persistent asthma with elevated eosinophil levels. N Engl J Med 2013;368:2455–66.
98. Beck LA, Thaci D, Hamilton JD, et al. Dupilumab treatment in adults with moderate-to-severe atopic dermatitis. N Engl J Med 2014;371:130–9.
99. Gauvreau GM, O'Byrne PM, Boulet LP, et al. Effects of an anti-TSLP antibody on allergen-induced asthmatic responses. N Engl J Med 2014;370:2102–10.
100. Gauvreau GM, Boulet LP, Leigh R, et al. A non-steroidal glucocorticoid receptor agonist inhibits allergen-induced late asthmatic responses. Am J Respir Crit Care Med 2014. http://dx.doi.org/10.1164/rccm.201404-0623OC.
101. Akdis CA. Therapies for allergic inflammation: refining strategies to induce tolerance. Nat Med 2012;18:736–49.
102. Oh CK, Leigh R, McLaurin KK, et al. A randomized, controlled trial to evaluate the effect of an anti-interleukin-9 monoclonal antibody in adults with uncontrolled asthma. Respir Res 2013;14:93.
103. Ding C, Li J, Zhang X. Bertilimumab Cambridge Antibody Technology Group. Curr Opin Investig Drugs 2004;5:1213–8.
104. Blanchard C, Wang N, Stringer KF, et al. Eotaxin-3 and a uniquely conserved gene-expression profile in eosinophilic esophagitis. J Clin Invest 2006;116:536–47.
105. Caldwell JM, Collins MH, Stucke EM, et al. Histologic eosinophilic gastritis is a systemic disorder associated with blood and extragastric eosinophilia, TH2

immunity, and a unique gastric transcriptome. J Allergy Clin Immunol 2014;134: 1114–24.

106. Available at: http://ir.kalobios.com. ReleaseID-5821931. Accessed May 30, 2015.

107. Groopman JE, Mitsuyasu RT, DeLeo MJ, et al. Effect of recombinant human granulocyte-macrophage colony-stimulating factor on myelopoiesis in the acquired immunodeficiency syndrome. N Engl J Med 1987;317:593–8.

108. Bochner BS, Friedman B, Krishnaswami G, et al. Episodic eosinophilia-myalgia-like syndrome in a patient without L-tryptophan use: association with eosinophil activation and increased serum levels of granulocyte-macrophage colony-stimulating factor. J Allergy Clin Immunol 1991;88:629–36.

109. Divekar RD, Samant S, Rank MA, et al. Immunological profiling in chronic rhinosinusitis with nasal polyps reveals distinct VEGF and GMCSF signatures during symptomatic exacerbations. Clin Exp Allergy 2015;45(4):767–78.

110. Gauvreau GM, Boulet LP, Cockcroft DW, et al. Antisense therapy against CCR3 and the common β chain attenuates allergen-induced eosinophilic responses. Am J Respir Crit Care Med 2008;177:952–8.

111. Gauvreau GM, Pageau R, Seguin R, et al. Dose-response effects of TPI ASM8 in asthmatics after allergen. Allergy 2011;66:1242–8.

112. Imaoka H, Campbell H, Babirad I, et al. TPI ASM8 reduces eosinophil progenitors in sputum after allergen challenge. Clin Exp Allergy 2011;41:1740–6.

113. Roufosse FE, Kahn JE, Gleich GJ, et al. Long-term safety of mepolizumab for the treatment of hypereosinophilic syndromes. J Allergy Clin Immunol 2013;131:461–7.

114. Haldar P, Brightling CE, Singapuri A, et al. Outcomes after cessation of mepolizumab therapy in severe eosinophilic asthma: a 12-month follow-up analysis. J Allergy Clin Immunol 2014;133:921–3.

115. Kim YJ, Prussin C, Martin B, et al. Rebound eosinophilia after treatment of hypereosinophilic syndrome and eosinophilic gastroenteritis with monoclonal anti-IL-5 antibody SCH55700. J Allergy Clin Immunol 2004;114:1449–55.

116. Gleich GJ, Klion AD, Lee JJ, et al. The consequences of not having eosinophils. Allergy 2013;68:829–35.

117. Klion AD, Robyn J, Maric I, et al. Relapse following discontinuation of imatinib mesylate therapy for FIP1L1/PDGFRA-positive chronic eosinophilic leukemia: implications for optimal dosing. Blood 2007;110:3552–6.

118. Furuta GT, Kagalwalla AF, Lee JJ, et al. The oesophageal string test: a novel, minimally invasive method measures mucosal inflammation in eosinophilic oesophagitis. Gut 2013;62:1395–405.

119. Lukawska JJ, Livieratos L, Sawyer BM, et al. Real-time differential tracking of human neutrophil and eosinophil migration in vivo. J Allergy Clin Immunol 2014;133:233–9.e1.

120. Farahi N, Loutsios C, Peters AM, et al. Use of technetium-99m-labeled eosinophils to detect active eosinophilic inflammation in humans. Am J Respir Crit Care Med 2013;188:880–2.

121. Wen T, Besse JA, Mingler MK, et al. Eosinophil adoptive transfer system to directly evaluate pulmonary eosinophil trafficking in vivo. Proc Natl Acad Sci U S A 2013;110:6067–72.

122. Loutsios C, Farahi N, Porter L, et al. Biomarkers of eosinophilic inflammation in asthma. Expert Rev Respir Med 2014;8:143–50.

123. Na HJ, Hamilton RG, Klion AD, et al. Biomarkers of eosinophil involvement in allergic and eosinophilic diseases: review of phenotypic and serum markers including a novel assay to quantify levels of soluble Siglec-8. J Immunol Methods 2012;383:39–46.

124. Mawhorter SD, Stephany DA, Ottesen EA, et al. Identification of surface molecules associated with physiologic activation of eosinophils - application of whole-blood flow cytometry to eosinophils. J Immunol 1996;156:4851–8.
125. Bochner BS. Systemic activation of basophils and eosinophils: markers and consequences. J Allergy Clin Immunol 2000;106:S292–302.
126. Jia G, Erickson RW, Choy DF, et al. Periostin is a systemic biomarker of eosinophilic airway inflammation in asthmatic patients. J Allergy Clin Immunol 2012; 130:647–54.
127. Nair P, Kraft M. Serum periostin as a marker of T(H)2-dependent eosinophilic airway inflammation. J Allergy Clin Immunol 2012;130:655–6.
128. Hijnen D, De Bruin-Weller M, Oosting B, et al. Serum thymus and activation-regulated chemokine (TARC) and cutaneous T cell-attracting chemokine (CTACK) levels in allergic diseases: TARC and CTACK are disease-specific markers for atopic dermatitis. J Allergy Clin Immunol 2004;113:334–40.
129. Wilson TM, Maric I, Shukla J, et al. IL-5 receptor α levels in patients with marked eosinophilia or mastocytosis. J Allergy Clin Immunol 2011;128:1086–92.
130. Nair P, Ochkur SI, Protheroe C, et al. Eosinophil peroxidase in sputum represents a unique biomarker of airway eosinophilia. Allergy 2013;68:1177–84.
131. Butterfield JH, Leiferman KM, Abrams J, et al. Elevated serum levels of interleukin-5 in patients with the syndrome of episodic angioedema and eosinophilia. Blood 1992;79:688–92.
132. Simon HU, Plotz SG, Dummer R, et al. Abnormal clones of T cells producing interleukin-5 in idiopathic eosinophilia. N Engl J Med 1999;341:1112–20.
133. Gevaert P, Lang-Loidolt D, Lackner A, et al. Nasal IL-5 levels determine the response to anti-IL-5 treatment in patients with nasal polyps. J Allergy Clin Immunol 2006;118:1133–41.

Printed and bound by CPI Group (UK) Ltd, Croydon, CR0 4YY

03/10/2024

01040491-0003